Clues for a Clear Head and the E-F-G Approach to Better Health

Clues for a
Clear Head and
the E-F-G Approach
to Better Health

LYNN SMITH

Tanga Breeze Publishing, LLC
P.O. Box 9283
Erie, Pennsylvania 16505

Printed in the United States of America

ISBN: 978-0-578-05742-2

Disclaimer: This publication is a reference of clues and information for clearer
thinking and better health and is not intended to be medical advice. It is not a
substitute for your physician or a medical practitioner's expertise. The methods
and strategies in this book are the opinions of the author and have not been evaluated by the Food and Drug Administration. Readers should consult their physician
or medical practitioner before using the methods and strategies in this book. The
author/publisher/distributors disclaim any liability from the direct or indirect use
of this publication. Any health benefits received are incidental to the recommended
methods and strategies and are not to be construed as medical advice. Have fun as
you learn new ways to improve your life and the lives of those you love.

Contents

Dedication

To all of you out there—trying to do what is right, living as honestly as you can, even when its difficult, being fair, and helping one another—thank you for making our world a better place.

Preface

SMASH! The sound of broken glass falling to the floor was loud. The glass-framed plaque on the wall that held my professional engineer's license was the object of my anger. I had lost control of myself and flung an object at it. I sat at my desk in a room upstairs, feeling frustrated and broken, just like the broken pieces of glass that had just rained down on the floor. I was ashamed at losing my temper. Yet the frustration remained: how could I go through 4 years of engineering school, plus extra years of graduate courses, plus be able to pass the difficult engineer's licensing exam, but not excel at work? Were all those years of hard work a total waste? Why did my brain seem foggy and my memory poor? Why couldn't I use my abilities and education to get ahead in life? Why couldn't I get more work done? Why couldn't I speak clearly without stuttering? Why did I have continual sinus infections and congestion all winter long? What caused the squeezing in my head and the ringing in my ears? Was the fogged-in feeling from sinus infections, migraines, or a combination of several things? Why was I tired all the time? Why was life so difficult?

It finally makes sense! After multiple career changes and trying to function for 25 years with degraded mental abilities, I almost lost all hope of feeling normal. I tried vitamins, supplements, blood tests, allergy tests—and finally, a breakthrough ... I slowly came out of the tiredness and mental fog to reclaim my life and get my energy back. Nine years of intensive research have been whittled down to *7 clues and 3 simple food groups we need to be aware of to help sharpen our minds and improve our health.* This book provides simple explanations to address some complex and overlooked conditions that can degrade our mental abilities and our health. Automobile analogies are included.

Life does not need to be so difficult. The clues will provide guidance as you discuss various conditions with your medical practitioner and a strategy to help you perform up to your natural potential.

PART I

Clues

DO YOU SEE SOME WARNING LIGHTS?

Quick Summary: ABCs and Automobile Analogy

AUTHOR'S definition of a clear head: *The ability to use your thinking and reasoning skills to your inherited potential on a consistent basis.*

The object of this book is to make you aware of many factors that can lead to mental fog, degrade our mental abilities, and open the way to illness. Use the letters A through G as a reminder of some of the clues, concepts, and three food groups that can improve our mental abilities, our health and our overall quality of life!

A ... Antibiotics, alcohol abuse, overuse of nonsteroidal anti-inflammatory drugs (NSAIDs) and a bad diet can harm the digestive tract, weaken our immune system and by a series of subtle, complex events, allow mental fog and other illness to set in.

Undisputed evidence shows that the overuse of broad-acting antibiotics can lead to health problems in addition to those they were intended to treat. Broad-acting antibiotics are effective at killing off infections in our bodies caused by bad bacteria however, these same antibiotics also kill off the good bacteria in our digestive tract called beneficial bacteria. This beneficial bacteria acts as a protective shield, but when damaged and disturbed, allows bad bacteria, toxins and tiny, undigested food particles to enter our bloodstream. Our immune system can become overloaded followed by mental fog and eventual illness.

In a similar way, overuse of alcohol and NSAIDs (ibuprofen is the most common) can also harm the digestive tract, overload the immune system and lead to mental fog and illness.

Other factors that can lead to mental fog and illness are: high levels of certain heavy metals in our body, such as mercury; exposure to toxins, pollution, cigarette smoke and various infections. A bad diet with large amounts of sugar, white flour and bad fats places extra stress on our body, promotes unhealthy inflammation and will lead to problems later in life. All these and other things we may not even be aware of can weaken our immune system, degrade our mental abilities, and harm our health.

> *Automobile analogy: We pay attention when our car spits and sputters or when warning lights come on and we know maintenance and repairs are needed. Likewise, we need to listen to what our bodies are telling us and be aware that things like antibiotics, alcohol abuse, infections, and toxins can cause our bodies to spit and sputter. We must pay attention to "warning lights" telling us that maintenance and repairs are needed.*

B... **Beneficial bacteria** (the good bacteria in the digestive tract) is an important component of our immune system. This beneficial bacteria also produces vitamins and anticancer chemicals that help protect our bodies and aid in good digestion. An unhealthy digestive tract may become inflamed, allowing undigested food particles and harmful toxins and bacteria to leak into the bloodstream. This condition is called leaky gut syndrome (LGS). When too much beneficial bacteria becomes disturbed or destroyed, it may no longer keep in check a potentially harmful yeast called *Candida* albicans, commonly called *Candida*.

> *Beneficial bacteria in the digestive tract is like having the best motor oil, the best oil filter, the best air filter, and the best fuel filter all working together to provide the best protection for your car's engine.*

C... Candida is the most common yeast to overtake the digestive tract. It is very sneaky and can change into several different forms. One form is an aggressive fungus that can grow tentacles that poke holes through the wall of the digestive tract. This also harms our digestion and can cause LGS. Candida also gives off its own harmful toxins, which can leak into the bloodstream and cause a wide range of psychological symptoms and physical illnesses that vary from person to person. Candida's stealthiness and its wide range of effects make it very difficult to recognize and diagnose.

In the 1980s, Japanese researchers discovered a condition called "drunk disease," which occurs when *Candida* overgrowth in the digestive tract produces alcohol within the body, causing actual drunkenness even though no alcohol is consumed.

Some psychological symptoms of *Candida* overgrowth may include degraded mental and physical abilities and abnormal or irrational behaviors. In the past, *Candida* overgrowth was not recognized by many physicians as an illness and often went undetected. (The reasoning was that everybody has *Candida*, therefore it must be harmless.) However, as we will find out, certain heavy metals in our body can weaken our immune system and allow *Candida* to overgrow and degrade our quality of life. *Candida* overgrowth can harm our mental and physical abilities, hold us back in our careers, and significantly reduce our quality of life. This condition is discussed in chapter 14.

> *Candida overgrowth in the body is like dirty, filthy oil that sludges up your car's engine along with old, dirty, rusty gasoline. The car will run but will have degraded performance as it spits and sputters along.*

D... Digestion is extremely important to our mind and body. When undigested food particles enter the bloodstream, our immune system kicks into action and attacks them as if they were foreign invaders. This reaction produces products called immune complexes, which can end up in the synovial fluid in the joints and can cause inflammation as seen in rheumatoid arthritis. Inflammation also occurs in other parts of the body—including the digestive tract, which can lead to LGS (or a worsening of LGS). The problem is further compounded when harmful bacteria and other toxins enter the bloodstream. High levels of toxins in our tissues reduce our cells' ability to produce necessary energy. This is seen in chronic fatigue syndrome (CFS). The liver may become overloaded and unable to do its job of removing harmful toxins and waste products from the blood. For some people, a condition of mental fog and fatigue becomes a constant struggle, making life very difficult.

Some people may not produce enough digestive enzymes for proper digestion. Heredity and low levels of hydrochloric acid in the stomach are other important factors. Poor digestion can allow the immune system to become stressed beyond its ability to defend the body against other illnesses. All these factors can degrade our mental abilities.

When digestion becomes disturbed, a chronic cycle of inflammation can set in, which can take many months and a great deal of effort to overcome.

> *Digestion is a normal process, like starting our car and driving somewhere. LGS in the body is like leaky gaskets in our car's engine—coolant leaks into the motor oil, performance is degraded, and additional problems will likely arise.*

> *Think of chronic inflammation as a car engine that overheats. Engines do not run well when they overheat. Continuous overheating will cause major engine damage. Likewise, chronic inflammation will eventually cause damage in our body.*

The aforementioned **A-B-C-D** summary provides some issues to explore with your health practitioner. The **E-F-G** approach consists of simple and inexpensive things you can do right away to get started on the path to increased mental sharpness, increased energy, and better health. You may want to know that this approach is anti-inflammatory (reduces swelling) and also has some interesting anticancer actions as well. Some health problems may go away as you use the **E-F-G** approach and you become healthier and stronger.

E... Enzymes and plant phytochemicals. Enzymes either start up or speed up the billions of chemical reactions in our bodies and in every other living plant or animal. Our body contains over 3000 different enzymes and more are being discovered as researchers learn more about how the human body works. Digestive enzymes are secreted by the salivary glands, stomach, intestines, and pancreas and are required for digestion. A deficiency of digestive enzymes is a likely cause of poor digestion. Enzyme supplements are available in the form of capsules and tablets. When taken with a meal, digestive enzyme supplements can help break down foods for improved digestion.

Special enzyme supplements can help reduce and control inflammation. These enzyme supplements are used by some athletes to reduce inflammation and promote faster healing of pulled muscles and other inflammatory injuries. These special enzyme supplements have an enteric coating, which protects the enzymes from stomach acids, so they enter the intestine intact and become absorbed into the bloodstream. (*Enteric* means *in the intestine*). Enteric-coated enzymes are readily available and have been shown to help various inflammatory conditions such as arthritis and pain. Enteric-coated enzymes are taken between meals to maximize absorption into the bloodstream. Refer to the Web sites www. buywobenzym.com and www.doctormurray.com for more information.

Each fresh, uncooked fruit or vegetable comes prepackaged with the exact enzymes needed to digest it—all we have to do to release these enzymes is chew up the fruit or vegetable. Cooking destroys these important food enzymes. When we eat cooked food, our body must produce extra digestive enzymes in order to carry out digestion since cooked food has no enzymes. This requirement places a heavy demand on our body.

Fruits and vegetables also contain important vitamins, minerals, and some very special phytochemicals (plant chemicals with special properties), which can help our body fight off infection and disease. Enzymes and phytochemicals are discussed in chapter 15.

Enzymes and phytochemicals in our body are like our car's electronic engine controls, spark plugs, and fuel injectors, which make our car's engine run smoothly and reliably.

F... Fish oil and flaxseed oil contain special types of essential fatty acids (EFAs), which are the building blocks of our cells' membranes. Certain EFAs (especially omega-3) are extremely important for proper cell-to-cell signaling and also have anti-inflammatory actions. We all must make a conscious effort to include omega-3 EFAs in our diet because our body cannot produce them—hence the name "essential." The Western diet is seriously lacking in omega-3 EFAs.

Certain oily fish contain the final forms of omega-3 EFAs called EPA and DHA, which are extremely important for proper function of our brain and nerve cells as well as controlling inflammation. These two nutrients have very long names and will be discussed in chapters 3 and 13.

Flaxseed oil is one of nature's richest sources of another omega-3 EFA—called ALA (alpha-linolenic acid)—and our body can transform a portion of it into final forms of omega-3 EFAs (EPA and DHA).

The late Dr. Johanna Budwig, world-renowned researcher, biologist, pharmacologist, and medical doctor, discovered that when flaxseed oil is mixed with a sulfurated protein (sulfur-containing protein) such as cottage cheese or yogurt, the flaxseed oil becomes water soluble and is easily absorbed by our body. Flaxseeds must be ground up in order to release the omega-3 EFAs (a blender works fine), after which you should immediately mix the ground seeds with cottage cheese or yogurt. It is important to note that omega-3 EFAs are highly reactive and begin to deteriorate after being ground up and exposed to air, light or heat.

Dr. Budwig wrote about the many benefits of flaxseed oil in her book *Flax Oil as a True Aid Against Arthritis, Heart Infarction, Cancer and Other Diseases*, Apple Publishing Co. Ltd. 1994. Note that commercially produced flaxseed oil is processed in the absence of heat, light, and oxygen in order to protect the omega-3 EFAs from deteriorating. I enjoy making delicious fruit-flax smoothies (the recipe is in chapter 22).

Omega-3 EFAs in our body are like frequent oil changes for our car, complete with new oil filters, new air filters, and high-grade fuel.

G... Ginger, garlic, and turmeric can do amazing things in our body. Fresh ginger is one of nature's richest sources of proteolytic (protein-digesting) enzymes. When taken with a meal, fresh ginger's enzymes start breaking down food proteins, improving digestion. Fresh ginger is eaten as a vegetable in some countries. Confucius, the great Chinese philosopher and administrator known for his wise sayings, was known to eat a slice of fresh ginger with every meal.

It was shown in 1935 that undigested food proteins in the bloodstream can cause certain allergies, and ginger can help protect against this. Fresh ginger also has significant anti-inflammatory actions and can benefit our health many other ways. Dried ginger powder also has some anti-inflammatory actions and is available in capsules and tablets; however, the dose must be limited because too much can over-thin the blood. Do not use dried ginger powder if you are taking blood-thinning medications, have gallstones, or have blood-clotting disorders. See chapter 10 for cautions when taking ginger.

Turmeric is a botanical cousin of ginger and also has anti-inflammatory actions. Curcumin, a compound in turmeric, is currently being studied as a possible medication for treating Alzheimer's disease. Turmeric powder may already be in your kitchen cupboard.

Garlic is known to kill off a wide variety of harmful bacteria, viruses, and other microbes and also has anti-inflammatory actions. For those who cannot eat garlic, aged garlic extract is easy to take and has many of the important actions of fresh garlic but without the odor.

*The multiple, protective actions of ginger, garlic, turmeric and
omega-3 EFAs in our bodies can be compared to a car engine's
radiator and cooling system, which protects the engine from
overheating, allowing it to run properly and reliably.*

Out of deep respect to you, the reader, I have attempted to reduce
vast amounts of information down to 7 helpful clues and 3 health-
boosting food groups for which our Western diet comes up short. I call
these 3 food groups the E-F-G approach. This approach is very simple
(because it uses foods and some supplements), will enhance your mind
and body but does not cost a lot of money. The clues that follow will
quickly introduce some major issues to consider while more detailed
explanations and practical steps are presented in later chapters.

Mental and psychological symptoms are printed in *italics* for easy
recognition.

*Remember to ask yourself: How can I include the E-F-G
approach into each meal or snack every day?*

CHAPTER 2

Digestion and Antibiotics

HELP! *Helfen! Socorro! You try as hard as you can to succeed in life, yet it seems so difficult—like you're dragging around an invisible ball and chain.*

Do you feel like something has been holding you back in life, dragging you down, but you don't know what it is?

Do you feel like you've missed out on opportunities and achievements that could have been yours, if only you had been thinking clearly and had more "get up and go."

When you wake up, are you more tired than when you went to bed?

Does your world improperly appear as two-dimensional, with distorted feeling and emotions?

Are you tired of feeling drained, exhausted, and unable to cope with life? Are you tired of being tired? What's wrong?

CLUE #1: Three keys to good health: Digestion! Digestion! Digestion! How important is digestion? When your digestion is good, you will most likely feel good and, in turn, will have more energy to exercise and prepare healthy foods to eat. The benefits of good digestion are enormous. Ignoring it can have a very high cost. A 1985 study by the U.S. Department of Health and Human Services estimates that *at least 26% of Americans have been diagnosed with some type of digestive illness.*[1]

Improper digestion can be a huge contributor to *fuzzy thinking and other symptoms, including anxiety, confusion, aggressive behavior, mood swings, nervousness, poor memory, fatigue, and malaise.*[2] Here's how it happens: The digestive tract can leak undigested food particles into the bloodstream. Next, the immune system kicks into action and tags these particles as foreign invaders, resulting in inflammation in various tissues of the body. Inflammation of the digestive tract increases its leakiness, sending even more undigested food particles and bacteria into the bloodstream.[3] This condition is called leaky gut syndrome (LGS). LGS causes extra stress on the immune system and can leave us feeling tired and run down. LGS can also *degrade our mental and physical abilities.*

LGS is seen in other illness and diseases such as rheumatoid arthritis (inflammation of the joints),[4] food allergy, Crohn's disease, various skin problems, migraine headaches, and certain mental problems including schizophrenia.[5] With LGS, our immune system is forced to fight against the food we eat. LGS is discussed in detail in chapter 12.

Although ginger has been used throughout history to improve digestion, fresh ginger can also help fight inflammation.[6] This is especially important since inflammation of the digestive tract is a major cause of LGS, which, in turn, causes more inflammation to the digestive tract and other parts of the body. This sets up a vicious cycle that must be stopped. Chapter 16 tells more about ginger's potent anti-inflammatory actions.

Fresh ginger improves digestion because it is one of nature's richest sources of proteolytic (protein-digesting) enzymes.[7] Proteolytic enzymes break down food proteins and have many other benefits, as discussed in chapter 15. Juice from fresh, crushed ginger is a potent meat tenderizer when used as a marinade for raw meat. Another advantage of eating fresh ginger is the presence of gingerols, the compounds most responsible for ginger's pungent taste, its potent anti-inflammatory actions and many other healthful benefits. Upon drying, the gingerols are transformed into another compound called shogaols, which have aspirin-like properties. The benefits of fresh ginger and dried ginger will be discussed in upcoming chapters.

CLUE #2: If you were a child during the 1970s or later, you are of "the antibiotic generation" meaning you have probably received antibiotics several times.[8] Unfortunately, as we now know, the same antibiotics that kills the harmful bacteria in our body can also destroy the beneficial bacteria in our digestive tract. This beneficial bacteria is a major part of our body's immune system, forming a protective shield that is *extremely important* to our health. When much of the beneficial bacteria is destroyed and the immune system is weak, a condition called *Candida* overgrowth can set in, as described in *The Missing Diagnosis* by Dr. C. Orian Truss,[9] *The Yeast Syndrome* by Dr. John Parks Towbridge,[10] *The Yeast Connection* by Dr. William Crook,[11] and many other sources.[12] *Candida* overgrowth is a yeast infection that can cause *mental fog, depression, anxiety, headaches, loss of self-confidence, memory loss, difficulty concentrating and reasoning,*[13] *and degrading of our mental and physical abilities.* A double whammy occurs as certain antibiotics can actually promote the growth of *Candida,*[14] and, in turn, *Candida* wreaks more havoc by further weakening the immune system.[15] Clinical research studies indicate that *Candida* overgrowth may be a cause of LGS.[16] A vicious cycle is started and our health spirals downward.

It is known that *Candida* spews out dozens of toxins, some of which are quite harmful.[17] With these toxins circulating in our body, our immune system is forced to fight a constant battle. It is no wonder chronic fatigue often sets in.

From treating many patients, Dr. C. Orian Truss describes how *Candida* overgrowth can contribute to various psychological problems, including *depression* and *"explosive irritability"* in women. For men, he reports seeing *"chronic ill temper"* and *"low-grade depression."*[18] A well-known psychologist writes that "fatigue produces irritability—and irritability produces indifference."[19] With these conditions straining a marriage, there is little hope of a happy union and the marriage is more likely to fail. It is said that marriage is not about marrying the right person but about *becoming* the right person. How can we become the right person when our thinking is fuzzy and our emotions out of touch? With no logical explanation for our negative feelings, it is easy to blame other people and circumstances for our life struggles.

In children, it is known that *Candida* overgrowth can cause *"hyperactivity, irritability, learning problems, behavior problems, recurrent ear infections,"*[20] and many other symptoms.

Here are a few more symptoms of *Candida* overgrowth that you may consider as warning lights that your body is in need of a major tune-up. Some psychological symptoms may include the following:

- *Irritability, anxiety, depression, fearfulness, nervousness, and nervous habits*
- *Feelings of despair, low self-esteem*
- *Feeling out of touch with yourself, out of touch with others, and out of touch with life in general*
- *Feeling out of place in this world, like you don't belong*

Physical symptoms may include the following:

- Frequent headaches and sinus infections, achiness, feeling sick all over
- A "squeezing" feeling in the head, like a band around your head with two strong men pulling the band tighter and tighter
- Sensitivities and allergies to molds, smoke, odors, and certain foods

The symptoms and effects are physical and psychological, and they go hand in hand, making life extremely difficult. They affect everything—your job, your family, your marriage, your outlook on life, how you relate to others—your whole life. Regretfully, for many of us, life has become unnecessarily difficult because we do not understand our condition, cannot describe it to our medical provider, or are not aware of the steps to overcome it. *Candida* overgrowth is discussed in chapter 14.

You always knew something was wrong inside your body, but did not know what it was or even how to describe it.

REFERENCES FOR CHAPTER 2

1a.   *Digestive Diseases in the United States: Epidemiology and Impact.* US Department of Health and Human Services. National Institutes of Health. National Digestive Diseases Data Working Group. James E. Everhart, M.D., M.P.H. Editor. NIH Publication No. 94-1447. May 1994. "Table 1.-Burden of selected digestive diseases in the United States, 1985." p.x.

1b.   "Historical National Population Estimates: July 1, 1900 to July 1, 1999" Web site: U.S. Census Bureau. Accessed 2/15/2008. <http://www.factfinder.census. gov/popest/archives/1990s/popclockest.txt>.

2.   Galland L. "Solving the Digestive Puzzle". (conference manual), Great Smokies Diagnostic Laboratory / HealthComm International Inc. San Francisco, May 1995, p.10. (Cited by Elizabeth Lipski, M.S., C.C.N. *Leaky Gut Syndrome.* Keats Publishing, Inc., New Canaan, Connecticut. 1998, p.9).

3.   Pironi L, Miglioli M, Ruggeri E, Levorato M, Dallasta MA, Corbelli C, Nibali MG, Barbara L. "Relationship between intestinal permeability to [51Cr] EDTA and inflammatory activity in asymptomatic patients with Crohn's disease." *Dig Dis Sci* 1990, 35(5):582-8.

4a.   Smith MD, Gibson RA, Brooks PM. "Abnormal bowel permeability in anky- losing spondylitis and rheumatoid arthritis." *J Rheumatol* 1985;12(2):299-305.

4b.   Katz KD, Hollander. "Intestinal mucosal permeability and rheumatological diseases." D. *Bailliere's Clin Rheumatol* 1989;3(2):271-84.

5.   "Symptoms of Leaky Gut", "Conditions linked with LGS" Web site: Leaky Gut Syndrome. Accessed 4/16/2009. <http://www.leakygut.co.uk/symptoms. htm>.

6.   Jolad SD, Lantz RC, Chen GJ, Chen GJ, Bates RB, Timmermann BN. "Commercially processed dry ginger (Zingiber officinale): composition and effects on LPS-stimulated PGE2 production." Phytochemistry. 2005 Jul;66 (13):1614-35.

7.   Thompson EH, Wolf ID, Allen CE. "Ginger Rhizome: A New Source of Proteolytic Enzyme." Meat Science Lab, Dept. of Animal Sci., Univ. of Minnesota, St. Paul, MN 55101.

8.   Truss CO, MD. *the Missing Diagnosis.* The Missing Diagnosis, Inc. PO Box 26508, Birmingham, AL 35226. 1985. p.144.

9.   Franco A. Ferrari, Ambrogio Pagani, Massimo Marconi, Renzo Stefanoni,

and Antonio G. Siccardi. "Inhibition of Candidacidal Activity of Human Neutrophil Leukocytes by Aminoglycoside Antibiotics" *Antimicrobial Agents and Chemotherapy.* Jan. 1980. p.87-88.

10. Towbridge JP, MD, Walker, M DPM. *The Yeast Syndrome.* Bantam Books, New York, NY 10103. 1986.

11. Crook W. *The Yeast Connection Handbook*, Professional Books, Inc., Box 3246, Jackson, TN, Copyright 2000.

12a. Ruiz-Sanchez D, Calderon-Romero L, Sanchez-Vega JT, Tay J. "Intestinal candidiasis. A clinical report and comments about this opportunistic pathology." *Mycopathologia.* 2003;156(1):9-11.

12b. Still JM Jr, Law EJ, Belcher KE, Spencer SA. "A comparison of susceptibility to five antifungal agents of yeast cultures from burn patients." *Burns.* 1995 May;21(3):167-70.

12c. Saadia R, Lipman J. "Antibiotics and the gut." *Eur J Surg Suppl.* 1996;(576):39-41.

12d. Berg RD. "Bacterial translocation from the gastrointestinal tract." *J Med* 1992;23(3-4):217-44.

12e. Kennedy MJ, Volz PA. "Ecology of Candida albicans gut colonization: inhibition of Candida adhesion, colonization, and dissemination from the gastrointestinal tract by bacterial antagonism." *Infect Immun.* 1985 September; 49(3):654-663.

13. Truss CO, MD. *the Missing Diagnosis.* The Missing Diagnosis, Inc., PO Box 26508, Birmingham, AL 35226, 1985, p.15.

14a. Towbridge JP, MD, Walker, M DPM. *The Yeast Syndrome.* Bantam Books, New York, NY 10103, 1986 pp.42-53.

14b. Franco A. Ferrari, Ambrogio Pagnani, Massimo Marcone, Renzo Stefanoni and Antonio G. Siccardi. "Inhibition of Candidacidal Activity of Human Neutrophil Leukocytes by Aminoglycoside Antibiotics" *Antimicrobial Agents and Chemotherapy*, Jan. 1980, p.87-88.

14c. Brajtburg A, Elberg S, Medoff G, Kobayashi GS. "Increase in colony-forming units of Candida albicans after treatment with polyene antibiotics," *Antimicrobial Agents and Chemotherapy.* 1981 Jan;19(1):199-200.

14d. Seelig MS. "The role of antibiotics in the pathogenesis of Candida infections." *Am J Med.* 1966 Jun;40(6):887-917.

15a. Bartizal KF, Salkowski C, Balish E. "The influence of a gastrointestinal micro-flora on natural killer cell activity," *Journal of the Reticuloendothelial Society.* 1983 May; 33(5):381-90.

15b. Iwata K., Uchida K., "Cellular Immunity in Experimental Fungus Infections in Mice: The influence of infections in treatment with a candida toxin on spleen lymphoid cell." *Mykosen, Suppl.* 1, 72-81 (1978), Symposium Medical Mycology, Flims, January 1977.

15c. Iwata k., Yamamoto Y., "Glycoprotein Toxins Produced by Candida Albicans."

Proceedings of the Fourth International Conference on the Mycoses, June, 1977, PAHO Scientific Publication #356.

16. Crook W, *The Yeast Connection Handbook*, Professional Books, Inc., Box 3246, Jackson, TN, Copyright 2000, p.11.

17a. Towbridge JP, MD, Walker, M DPM. *The Yeast Syndrome*. Bantam Books, New York, NY 10103, 1986 pp.37-39.

17b. Truss CO, "Metabolic abnormalities in patients with chronic candidiasis: the acetaldehyde hypothesis." *Journal of Orthomolecular Psychiatry*, 1984;13:66-93.

17c. Hasumura Y, Teschke R, Lieber CS, "Characteristics of acetaldehyde oxidation in rat liver mitochondria," *J Biol Chem*. 1976 Aug 25;251(16):4908-13.

17d. Aberle II NS, Rn J. "Experimental Assessment of the Role of Acetaldehyde in Alcoholic Cardiomyopathy." Biol Proceed Online. 2003;5:1-12. Epub 2003 Feb 17.

17e. Tuma Dean J, Ph.D., Casey, Carol A. Ph.D. "Dangerous Byproducts of Alcohol Breakdown-Focus on Adducts." National Institute on Alcohol Abuse and Alcoholism. Accessed 8/28/05. <http://www.niaaa.nih.gov/publications/arh27-4/285-290.htm.>.

18. Truss CO, MD, *the Missing Diagnosis*, The Missing Diagnosis, Inc., PO Box 26508, Birmingham, AL 35226, 1985, pp.17, 29, 38.

19. Dr. James Dobson. *What wives wish their husbands knew about women*. Tyndale House Publishers, Inc. Wheaton, IL. 1984. p.50.

20. Truss CO, MD, *the Missing Diagnosis*, The Missing Diagnosis, Inc., PO Box 26508, Birmingham, AL 35226, 1985, front cover.

CHAPTER 3

Omega-3 EFA Deficiency

CLUE #3: Essential fatty acids are required for proper function of the brain and nerves. EFAs are important building blocks for the outer skin (membrane) of our body's cells. A special type of EFA, called omega-3s because of their unique chemical structure, are especially important to our nerve cells and brain cells and how well they communicate with each other. Omega-3 EFAs also have anti-inflammatory actions. *We do not get enough omega-3 EFAs in our modern diet. It is estimated that 80% of Americans are deficient in omega-3 EFAs.*[1]

Fish oil and flaxseed oil are nature's richest sources of omega-3 EFAs. Both are available in capsules as supplements.

I enjoy using flaxseeds in fruit smoothies—see my recipe in chapter 22. Ground flaxseeds or flaxseed oil should be mixed with cottage cheese or yogurt, which make the EFAs water soluble so our body can easily absorb them. Flaxseed oil has some amazing actions against three major killers—heart disease, cancer, and stroke—as demonstrated by seven-time Nobel Prize nominee Dr. Johanna Budwig in her scientific research and medical practice.[2]

EFAs from many natural foods were once part of our diet a hundred years ago when we ate more foods in their natural form. Now, however, our modern diet contains large amounts of animal fats, too much omega-6 EFAs (another type of EFA from grains and animal meats and fats), and trans fats. Trans fats are oils that have been chemically altered to become solid at room temperatures by hydrogenation (forcing hydrogen molecules into vegetable oils to make them solid at room temperature). Trans fats have been widely used in many snack foods because of their long shelf life and resistance to breakdown and spoiling. Because trans fats are so durable, our body cannot break them down. Trans fats become part of a cell's membrane, making the membrane less flexible, which interferes with the cell's function. Trans fats also can clog our blood vessels.

One of the largest studies ever conducted involved over 48,000 women over an eight-year period and came to a surprising conclusion: a low-fat diet showed no significant benefits for protecting against breast cancer, colorectal cancer, heart attack, stroke, and cholesterol levels.[3] The U.S. Institute of Medicine and the U.S. Dietary Guidelines Committee have concluded that the *type of fat is far more important than the amount of fat* for the prevention of disease and that "replacing saturated and trans fats with natural vegetable oils can greatly reduce the risk of heart disease and diabetes."[4]

As of 2005, it was estimated that about 40% of supermarket foods contained trans fats.[5] Finally, trans fats are gradually being removed from foods on our grocery store shelves. EFAs are discussed in more detail in chapter 13.

REALITY CHECK

My wife and I teach Sunday School for 1st & 2nd grade children. I volunteered to take over a group of boys who could not be in the regular class due to various problems with behavior, anger, ADHD and autism. I believed every boy was assigned a TSS in their public school. (TSS is short for Therapeutic Staff Support; often a staff member is assigned to work one-on-one to keep child on task, promote good behavior and monitor progress). Here I was, in a room with 5 of 6 of these boys, with no formal training in the areas of childhood education, attention deficit hyperactivity disorder, anger management or autistic spectrum disorder. One of the boys even ran out the door and into the parking lot and kept on running. Fortunatley, I was able to out run him and bring him back to our room and continue our class. (Forgive me if I was too busy to notice, but I didn't recall seeing people lined up and ready to volunteer with this class). Somehow, it is in these difficult situations when we discover how much we can help others—if we choose to. I was determined to stick with the class. The parents deserved a break and the children needed love and nurturing. Besides, my past training as an engineer helped me to take research and apply it to the real world—that's what engineers do. Based on my research of omega-3s and their importance for proper function of the brain and nerves, I offered some parents a bottle of fish oil capsules to give their boys during the week. Several months later, here are the results:

A single mother of 3 boys and 1 daughter (2 of her boys were in my class and would often pick fights with each other) reported that their school re-evaluated her boys and recommended that all 3 be mainstreamed with their peers. Tears of joy flowed from her eyes as she told of her boys' amazing progress. Her youngest boy now comes to our regular Sunday School class, sits down, and starts coloring. His next older brother moved on to the next class and is doing well.

A father reported that he took his son to a baseball game and noticed that his son looked him in the eye when talked to, interacted together and they both enjoyed the game. Prior to this, his behavior was good but he often wanted to lie down under a table and be in his own little world. Being adopted, he had displayed some separation anxiety when his mom and dad were out of sight. He often wanted to sit on my lap during class time. He also had difficulty focusing on the lesson and participating in class activities. I did notice some dry patches on his skin, a symptom of omega-3 deficiency. He also has moved on to the next class and is doing well.

Several recent studies indicate omega-3 EFAs may be a possible treatment for ADHD (Attention Deficit/Hyperactivity Disorder) although more detailed studies are needed.[6]

TAKE A COUPLE SPOONFULS OF
EXTRA VIRGIN OLIVE OIL EVERY DAY

Although olive oil does not contain omega-3 EFA's like fish and flaxseed oil, this oil also has some amazing actions, so I wanted to alert you of its benefits right away. Virgin olive oil is a major component of the Mediterranean diet, which seems to show a reduced risk of cardiovascular disease and other diseases.[7] Olive oil also has some slight blood-thinning actions, which is healthy for our circulatory system,[8] as well as antioxidant and anti-inflammatory actions.[9] It was recently discovered that virgin olive oil contains small amounts of a painkiller similar to ibuprofen. (Interestingly, a research expert attending a conference in Sicily tasted some freshly squeezed olive oil and immediately recognized the slight stinging in the back of his throat as similar to that of ibuprofen, which acts like aspirin.)[10] My kids willingly take a couple of spoonfuls from time to time. My wife saw a man on TV who breaks slabs of marble with his hand. The man said he drinks about two cups of extra virgin olive oil a day. This was very inspirational to my kids. There are many ways that virgin olive oil can benefit our health as discussed in chapter 13. I enjoy mixing olive oil with crushed fresh garlic and spreading it on top of toasted bread as a way to get both garlic and olive oil in my diet. Adding parmesan cheese on top takes some of the bite out of the garlic and tastes good.

REFERENCES FOR CHAPTER 3

1.   Bionatures Flaxseed Oil Products: Frequently Asked Questions. Accessed 6/7/06. <http://www.budwigflax.com/FAQs/questions.htm>.

2.   Budwig, Johanna. *Flax Oil as a True Aid Against Arthritis, Heart Infarction, Cancer and Other Diseases*. Apple Publishing Co. Ltd. 1994.

3.   Prentice RL, Caan B, Chlebowski RT, Patterson R, Kuller LH, et al. "Low-Fat Dietary Pattern and Risk of Invasive Breast Cancer: The Woman's Health Initiative Randomized Controlled Dietary Modification Trial." JAMA 2006; 295:629-642.

4.   "Low-Fat Diet Not a Cure-All." Harvard School of Public Health. Accessed 10/31/2006. <http://www.hsph.harvard.edu/nutritionsource/low_fat.html>.

5.   Enig M, Ph.D, "The Deadliest Fats - Easy ways to eliminate them from your diet." *Bottom Line/Health*. Sept. 2005 p.4.

6a. Gow RV, Matsudaira T, Taylor E, Rubia K, Crawford M, Ghebremeskel K, Ibrahimovic A, Vallée-Tourangeau F, Williams LM, Sumich A. "Total red blood cell concentrations of omega-3 fatty acids are associated with emotion-elicited neural activity in adolescent boys with attention-deficit hyperactivity disorder." *Prostaglandins Leukot Essent Fatty Acids*. 2009 Feb-Mar;80(2-3): 151-6. Epub 2009 Feb 20.

6b. Frölich J, Döpfner M. "[The treatment of Attention-Deficit/Hyperactivity Disorders with polyunsaturated fatty acids – an effective treatment alternative?]" *Z Kinder Jugendpsychiatr Psychother*. 2008 Mar;36(2):109-16.

7.   "Olive oil, extra virgin". Web site: www.whfoods.com. George Mateljan Foundation. Accessed 5/26/2009. <http://www.whfoods.com/genpage.php?tname=foodspice&dbid=132>.

8a. Larsen LF, Jaspersen J, Marckmann P. "Are olive oil diets antithrombotic? Diets enriched with olive, rapeseed, or sunflower oil affect postprandial factor VII differently." *The American Journal of Clinical Nutrition*. 70(6), 1999, pages 976-982. Obtained from web site: Atkins.com Accessed 2/5/2004. <http://atkins.com/Archive/20026/20-65315.html>.

8b. Oosthuizen W, Vorster HH, Jerling JC, Barnard HC, Smuts CM, Silvis N, Kruger A, Venter CS. "Both fish oil and olive oil lowered plasma fibrinogen in women with high baseline fibrinoben levels." *Thromb Haemost*. 1994 Oct;72(4):557-62.

9.   "Olive oil, extra virgin". Web site: www.whfoods.com. George Mateljan Foundation. Accessed 5/26/2009. <http://www.whfoods.com/genpage.php?tname=foodspice&dbid=132>.

10a. Beauchamp GK, Keast RS, Morel D, Lin J, Pika J, Han Q, Lee CH, Smith AB, Breslin PA. "Phytochemistry: ibuprofen-like activity in extra-virgin olive oil. *Nature*. 2005 Sep 1;437(7055):45-6.

10b. "Olive Oil Contains Natural Anti-inflammatory Agent" ScienceDaily. Accessed 5/26/2009. <http://www.sciencedaily.com/releases/2005/09/050906075427.htm>.

CHAPTER 4

Infections, Inflammation and The "Ginger Effect"

CLUE #4: Infections from bacteria, viruses, parasites, and other microbes (such as *Candida*) can degrade our mental abilities and harm our health by giving off toxins and causing inflammation. Ginger can help fight against infections as well as help fight inflammation, detoxifiy our body and do a lot of other things. I call these many mutiple actions the "Ginger Effect."

Forgive me for my excitement about ginger; however, ginger was key to ending a several-decade-long mystery illness that had wreaked havoc in my life for many years. Since ginger is the "new kid on the block" in our Western diet when eaten by the slice or the squeezed juice used in tea, I have devoted several chapters later in this book to showcase its multiple beneficial actions, especially in the areas of improving digestion and reducing inflammation. Why not be like Confucius and eat a slice or two with every meal? I also enjoy chewing on a slice of fresh ginger after eating a meal, as it helps clean the teeth like a natural toothbrush (yes, I enjoy eating ice cream and other treats from time to time, too). You can even take some along on picnics and trips to help clean your teeth after eating and also first thing in the morning as a breath freshener. Forgive me again, I get carried away.

This is my story. Throughout my 20s and 30s, my brain would not work right. I did well in engineering school but for some reason could not use my full potential at work after graduating from college.

Chronic fatigue, mental fog, headaches, and sinus infections—all winter long—became a way of life. Working in smoke-filled offices seemed to aggravate my "mystery illness." This was in the 1980s, before smoking rules were in place. I ended up making several career changes, which added to the disruptions to my family and compounded the stress, anxiety and frustration. Medical exams, blood tests, and allergy testing did not produce any clear diagnosis other than that my body had no resistance to *Candida*. I was given a choice to receive allergy shots. I was told my slight allergies were due to immune system overload, so I spent a lot of money on air purifiers, allergenic mattress covers, and pillow covers; even scrubbed out the duct work in our house (from thirty years of smoking by the previous owner); and had many discussions with my wife over what to do next. What I did not know was that *Candida* over-growth and improper digestion can lead to many health problems, often in other parts of the body, and often have no obvious symptoms that fit into a nice, neat box.

As I mentioned, fatigue, mental fog, continual sinus infections, and a dull headache became a way of life for me. Some days, especially in the wintertime, I had tremendous difficulty concentrating, and I was often stressed out and completely exhausted at the end of the workday. Sometimes, I felt almost too tired to drive home from work—one woman even accused me of drunk driving. Sleep became an escape from life rather than a source of renewed energy. I was more tired in the morning than when I went to bed, and I dreaded hearing the sound of the alarm each morning. Sunday nights were especially depressing knowing that another rigorous week was about to begin. I forgot what it was like to feel good. I felt hopeless and depressed, like I was dying a slow, miserable death. I desperately wanted to get to the root of my illness rather than cover it up with medications and allergy shots. I knew that if I did not get better, I would probably live a shorter life than my father, who passed away from a brain aneurysm at the age of fifty-one. (An aneurysm occurs when a blood vessel stretches like a balloon and suddenly bursts, which is often fatal.) My heart ached for my seven-year-old son, whose headaches lasted two weeks or more and were seriously affecting his school performance and social development. He would often say his head "felt like a balloon" and would have fits of anger he could not explain. I was tired of living in the valley of the shadow of death and wanted to get my life back and be able to help others avoid this dreadful and unnecessary misery.

One day, hope came in a very small way. I remember walking through the produce aisle at our local grocery store when one of my kids said, "Hey, Daddy, there's ginger root, let's get some." (They knew I was taking dried ginger powder because it seemed to help my headaches somewhat.) I replied, "I don't know, I don't have much money, and I don't know how to use fresh ginger root." They insisted. "Come on, Daddy, get some." That small piece of ginger ended up costing about seventy-five cents. When we got home, I cut off a small slice and placed it in my mouth. Within minutes, my sinuses began to drain as some of the pressure in my head went away! I gave some to my son, who also said the ginger seemed to help his head feel better too. It was several years later that I figured out that the fresh ginger had killed off the *Candida* overgrowth and helped detoxify my body. I also learned that fresh ginger's antifungal, anti-inflammatory, antioxidant, and detoxi-fication actions must have promoted a lot of healing in my digestive tract, which helped restore my energy, my mental abilities, and my life! Looking back, it appears the chronic, dull ache within my head could have been caused by swelling, or squeezing of the brain, which has been associated with patients suffering from chronic fatigue.[1]

Years later (now in my late forties), I feel healthier and stronger than I ever thought possible—even stronger than when I was eighteen. My goal in writing this book is to pass on valuable knowledge and some very simple and inexpensive things you can do right away to improve your mental alertness, your health, and, in turn, have a better quality of life.

THE "GINGER EFFECT"

The "Ginger Effect" is an amazing synergy of healing actions: ginger contains over 477 known compounds,[2] many of which interact to help "tune up" the mind and body. Synergy means the combined effect is much greater than the effects of each individual compound. It's like having a designer food supplement that does many different things, all of which are great for your health! Let's look at 10 major actions of ginger that help bring about a clear head and better health:

1. Fresh ginger loosens stuck mucous and produces a head-clearing effect.
2. Fresh ginger's potent enzymes improve digestion (chapter 15).
3. Ginger's anti-inflammatory actions can help reduce and prevent chronic, low-grade inflammation and swelling (chapter 16).
4. Ginger is a potent antioxidant (chapter 17).
5. Ginger's antibiotic, antiviral, and antifungal actions can help fight infections. Potent anti-*Candida* properties rival those of some prescription antifungal medications.[3]
6. Ginger can kill parasites and their larvae (chapter 18).
7. Ginger improves blood circulation and can help reduce cholesterol and blood pressure (chapter 19).
8. Ginger increases the pumping action of the heart (chapter 19).
9. Ginger helps detoxify the body by increasing sweating.[4] In animal studies, ginger has been shown to stimulate the flow of bile into the intestine[5] and help detoxify the liver.[6] (Bile is secreted by the liver into the small intestine and acts to break down fats and remove wastes. The liver is the largest internal organ and it has a big job—to detoxify the food we eat and to detoxify pollutants that are breathed in or absorbed by the skin. The liver also breaks down fats, carbohydrates, and proteins and performs many other functions that regulate and protect our body).
10. Fresh ginger contains significant amounts of phosphorous, calcium, and magnesium,[7] which work together for proper nerve transmission, muscle contraction, and bone formation.

As an added bonus, ginger is very user-friendly, with a long history of safety and no adverse effects,[8] and is one of the three most researched plants in the world.[9] The other two are garlic and ginseng. Ginger requires no prescription (because it is a food) and is used in over 25 countries.[10] Ginger is eaten as a vegetable in some countries[11] and can be quickly and easily added to your lifestyle.

Here are some more interesting actions of ginger. Note that most studies involve animals, not humans. These studies give us more insight into ginger's wide range of potential actions:

1. Stimulates the immune system[12] and may help detoxify the body from harmful chemicals and toxins[13]
2. Antitumor actions[14]
3. Anticancer actions[15]
4. Reduced symptoms of radiation sickness in mice when given ginger extract *before* exposure to large doses of radiation[16].
5. May inhibit (prevent) DNA damage[17] (DNA contains the code of instructions for each cell to reproduce and grow)
6. Improved performance learning in rat studies[18]
7. Antiulcer actions[19]
8. Anti-diabetic actions by enhancing insulin sensitivity,[20] increasing insulin levels, and decreasing blood glucose levels[21] (omega-3 EFAs can also improve insulin sensitivity—see chapter 13)
9. Antiobesity actions[22] and may help inhibit absorption of dietary fat[23] (In one animal study, fresh ginger extract was shown to increase oxygen uptake and metabolism,[24] the burning of calories by our body's cells to produce energy; interestingly, another animal study showed that feeding a high-fat diet plus ginger did *not* result in weight gain.[25] Omega-3 EFAs also can help our body burn off calories and are discussed in chapter 13).

10. Helped reduce death of nerve cells following spinal injury[26] (6-shogaol from dried ginger was used)
11. Helped prevent kidney damage from large doses of the chemotherapy drug cisplatin[27] (6-gingerol from fresh ginger was used)
12. Has some antiwrinkle actions when used on skin against damage from ultraviolet light[28] (extract from fresh ginger was used).

As you can see, ginger has much to offer and can provide a great start on your journey back to wellness. As you begin to feel better and gain understanding of your particular condition, you will have the confidence to discuss a plan of action with your health practitioner.

EXPERIENCING FRESH GINGER

I still remember when I ate that first slice of ginger. It was dramatic; the pressure and tightness in my head began to melt away—within minutes! The warm, soothing, lemony vapors had a pronounced head-clearing effect like I had never felt before. It is amazing how a clear head can enhance our mood, our abilities, our confidence, and our productivity. It became an exciting adventure to discover the many, many health benefits packed into just one food! With many other food supplements, it takes weeks before you know if they are helping you or not. *With fresh ginger, you should feel a clearing effect in your head and throat within minutes.*

One of the first things you may notice when taking fresh ginger on a regular basis is that you will not have to clear your throat nearly as often. Your voice will be clearer. Ginger thins mucus and gets it moving, helping the throat and sinuses drain naturally. This action also can help prevent infections from setting in.

Friends and acquaintances with sore throats who were willing to slowly chew small slices of fresh ginger were surprised how quickly the soreness went away.

TRY IT BY THE SLICE

Here's a simple way to take fresh ginger and feel its head-clearing effect:

1. Using a serrated knife, carve off a thin slice of ginger root about the size of a penny or nickel.
2. Place it in your mouth like a lozenge, chewing slightly from time to time to release more flavor and vapors as desired. These vapors can help clear your head. (If you chew it up all at once, the sudden warmth may be overwhelming!)
3. Slowly exhale through your nose, allowing the soothing vapors to rise up into the passageways of your head. Inhaling through your mouth and slowly exhaling out your nose will allow the vapors to flow into the sinuses.

TRY FRESH GINGER TEA

A great way to get more fresh ginger in your diet is to make a quick and delicious tea. First, heat a cup of water to less than 140°F (60°C). Next, place a chunk of fresh ginger in a garlic press and squeeze the juice into the warm water. Add some honey for sweetness if you like. It is important to keep the water less than 140°F so the delicate yet powerful enzymes are not destroyed. The importance of enzymes are discussed in chapter 15.

REALITY CHECK

An acquaintance who was an alcoholic of 20 years frequently stopped by our office building to help do some outdoor yard work to earn some money. I am not that familiar with alcoholism but I do believe he was a fully addicted alcoholic. One morning I came in to work and noticed him sleeping in the back lawn, with his jacket under his head. Another morning, I came in and observed him sitting in his car, asleep in the front seat, driver's door open and engine still running. I shut off the car and went in the building to work. He later lost his license for driving under the influence. He owned only the clothes on his back, a few other items and had to return his leased car. One day he showed up at the office drunk and I told him if he showed up that way again, I would call the police.

One day hope came in a small way. His throat had been very sore for over a month and he pretty much lost his voice. He also smoked and hung out in smokey places. I cut off a slice of fresh ginger and gave it to him. Then he wanted more. And more the next day. And the next. He ate chunks of it like it was candy. He would say in his gruff voice: "I don't know what this stuff does, but it does something." His sore throat cleared up in a week. Some time later, he finally took our recommendation to enter a rehabilitation program for alcoholics and has stayed dry ever since. That was about 5 years ago. He is now busy rebuilding his life and a career.

Did the fresh ginger help detoxify his body, giving him a clear enough head to want to quit drinking? I believe it did this and much more, like killing off *Candida* overgrowth which thrives on alcohol. We will cover this in chapter 14. Coincidence? I don't think so. A recent study using mice stated that extracts of ginger and the herb thyme can "detoxify the injuries of alcohol abuse on liver and brain of mice."[29]

OTHER FOODS AND SUPPLEMENTS

If you don't like the taste of fresh ginger, don't worry; there are some other helpful foods and supplements, some of which are discussed in following chapters, including:

Dried ginger powder has properties both similar to and different from fresh ginger and can be taken along with fresh ginger. Dried ginger powder is available in capsules.

Enzyme supplements can improve digestion. Special enteric-coated enzymes have anti-inflammatory properties and are discussed in chapter 15.

Quercetin is a supplement with natural antihistamine actions and is discussed in a later chapter. Antihistamines help reduce allergy-related reactions such as sneezing, itching, and runny nose. Popular antihistamine medications include Claritin and Alavert (loratadine), Allegra (fexofenadine), and Zyrtec (cetirizine) and are very helpful to many people.

Turmeric contains a phytochemical called curcumin, which has some amazing actions. Turmeric is a nonpungent cousin of ginger and is often used as a natural food coloring. It gives a bright yellow color to mustard and other foods. Turmeric and curcumin have many actions common to ginger, such as anti-inflammatory,[30] antioxidant,[31] antibiotic[32] (like ginger, turmeric is effective at killing *Helicobacter pylori*, the bacteria most responsible for stomach ulcers),[33] antitumor,[34] anticancer,[35] cholesterol-lowering,[36] and several other important actions.[37]

Curcumin, the phytochemical in turmeric responsible for its many beneficial actions (and its bright yellow color), is receiving a lot of attention for its actions against Alzheimer's disease.[38] It is interesting to note that ginger and turmeric are widely consumed in India, which has a very low rate of Alzheimer's disease among the elderly.[39] Alzheimer's is the fourth leading cause of death among the elderly in industrialized nations after heart disease, cancer, and stroke. (Ginger also has anti-Alzheimer's actions.[40]) One study suggests the shogaols (which are abundant in dried ginger powder) may also have some protective properties against Alzheimer's.[41] Ethnic background[42] and diet[43] are other important factors in Alzheimer's disease.

Curcumin is very similar in function to 6-gingerol, the phytochemical in fresh ginger[44] that gives ginger its pungent taste and many of its amazing actions. Turmeric can be taken as a supplement; however, it contains only about 5 percent curcumin,[45] and curcumin is also available in capsules.

A recommended dose of dried turmeric powder is 1,000 to 3,000 milligrams per day. A recommended dose of standardized curcumin powder is 400 to 600 milligrams, three times a day. These doses are for a 150-pound adult and should be reduced proportionally for children.[46] For example, a 75-pound child could be given one-half the dose of an adult. I frequently give my wife and kids 1 turmeric capsule one day and 1 dried ginger capsule the next day, alternating each day.

Turmeric and curcumin are fairly well tolerated by most people at the recommended doses; however, both should be avoided by individuals with the following conditions:

- Gall bladder disease
- Gallstones or obstruction of the bile passages[47]
- Undergoing chemotherapy or any other cancer therapy unless taken under the direct care of a physician[48]

Consult your physician before taking curcumin or turmeric if you are pregnant, taking blood-thinning medications, or before taking higher medicinal/therapeutic doses.

Visit the Web site www.turmeric-curcumin.com for more information about turmeric and curcumin.

Garlic has antifungal actions,[49] antibiotic actions,[50] anticancer actions,[51] cholesterol-lowering actions,[52] and can significantly reduce the formation of harmful toxins in the body.[53] When using garlic, you must first crush it using a garlic press then let it sit for 10 minutes so the phytochemicals have time to mix and reach their full effectiveness. Remember that cooking garlic (and microwaving) destroys many of its beneficial properties.[54] Refer to chapter 22 for recipe suggestions. Aged garlic extract is claimed to have many of the actions of fresh garlic but without the odor.

REFERENCES FOR CHAPTER 4

1.   Dr. Charles W. Lapp. "THE TREATMENT OF CHRONIC FATIGUE SYNDROME (CFS) THE PERSPECTIVE OF A PRIVATE SPECIALTY PRACTICE IN CHARLOTTE, NC.", Lecture given in Nashville, TN, April 1997 (translated by Angela). Accessed 2/13/2008. <http://www.co-cure.org/Lapp.htm>.

2.   Schulick, P. *Ginger: Common Spice & Wonder Drug.* 3rd ed. Prescott, AZ. Hohm Press, 1996, pp.112-125.

3a. Ficker C, Smith ML, Akpagana K, Gbeassor M, Zhang J, Durst T, Assabgui R, Arnason JT. "Bioassay-guided isolation and identification of antifungal compounds from ginger." *Phytotherapy Research.* 2003, Volume 17, Issue 8, pp.897-902.

3b. Ficker CE, Amason JT, Vindas PS, Alvarez LP, Akpagana K, Gbeassor M, De Souza C, Smith ML. "Inhibition of human pathogenic fungi by ethnobotanically selected plant extracts." *Mycosis* 2003; February 46:29

4.   Fulder S, Ph.D. *The Ginger Book.* Avery Publishing Group, Garden City Park, New York. pp.38-39.

5a. Fulder S, Ph.D. *The Ginger Book.* Avery Publishing Group, Garden City Park, New York. p.42.

5b. Yamahara J, Miki K, Chisaka T, et al. "Cholagogic effect of ginger and its active constituents." *J Ethnopharmacol* 1985; 13:217-25.

6.   Hikino H, Kiso Y, Kato N, Hamada Y, Shioiri T, Aiyama R, Itokawa H, Kiuchi F, Sankawa U. "Antihepatotoxic actions of gingerols and diarylheptanoids." *J Ethnopharmacol.* 1985 Sep;14(1):31-9.

7.   Schulick, P. *Ginger: Common Spice & Wonder Drug.* 3rd ed. Prescott, AZ. Hohm Press, 1996, pp.112-125.

8.   Schulick, P. *Ginger: Common Spice & Wonder Drug.* 3rd ed. Prescott, AZ. Hohm Press, 1996, p.83.

9.   Statement by Norman Farnsworth, Ph.D., Senior university scholar of pharmacognosy and director of the World Health Organization Collaborating Centre for Traditional Medicine at the University of Illinois-Chicago College of Pharmacy.

10. Schulick, P. *Ginger: Common Spice & Wonder Drug.* 3rd ed. Prescott, AZ. Hohm Press, 1996, pp.28-29.

11. Puri HS, and Pandey G, "Glimpses into the crude drugs of Sikkim." *Bulletin Medical Ethnobotany Research* 1 (1980):55-71.

12a. Tan BK, Vanitha J. "Immunomodulatory and antimicrobial effects of some traditional Chinese medicinal herbs: a review." *Curr Med Chem.* 2004 Jun;11(11):1423-30.

12b. Dugenci SK, Arda N, Candan A. "Some medicinal plants as immunostimulant for fish." *J Ethnopharmacol.* 2003 Sep;88(1):99-106.

12c.   Puri A, Sahai R, Singh KL, Saxena RP, Tandon JS, Saxena KC.
       "Immunostimulant activity of dry fruits and plant materials used in Indian
       traditional medical system for mothers after child birth and invalids." *J
       Ethnopharmacol.* 2000 Jul;71(1-2):89-92.

13.   Shri J.N. Mathur. ICMR BULLETIN. "GINGER: ITS ROLE ON
       XENOBIOTIC METABOLISM." Vol. 33, No. 6, June 2003.

14a.   Manju V, Nalini N. "Chemopreventive efficacy of ginger, a naturally occurring
       anticarcinogen during the initiation, post-initiation stages of 1,2 dimethylhy-
       drazine-induced colon cancer. *Clin Chim Acta.* 2005 Aug;358(1-2):60-7.

14b.   Kim SO, Chun KS, Kundu JK, Surh YJ. "Inhibitory effects of [6]-gingerol
       on PMA-induced COX-2 expression and activation of NF-kappaB and p38
       MAPK in mouse skin." *Biofactors.* 2004;21(1-4):27-31.

14c.   Nagasawa H, Watanabe K, Inatomi H. "Effects of bitter melon
       (Momordica charantia l.) or ginger rhizome (Zingiber officinale rosc) on
       spontaneous mammary tumorigenesis in SHN mice." *Am J Chin Med.*
       2002;30(2-3):195-205.

14d.   Surh YJ. "Anti-tumor promoting potential of selected ingredients with anti-
       oxidative and anti-inflammatory activities: a short review." *Food Chem Toxicol.*
       2002 Aug;40(8):1091-7.

14e.   Surh YJ, Park KK, Chun KS, Lee LJ, Lee E, Lee SS. "Anti-tumor-promoting
       activities of selected pungent phenolic substances present in ginger." *J Environ
       Pathol Toxicol Oncol.* 1999;18(2):131-9.

14f.   Surh Y. "Molecular mechanisms of chemopreventive effects of selected
       dietary and medicinal phenolic substances." *Mutant Res.* 1999 Jul
       16;428(1-2):305-27.

14g.   Park KK, Chun KS, Lee JM, Lee SS, Surh YJ. "Inhibitory effects of
       [6]-gingerol, a major pungent principal of ginger, on phorbol ester-induced
       inflammation, epidermal ornithine decarboxylase activity and skin tumor
       promotion in ICR mice." *Cancer Lett.* 1998 Jul 17;129(2):139-44.

14h.   Katiyar SK, Agarwal R, Mukhtar H. "Inhibition of tumor promotion in
       SENCAR mouse skin by ethanol extract of Zingiber officinale rhizome.
       Cancer Res. 1996 Mar 1;56(5):1023-30.

14i.   Unnikrishnan MC, Kuttan R. "Cytotoxity of extracts of spices to cultured
       cells." *Nutr Cancer.* 1988;11(4):251-7.

15a.   Shukla Y, Singh M. "Cancer preventive properties of ginger: a brief review."
       Food Chem Toxicol. 2007 May;45(5):683-90. Epub 2006 Nov 12.

15b.   Rhode J, MD, Liu R, MD, Huang J, Fogoros S, Tan L, Zick S. "Ginger causes
       ovarian cancer cells to die." News release by University of Michigan, American
       Association for Cancer Research 97th annual meeting, April 1-5, 2006,
       Washington, D.C. Accessed 9/3/2006. <http://www.med.umich.edu/opm/
       newspage/2006/ginger.htm>.

15c.   Hsu MH, Kuo SC, Chen CJ, Chung JG, Lai YY, Huang LJ.

"1-(3,4-dimethoxyphenyl)-3,5-dodecenedione (I6) induces G1 arrest and apoptosis in human promyelocytic leukemia HL-60 cells. *Leuk Res.* 2005 Dec;29(12):1399-406. Epub 2005 May 31.

15d.   Manju V, Nalini N. "Chemopreventive efficacy of ginger, a naturally occurring anticarcinogen during the initiation, post-initiation stages of 1,2 dimethylhydrazine-induced colon cancer. *Clin Chim Acta.* 2005 Aug;358(1-2):60-7.

15e.   Wang CC, Chen LG, Lee LT, Yang LL. "Effects of 6-gingerol, an antioxidant from ginger, on inducing apoptosis in human leukemic HL-60 cells." *In Vivo.* 2003 Nov-Dec;17(6):641-5.

15f.   Miyoshi N, Nakamura Y, Ueda Y, Abe M, Ozawa Y, Uchida K, Osawa T. "Dietary ginger constituents, galanals A and B, are potent apoptosis inducers in Human T lymphoma Jurkat cells." *Cancer Lett.* 2003 Sep 25;199(2):113-9.

15g.   Leal PF, Braga ME, Sato DN, Carvalho JE, Marques MO, Meireles MA. "Functional properties of spice extracts obtained via supercritical fluid extraction." *J Agric Food Chem.* 2003 Apr 23;51(9):2520-5.

15h.   Bode AM, Ma WY, Surh YJ, Dong Z. "Inhibition of epidermal growth factor-induced cell transformation and activator protein 1 activation by [6]-gingerol." *Cancer Res.* 2001 Feb 1;61(3):850-3.

15i.   Schulick, P. *Ginger: Common Spice & Wonder Drug.* 3rd ed. Prescott, AZ. Hohm Press, 1996, pp.112-125. (Anti-cancer compounds include: alanine, aromadendrin, ascorbic-acid (vitamin C), beta-carotine, caffeic-acid, camphor, citral, p-coumaric-acid, custeine, fiber, geraniol, gingerol, glycine, beta-ionone, limonene, linalol, linoleic-acid, alpha-linolenic-acid, methionine, myristic-acid, niacin, oleic-acid, alpha-pinene, selenium, serine, tyrosine).

15j.   Lee W, Surh YJ. "Induction of apoptosis in HL-60 cells by pungent vanilloids, [6]-gingerol and [6]-paradol." *Cancer Lett.* 1998 Dec 25;134(2):163-8.

16a.   Hacksar A, Sharma A, Chawla R, Kumar R, Arora R, Singh S, Prasad J, Gupta M, Tripathi RP, Arora MP, Islam F, Sharma RK. "Zingiber officinale exhibits behavioral radioprotection against radiation-induced CTA in a gender-specific manner." *Pharmacol Biochem Behav.* 2006 Jun;84(2):179-88. Epub 2006 Jun 21.

16b.   Jagetia G, Baliga M, Venkatesh P. "Ginger (Zingiber officinale Rosc.), a dietary supplement, protects mice against radiation-induced lethality: mechanism of action." *Cancer Biother Radiopharm.* 2004 Aug;19(4):422-35.

17a.   Lu P, Lai BS, Liang P, Chen ZT, Shun SQ. "[Antioxidation activity and protective effection of ginger oil on DNA damage in vitro]" *Zhongguo Zhong Yao Za Zhi,* 2003 Sep;28(9):873-5.

17b.   Unnikrishnan MC, Kuttan R. "Cytotoxicity of extracts of spices to cultured cells." *Nutr Cancer.* 1988;11(4):251-7.

18a.   Topic B, Hasenohrl RU, Hacker R, Huston JP. "Enhanced conditioned inhibitory avoidance by a combined extract of Zingiber officinale and Ginkgo biloba." *Phytother Res.* 2002 Jun;16(4):312-5.

18b. Topic B, Tani E, Tsiakitzis K, Kourounakis PN, Dere E, Hasenohrl RU, Hacker R, Mattern CM, Huston JP. "Enhanced maze performance and reduced oxidative stress by combined extracts of zingiber officinale and ginkgo biloba in the aged rat." *Neurobiol Aging.* 2002 Jan-Feb;23(1):135-43.

19a. Yoshikawa M, Yamaguchi S, Kunimi K, Matsuda H, Okuno Y, Yamahara J, Murakami N. "Stomachic principals in ginger. III. An anti-ulcer principle, 6-gingesulfonic acid, and three monoacyldigalactosylglycerols, gingerglyco-lipids A, B, and C, from Zingiberis Rhizoma originating in Taiwan." *Chem Pharm Bull* (Tokyo). 1994 Jun;42(6):1226-30.

19b. Yoshikawa M, Hatakeyama S, Taniguchi K, Matuda H, Yamahara J. "6-Gingesulfonic acid, a new anti-ulcer principle, and ginger-glycolipids A, B and C, three new monoacyldigalactosylglycerols from Zingiberis rhizoma originating in Taiwan." *Chemical and Pharmaceutical Bulletin* 40, no. 8 (1992):2239-41.

19c. Yamahara J, Hatakeyama S, Taniguchi K, Kawamura M, Yoshikawa M. "Stomachic principals in ginger. II. Pungent and anti-ulcer effects of low polar constituents isolated from ginger, the dried rhizoma of *Zingiber officinale Roscoe* cultivated in Taiwan. The absolute stereostructure of a new diarylhep-tanoid." *Yakugaku Zasshi* 1992; 112:645-55.

19d. al-Yahya MA, Rafatullah S, Mossa JS, Ageel AM, Parmar NS, Tariq M. "Gastroprotective activity of ginger zingiber officinale rosc., in albino rats. *Am J Chin Med* 1989; 17:51-6.

19e. Yamahara J, Mochizuki M, Rong HQ, Matsuda H, Fujimura H. "The anti-ulcer effect in rats of ginger constituents. *J Ethnopharmacol* 1988; 23:299-304.

19f. Shiba M, et al. "Antiulcer furanogermenone extraction from ginger." *Chemical Abstracts* 106, no. 6 (1987).

20a. Nammi S, Sreemantula S, Roufogalis BD. "Protective effects of ethanolic extract of Zingiber officinale rhizome on the development of metabolic syndrome in high-fat diet-fed rats." *Basic Clin Pharmacol Toxicol.* 2009 May;104(5):366-73.

20b. Goyal RK, Kadnur SV. "Beneficial effects of Zingiber officinale on goldthio-glucose induced obesity." *Fitoterapia.* 2006 Apr;77(3):160-3. Epub 2006 Feb 28.

20c. Kato A, Higuchi Y, Goto H, Okamoto T, Asano N, Hollinshead J, Nash RJ, Adachi I. "Inhibitory effects of Zingiber officinale Roscoe derived components on aldose reductase activity in vitro and in vivo." *J Agric Food Chem.* 2006 Sep 6;54(18):6640-4.

20d. Sekiya K, Ohtani A, Kusano S. "Enhancement of insulin sensitivity in adipo-cytes by ginger." *Biofactors.* 2004;22(1-4):153-6.

20e. Akhani SP, Vishwakarma SL, Goyal RK. "Anti-diabetic activity of Zingiber officinale in streptozotocin-induced type I diabetic rats." *J Pharm Pharmacol.* 2004 Jan;56(1):101-5.

20f.   Kar A, Choudhary BK, Bandyopadhyay NG. "Comparative evaluation of hypoglycaemic activity of some Indian medical plants in alloxan diabetic rats." *J Ethnopharmacol.* 2003 Jan;84(1):105-8.

20g.   Mascolo N, Jain R, Jain SC, Capasso F. "Ethnopharmacologic investigation of ginger (Zingiber officinale)." J Ethnopharmacol. 1989 Nov;27(1-2):129-40.

21a.   Al-Amin ZM, Thomson M, Al-Qattan KK, Peltonen-Shalaby R, Ali M. "Anti-diabetic and hypolipidaemic properties of ginger (Zingiber officinale) in streptozotocin-induced diabetic rats." *Br J Nutr.* 2006 Oct;96(4):660-6.

21b.   Goyal RK, Kadnur SV. "Beneficial effects of Zingiber officinale on goldthioglucose induced obesity." *Fitoterapia.* 2006 Apr;77(3):160-3. Epub 2006 Feb 28.

22a.   Nammi S, Sreemantula S, Roufogalis BD. "Protective effects of ethanolic extract of Zingiber officinale rhizome on the development of metabolic syndrome in high-fat diet-fed rats." *Basic Clin Pharmacol Toxicol.* 2009 May;104(5):366-73.

22b.   Goyal RK, Kadnur SV. "Beneficial effects of Zingiber officinale on goldthioglucose induced obesity." *Fitoterapia.* 2006 Apr;77(3):160-3. Epub 2006 Feb 28.

22c.   Han LK, Gong XJ, Kawano S, Saito M, Kimura Y, Okuda H. "Antiobesity actions of Zingiber officinale Roscoe." *Yakugaku Zasshi.* 2005 Feb;125(2):213-7. [Article in Japanese].

23a.   Han LK, Gong XJ, Kawano S, Saito M, Kimura Y, Okuda H. "Antiobesity actions of Zingiber officinale Roscoe." *Yakugaku Zasshi.* 2005 Feb;125(2):213-7. [Article in Japanese].

23b.   Eldershaw TP, Colquhoun EQ, Dora KA, Peng ZC, Clark MG. "Pungent principles of ginger (Zingiber officinale) are thermogenic in the perfused rat hindlimb." *Int J Obes Relat Metab Disord.* 1992 Oct;16(10):755-63.

24.   Eldershaw TP, Colquhoun EQ, Dora KA, Peng ZC, Clark MG. "Pungent principals of ginger (Zingiber officinale) are thermogenic in the perfused rat hindlimb." *Int J Obes Relat Metab Disord.* 1992 Oct;16(10):755-63.

25.   Ahmed RS, Sharma SB. "Biochemical studies on combined effects of garlic (Allium sativum Linn) and ginger (Zingiber officinale Rosc) in albino rats." *Indian J Exp Biol.* 1997 Aug;35(8):841-3.

26.   Kyung KS, Gon JH, Geun KY, Sup JJ, Suk WJ, Ho J. "6-Shogaol. a natural product, reduces cell death and restores motor function in rat spinal cord injury." *European Journal of Neuralscience.* Volume 24 Page 1042 - August 2006.

27.   Kuhad A, Tirkey N, Pilkhwal S, Chopra K. "6-Gingerol prevents cisplatin-induced acute renal failure in rats." BioFactors. Volume 26, Number 3 - 2006. Pages 189-200.

28.   Tsukahara K, Nakagawa H, Moriwaki S, Takema Y, Fujimura T, Imokawa G. "Inhibition of ultraviolet-B-induced wrinkle formation by an

elastase-inhibiting herbal extract: implication for the mechanism underlying elastase-associated wrinkles." Int J Dermatology. 2006 Apr;45(4):460-8.

29. Shati AA, Elsaid FG. "Effects of water extracts of thyme (Thymus vulgaris) and ginger (Zingiber officinale Roscoe) on alcohol abuse." *Food Chem Toxicol.* 2009 Aug;47(8): 1945-9. Epub 2009 May 18.

30a. Bengmark S. "Curcumin, An Antioxidant and Natural NF{kappa}B, Cyclooxygenase-2, Lipooxygenase, and Inducible Nitric Oxide Synthase Inhibitor: A Shield Against Acute and Chronic Diseases." *JPEN J Parenter Enteral Nutr.* 2006 Jan-Feb;30(1):45-51.

30b. Shishodia S, Sethi G, Aggarwal BB. "Curcumin: getting back to the roots." *Ann N Y Acad Sci.* 2005 Nov;1056:206-17.

30c. Chianani-Wu N. "Safety and anti-inflammatory activity of curcumin: a component of turmeric (Curcuma longa)" *J Altern Complement Med.* 2003 Feb;9(1):161-8.

30d. Surh YJ. "Anti-tumor promoting potential of selected spice ingredients with antioxidative and anti-inflammatory activities: a short review." Food Chem Toxicol. 2002 Aug;40(8):1091-7.

30e. Lin JK, Lin-Shiau SY. "Mechanisms of cancer chemoprevention by curcumin." *ProcNatl Sci Counc Repub China B.* 2001 Apr;25(2):59-66.

30f. Zhang F, Altorki NK, Mestre JR, Subbaramaiah K, Dannenberg AJ. "Curcumin inhibits cyclooxygenase-2 transcription in bile acid- and phorbol ester-treated human gastrointestinal epithelial cells." Carcinogenesis. Vol. 20, No. 3, 445-451, March 1999.

30g. Kawamori T, Lubet R, Steele VE, Kelloff GJ, Kaskey RB, RaoCV, Reddy BS. "Chemopreventive effect of curcumin, a naturally occurring anti-inflammatory agent, during the promotion/progression stages of colon cancer." *Cancer Res.* 1999 Feb 1;59(3):597-601.

30h. Ammon HP, et al. "Mechanism of Anti-inflammatory Actions of Curcumin and Boswellic Acids." *J Ethnopharmacol.* 1993;38:113.

30i. Deodhar SD, et al. "Preliminary Studies on Anti-Rheumatic Activity of Curcumin." *Ind J Med Res.* 1980;71:632.

31a. Bengmark S. "Curcumin, An Antioxidant and Natural NF{kappa}B, Cyclooxygenase-2, Lipooxygenase, and Inducible Nitric Oxide Synthase Inhibitor: A Shield Against Acute and Chronic Diseases." *JPEN J Parenter Enteral Nutr.* 2006 Jan-Feb;30(1):45-51.

31b. Sugiyama T, Nagata JI, Yamagishi A, Endoh K, Saito M, Yamada K, Yamada S, Umegaki K. "Selective protection of curcumin against carbon tetrachloride-induced inactivation of hepatic cytochrome P450 isozymes in rats." *Life Sci.* 2005 Nov 7.

31c. Tilak JC, Banerjee M, Mohan H, Devasagayam TP. "Antioxidant availability of turmeric in relation to its medicinal and culinary uses." *Phytother Res.* 2004 Oct;18(10):798-804.

31d.   Shukla PK, Khanna VK, Khan MY, Srimal RC. "Protective effect of curcumin against lead neurotoxicity in rat." *Hum Exp Toxicol.* 2003 Dec;22(12):653-8.

31e.   Jayaprakasha GK, Jena BS, Negi PS Sakariah KK. "Evaluation of antioxidant activities and antimutagenicity of turmeric oil: a byproduct from curcumin production." *Z Naturforsch [C].* 2002 Sep-Oct;57(9-10):828-35.

31f.   Surh YJ. "Anti-tumor promoting potential of selected spice ingredients with antioxidative and anti-inflammatory activities: a short review." Food Chem Toxicol. 2002 Aug;40(8):1091-7.

31g.   Surh Y. "Molecular mechanisms of chemopreventive effects of selected dietary and medicinal phenolic substances." *Mutat Res.* 1999 Jul 16;428(1-2):305-27.

31h.   Ruby AJ, Kuttan G, Babu KD, Rajasekharan KN, Kuttan R. "Anti-tumour and antioxidant activity of natural curcuminoids." *Cancer Lett.* 1995 Jul 20;94(1):79-83.

31i.   Weber WM, Hunsaker LA, Abcouwer SF, Deck LM, Vander Jagt DL. "Antioxidant activities of curcumin and related enones." *Bioorg Med Chem.* 2005 Jun 1;13(11):3811-20.

32a.   Leal PF, Braga ME, Sato DN, Carvalho JE, Marques MO, Meireles MA. "Functional properties of spice extracts obtained via supercritical fluid extraction." *J Agric Food Chem.* 2003 Apr 23;51(9):2520-5.

32b.   Mahady GB, Pendland SL, Yun G, Lu ZZ. "Turmeric (Curcuma longa) and curcumin inhibit the growth of Helicobacter pylori, a group 1 carcinogen." *Anticancer Res.* 2002 Nov-Dec;22(6C):4179-81.

33a.   O'Mahony R, Al-Khtheeri H, Weerasekera D, Fernando N, Vaira D, Holton J, Basset C. "Bactericidal and anti-adhesive properties of culinary and medicinal plants against Helicobacter pylori." *World J Gastroenterol.* 2005 Dec 21;11(47):7499-507.

33b.   Surh YJ. "Anti-tumor promoting potential of selected spice ingredients with antioxidative and anti-inflammatory activities: a short review." *Food Chem Toxicol.* 2002 Aug;40(8):1091-7.

34a.   Chauhan DP. "Chemotherapeutic potential of curcumin for colorectal cancer." *Curr Pharm Des.* 2002;8(19):1695-706.

34b.   Lin JK, Lin-Shiau SY. "Mechanisms of cancer chemoprevention by curcumin." *Proc Natl Sci Counc Repub China B.* 2001 Apr;25(2):59-66.

34c.   Churchhill M, Chadburn A, Bilinski RT, Bertagnolli MM. "Inhibition of intestinal tumors by curcumin is associated with changes in the intestinal immune cell profile." *J Surg Res.* 2000 Apr;89(2):169-75.

34d.   Han SS, Chung ST, Robertson DA, Ranjan D, Bondada S. "Curcumin causes the growth arrest and apoptosis of B cell lymphoma by downregulation of egr-1, c-myc, bcl-XL, NF-kappa B, and p53." *Clin Immunol.* 1999 Nov;93(2):152-61.

34e.   Kawamori T, Lubet R, Steele VE, Kelloff GJ, Kaskey RB, Rao CV, Reddy BS. "Chemopreventive effect of curcumin, a naturally occurring anti-inflammatory agent, during the promotion/progression stages of colon cancer." *Cancer Res.* 1999 Feb 1;59(3):597-601.

34f.   Verma SP, Goldin BR, Lin PS. "The inhibition of the estrogenic effects of pesticides and environmental chemicals by curcumin and isoflavonoids." *Environ Health Perspect.* 1998 Dec;106(12):807-12.

34g.   Mehta K, Pantazis P, McQueen T, Aggarwal BB. "Antiproliferative effect of curcumin (diferuloylmethane) against human breast tumor cell lines." *Anticancer Drugs.* 1997 Jun;8(5):470-81.

34h.   Huang MT, Newmark HL, Frenkel K. "Inhibitory effects of curcumin on tumorigenesis in mice." *J Cell Biochem Suppl.* 1997;27:26-34.

34i.   Ruby AJ, Kuttan G, Babu KD, Rajasekharan KN, Kuttan R. "Anti-tumour and antioxidant activity of natural curcuminoids." *Cancer Lett.* 1995 Jul 20;94(1):79-83.

34j.   Rao CV, Rivenson A, Simi B, Reddy BS. "Chemoprevention of colon carcinogenesis by dietary curcumin, a naturally occurring plant phenolic compound." *Cancer Res.* 1995 Jan 15;55(2):259-66.

35a.   Fujisawa S, Kadoma Y. "Anti- and pro-oxidant effects of oxidized quercetin, curcumin or curcumin-related compounds with thiols or ascorbate as measured by the induction period method." *In Vivo.* 2006 Jan-Feb;20(1):39-44.

35b.   Chen A, Xu J, Johnson AC. "Curcumin inhibits human colon cancer cell growth by suppressing gene expression of epidermal growth factor receptor through reducing the activity of the transcription factor Egr-1." *Oncogene.* 2006 Jan 12;25(2):278-87.

35c.   Sharma RA, Gescher AJ, Steward WP. "Curcumin: the story so far." *Eur J Cancer.* 2005 Sep;41(13):1955-68.

35d.   Baatout S, Derradji H, Jacquet P, Mergeay M. "Increased radiation sensitivity of an eosinophilic cell line following treatment with epigallocatechin-gallate, reservatol and curcuma." *Int J Mol Med.* 2005 Feb;15(2):337-52.

35e.   Cheng AL, Hsu CH, Lin JK, Hsu MM, Ho YF, Shen TS, Ko JY, Lin JT, Lin BR, Ming-Shiang W, Yu HS, Jee SH, Chen GS, Chen TM, Chen CA, Lai MK, Pu YS, Pan MH, Wang YJ, Tsai CC, Hsieh CY. "Phase I clinical trial of curcumin, a chemopreventive agent, in patients with high-risk or pre-malignant lesions." *Anticancer Res.* 2001 Jul-Aug;21(4B):2895-900.

35f.   Sharma RA, McLelland HR, Hill KA, Ireson CR, Euden SA, Manson MM, Pirmohamed M, Marnett LJ, Gescher AJ, Steward WP. "Pharmacodynamic and pharmacokinetic study of oral Curcuma extract in patients with colorectal cancer." *Clin Cancer Res.* 2001 Jul;7(7):1894-900.

35g.   Leal PF, Braga ME, Sato DN, Carvalho JE, Marques MO, Meireles MA. "Functional properties of spice extracts obtained via supercritical fluid extraction." *J Agric Food Chem.* 2003 Apr 23;51(9):2520-5.

35h. Aggarwal BB, Kumar A, Bharti AC. "Anticancer potential of curcumin: preclinical and clinical studies." *Anticancer Res.* 2003 Jan-Feb;23(1A):363-98.

35i. Chauhan DP. "Chemotherapeutic potential of curcumin for colorectal cancer." *Curr Pharm Des.* 2002;8(19):1695-706.

35j. Lin JK, Lin-Shiau SY. "Mechanisms of cancer chemoprevention by curcumin." *Proc Natl Sci Counc Repub China B.* 2001 Apr;25(2):59-66.

35k. Dorai T, Gehani N, Katz A. "therapeutic potential of curcumin in human prostate cancer. II. Curcumin inhibits tyrosine kinase activity of epidermal growth factor receptor and depletes the protein." *Mol Urol.* 2000 Spring;4(1):1-6.

35l. Kawamori T, Lubet R, Steele VE, Kelloff GJ, Kaskey RB, Rao CV, Reddy BS. "Chemopreventive effect of curcumin, a naturally occurring anti-inflammatory agent, during the promotion/progression stages of colon cancer." *Cancer Res.* 1999 Feb 1;59(3):597-601.

35m. Mehta K, Pantazis P, McQueen T, Aggarwal BB. "Antiproliferative effect of curcumin (diferuloylmethane) against human breast tumor cell lines." *Anticancer Drugs.* 1997 Jun;8(5):470-81.

36a. Asai A, Miyazawa T. "Dietary Curcuminoids Prevent High-Fat Diet-Induced Lipid Accumulation in Rat Liver and Epididymal Adipose Tissue." *J. Nutr.* 2001 131: 2932-2935.

36b. Babu PS, Srinivasan K. "Hypolipidemic action of curcumin, the active principle of turmeric (Curcuma longa) in streptozotocin induced diabetic rats." *Mol Cell Biochem.* 1997 Jan;166(1-2):169-75.

36c. Soni KB, Kuttan R. "Effect of oral curcumin administration on serum peroxides and cholesterol levels in human volunteers." *Indian J Physiol Pharmacol.* 1992 Oct;36(4):273-5.

36d. Hussain MS, Chandrasekhara N. "Effect of curcumin on cholesterol gall-stone induction in mice." *Indian J Med Res.* 1992 Oct;96:288-91.

36e. Srinivasan K, Sambaiah K. "The effect of spices on cholesterol 7 alpha-hydroxylase activity and on serum and hepatic cholesterol levels in the rat." *Int J Vitam Nutr Res.* 1991;61(4):364-9.

36f. Rao DS, et al. "Effect of curcumin on serum and liver cholesterol levels in the rat." *J Nutr.* 1970;100:1307-1316.

37a. Miquel J, Ramirez-Bosca A, Ramirez-Bosca JV, Alperi JD. "Menopause: A review on the role of oxygen stress and favorable effects of dietary antioxidants." *Arch Gerontol Geriatr.* 2006 Jan 25; [Epub ahead of print].

37b. Jagetia GC, Rajanikant GK. "Effect of curcumin on radiation-impaired healing of excisional wounds in mice." *J Wound Care.* 2004 Mar;13(3):107-9.

37c. Pandya U, Saini MK, Jin GF, Awasthi S, Godley BF, Awasthi YC. "Dietary curcumin prevents ocular toxicity of naphthalene in rats." Toxicol Lett. 2000 Jun 5;115(3):195-204.

37d. Park EJ, Jeon CH, Ko G, Kim J, Sohn DH. "Protective effect of curcumin in rat liver injury induced by carbon tetrachloride." *J Pharm Pharmacol.* 2000 Apr;52(4):437-40.

37e. Chuang SE, Kuo ML, Hsu CH, Chen CR, Lin JK, Lai GM, Hsieh CY, Cheng AL. "Curcumin-containing diet inhibits diethylnitrosamine-induced murine hepatocarcinogenesis." Carcinogenesis. 2000 Feb;21(2):331-5.

37f. Venkatesan N, Punithavathi D, Arumugam V. "Curcumin prevents adriamycin nephrotoxicity in rats." *Br J Pharmacol.* 2000 Jan;129(2):231-4.

37g. Hussain MS, Chandrasekhara N. "Effect on curcumin on cholesterol gallstone induction in mice." Indian J Med Res. 1992 Oct;96:288-91.

38a. Yang F, Lim GP, Begum AN, Ubeda OJ, Simmons MR, Ambegaokar SS, Chen PP, Kayed R, Glabe CG, Frautschy SA, Cole GM. "Curcumin inhibits formation of amyloid beta oligomers and fibrils, binds plaques, and reduces amyloid in vivo." *J Biol Chem.* 2005 Feb18;280(7):5892-901.

38b. Ono K, Hasegawa K, Naiki H, Yamanda M. "Curcumin has potent anti-amyloidogenic effects for Alzheimer's beta-amyloid fibrils in vitro." *J Neurosci Res.* 2004 Mar 15;75(6):742-50.

38c. Calabrese V, Butterfield DA, Stella AM. "Nutritional antioxidants and the heme oxygenase pathway of stress tolerance: novel targets for neuroprotection in Alzheimer's disease." *Ital J Biochem.* 2003 Dec;52(4):177-81.

38d. Frautschy SA, Hu W, Kim P, et al. "Phenolic anti-inflammatory antioxidant reversal of Abeta-induced cognitive deficits and neuropathology." *Neurobiol Aging.* 2001 Nov;22(6):993-1005.

38e. Lim GP, Chu T, Yang F, Beech W, Frautschy SA, Cole GM. "The curry spice curcumin reduces oxidative damage and amyloid pathology in an Alzheimer transgenic mouse. *J Neurosci.* 2001 Nov 1;21(21):8370-7.

39a. Chandra V, Pandav R, Dodge HH, Johnston JM, Belle SH, DeKosky ST, Ganguli M. "Incidence of Alzheimer's disease in a rural community in India: the Indo-US study. *Neurology* 2001; 57:985-9.

39b. Vas CJ, Pinto C, Panikker D, Noronha S, Deshpande N, Kulkarni L, Sachdeva S. "Prevalence of dementia in an urban Indian population." *Int Psychogeriatr.* 2001 Dec;13(4):439-50.

40. Grzanna R, Phan P, Polotsky A, Lindmark L, Frondoza CG. "Ginger extract inhibits beta-amyloid peptide-induced cytokine and chemokine expression in cultured THP-1 monocytes." *Altern Complement Med.* 2004 Dec;10(6):1009-13.

41a. Kim DS, Kim JY. "Side-chain length is important for shogaols in protecting neuronal cells from beta-amyloid insult." *Bioorg Med Chem Lett.* 2004 Mar 8;14(5):1287-9.

41b. Kim DS, Kim DS, Oppel MN. "Shogaols from Zingiber officinale protect IMR32 human neuroblastoma and normal human umbilical vein endothelial cells from beta-amyloid(25-35) insult." Planta Med. 2002 Apr;68(4):375-6.

42. Gerdes LU, Klausen IC, Sihm I, Faergeman O. "Apolipoprotein E

Polymorphism in a Danish Population Compared to Findings in 45 Other Study Populations Around the World. *Genet Epidemiol* 1992;9:155-67.

43. Grant WB. "Dietary links to Alzheimer's disease." *Alz Dis* Rev. 1997;2:42-55.

44. Shishodia S, Sethi G, Aggarwal B. "Curcumin: Getting Back to the Roots." Ann. N.Y. Acad. Sci. 1056: 206-217 (2005).

45. "What is Turmeric?" Accessed 10/22/06. <http://turmeric-curcumin.com/>.

46. University of Maryland Medical Center (web site). Turmeric - How to Take It. Accessed 10/26/06. <http://www.umm.edu/altmed/ConsHerbs/Turmericch.html>.

47. University of Maryland Medical Center (web site). Turmeric - Precautions. Accessed 10/26/06. <http://www.umm.edu/altmed/ConsHerbs/Turmericch.html.>.

48. Somasundaram S, et al. "Dietary curcumin inhibits chemotherapy-induced apoptosis in models of human breast cancer." *Cancer Res.* 2002;62:3868-75.

49. Yoshida S, Kasuga S, Hayashi N, Ushiroguchi T, Matsuura H, Nakagawa S. "Antifungal Activity of Ajoene Derived from Garlic." *Applied and Environmentsl Microbiology.* Mar 1987, p.615-617.

50. Johnson MG, Vaughn RH. "Death of Salmonella typhimurium and Escherichia coli in the Presence of Freshly Reconstituted Dehydrated Garlic and Onion." *Applied Microbiology.* June 1969, p.903-905.

51a. Ariga T, Seki T. "Antithrombotic and anticancer effects of garlic-derived sulfur compounds: a review." *Biofactors.* 2006;26(2):93-103.

51b. Milner JA. "A historical perspective on garlic and cancer." *J Nutr.* 2001 Mar;131(3s):1027S-31S.

51c. Lea MA. "Organosulfur compounds and cancer." *Adv Exp Med Biol.* 1996;401:147-54.

52. KT Aufusti, C Ashakumari, George Daniel, S Jaya, Sinu K Mathew, Sreerekhua and PK Joseph. "The beneficial effects of garlic oil and garlic cake on coconut oil fed rats." Journal of Medicinal Plants Research. Vol. 2(2), pp.034-038, February, 2008.

53. Milner JA. "A historical perspective on garlic and cancer." *J Nutr.* 2001 Mar;131(3s):1027S-31S.

54. "Garlic: Good...or Good for Nothing?" Bottom Line Natural Healing. June 2007 pp.4-5.

CHAPTER 5

Enzyme Deficiency

CLUE #5: Some people may not produce enough digestive enzymes for proper digestion. This is called pancreatic insufficiency and may result from past illness, injury, stress, sickness, exposure to chemicals, heredity, or aging. In addition, as we grow older, our body produces less and less enzymes.[1] Making matters worse, it is believed that the enzymes produced by an older person are weaker and less effective than those produced by a younger person.[2] As we age, poor digestion further weakens the immune system and stresses the body. The good news is that enzyme supplements are easy to take and have few if any side effects. Enzymes are an exciting new area of research.

The discovery of the science behind enzymes and their importance in sustaining life was such a huge breakthrough in the science of life that Eduard Buchner of Germany was awarded the Nobel Prize for Chemistry in 1907.[3] A growing number of athletes take enzyme supplements because of their powerful anti-inflammatory properties. When athletes suffer an inflammation injury (as they often do when training), it was found that having these extra enzymes in their bodies before the injury promoted faster recovery.[4]

It has been known for a long time that the pancreas and other organs secrete enzymes necessary for life itself. Enzymes are the spark plugs that either start up or speed up the many complex chemical reactions involved in every system in our body. Many researchers conclude that a shortage of enzymes hinders our body's ability to function, make repairs, and fight off disease. Enzyme deficiency has been blamed for slow recovery from injuries and the speeding of illnesses including arthritis, heart disease, cancer, and premature aging.[5] Enzymes are supplied from three sources: 1) secreted from organs within the body; 2) taken into the body by eating fresh, uncooked fruits and vegetables; and 3) by taking enzyme supplements.

Fresh, uncooked fruits and vegetables come prepackaged with natural supplies of their own enzymes. In most cases, every fruit or vegetable contains the exact enzymes needed to break down and digest it. The only thing we need to do is chew up fresh fruits and vegetables in order to release their enzymes. The bad news is that these enzymes are easily destroyed when the fruit or vegetable is cooked or heated above 118°F (48°C) for an extended time.[6] As you will read later, fresh ginger stands out among all other plants in that it contains an unusually high amount of proteolytic (protein-digesting) enzymes.

Our modern diet is filled with refined and processed foods and, for the most part, is sadly lacking in naturally occurring enzymes. If the food we eat has few or no enzymes, the pancreas is forced to steal enzyme components from other parts of the body in order to digest our food. In theory, this can create a shortage of enzymes in other parts of the body, enzymes that could have been used for such tasks as repairing an injury or running the immune system. Dr. Edward Howell, a pioneer in enzyme research, performed many animal studies showing how the pancreas of lab rats enlarges to produce extra enzymes needed for the digestion of a constant diet of cooked foods. When these rats were allowed to live until the end of their lifespan and then examined, he reported "an astonishing array of typically human degenerative diseases was revealed." Dr. Howell also studied the effects of enzyme deficiencies in other animals.[7]

If our diets are overloaded with bad fats, too much sugar, very little fiber, and a shortage of nutrients, our bodies are further stressed and our health suffers. Even more disturbing, *a government study estimated at least 35% of cancers are related to diet.*[8] Yes, it does take some effort to include fresh fruits and vegetables in our diet, but we need to do it. It helps to think of fresh fruits and vegetables as our medicine. I encourage you to have a garden if you are able. Most of us are fortunate to have a wide variety of fresh produce delivered to our grocery stores. We owe many thanks to those who grow, harvest, and transport the many fresh fruits and vegetables that end up on our dinner table and in our lunch boxes. Enzymes are discussed in more detail in chapter 15.

REFERENCES FOR CHAPTER 5

1a.   Cichoke A, Dr. *The Complete Book of Enzyme Therapy* 1999, Avery Publishing, New York, NY 10014 p.2.
1b.   Howell E, Dr. *Enzyme Nutrition* 1985 Avery Publishing, New York, NY pp. ix-xii, 12, 73-74, 153-155.
2.   Howell E, Dr. *Enzyme Nutrition* 1985 Avery Publishing, New York, NY pp.27-29.
3.   "The Nobel Prize in Chemistry 1946" Presentation Speech by Professor A. Tiselius, member of the Nobel Committee for Chemistry of the Royal Swedish Academy of Sciences. Web site accessed 6/14/2009. <http://nobelprize.org/nobel_prizes/chemistry/laureates/1946/press.html>.
4a.   Cichoke A, Dr. *The Complete Book of Enzyme Therapy* 1999, Avery Publishing, New York, NY 10014 pp.380-381.
4b.   "The Non-drug European Secret to Healing Sports Injuries Naturally." Accessed 7/8/2004. <http://www.buywobenzym.com>.
5a.   Howell E, Dr. *Enzyme Nutrition* 1985 Avery Publishing, New York, NY pp.x, 15.
5b.   Cichoke A, Dr. *The Complete Book of Enzyme Therapy* 1999, Avery Publishing, New York, NY 10014 pp.2,5,6.
6.   Howell E, Dr. *Enzyme Nutrition* 1985 Avery Publishing, New York, NY pp.xi.
7.   Howell E, Dr. *Enzyme Nutrition* 1985 Avery Publishing, New York, NY pp.27, 29, 80-84.
8.   R. Doll and R. Petro. "Cancer Rates and Risks." National Cancer Institute (Washington DC: 1985) *Journal of the National Cancer Institute.* 1981 66(6):1191-1308.

CHAPTER 6

Hydrochloric Acid Deficiency

CLUE #6: For many, the stomach may not produce enough hydrochloric acid (HCl). HCl is secreted by millions of special cells in the stomach lining (called parietal cells). Most high-protein foods need HCl for proper digestion because HCl creates an acidic condition in the stomach that activates pepsin, the stomach's main protein-digesting enzyme.[1] Dr. Atkins—physician, nutritionist, and author of *Dr. Atkins' Vita-Nutrient Solution*—writes that up to one-half of people over age 60 do not produce enough HCl.[2] Another physician who treated thousands of patients with heartburn reported almost no overacidity among patients over the age of 35.[3]

Researchers point out that the presence of certain bacteria, especially *Helicobacter pylori,* causes large decreases of HCl production in older people.[4] You will learn in chapter 18 that ginger can inhibit *Helicobacter pylori.* Just this one action alone may greatly improve digestion and health.

Here are two more ways ginger improves digestion:

1. Fresh ginger's potent proteolytic enzymes act to break down food proteins.[5]
2. Ginger ranks highest among 14 spices for enhancing the secretion of trypsin, another protein-digesting enzyme[6] (the enzyme trypsin is secreted by the pancreas and enters the small intestine).

Listed here are some illnesses Dr. Atkins believes are caused or aggravated by HCl deficiency and improper digestion of proteins:[7]

- *Candida* overgrowth and other intestinal infections
- Asthma
- Diabetes
- Food allergies
- Osteoporosis (bone loss in older people)
- Rheumatoid arthritis (inflammation of the joints and surrounding tissues, caused by the body attacking itself)
- Iron-deficiency anemia (a decreased number of red blood cells which results in a shortage of oxygen throughout the body, leading to fatigue, weakness, and shortness of breath)
- May increase risk of gastric cancer

Dr. Atkins writes that many skin conditions may be linked to low levels of HCl, including the following:[8]

- Acne (other studies show acne can also result from deficiency of folic acid, vitamin B12,[9] and pantothenic acid,[10] also known as vitamin B5; taking these supplements may be helpful)
- Eczema (scaly, itchy patches of skin caused by inflammation; long-term may have thick, leather-like appearance)
- Psoriasis (patches of thick, red skin that are often covered with silvery-white scales)
- Dermatitis (inflammation of the skin; appearance varies but may appear as redness, a rash, swelling, pimples, blisters, resembling a burn, etc.)
- Hives (raised, itchy red spots on the skin caused by an allergic reaction)
- Vitiligo (loss of pigment in the skin resulting in white patches; caused by the body attacking itself)

Adelle Davis, author of *Let's Get Well*, had tremendous insight back in 1965 when she wrote that "too little hydrochloric acid impairs protein digestion and vitamin-C absorption, allows the B vitamins to be destroyed, and prevents minerals from reaching the blood to the extent that anemia can develop and bones crumble." She also tells of an orthopedic (bone) specialist who tested all of his patients for low stomach acid and consistently found them to be deficient. He then prescribed HCl supplements to ensure proper healing of the bones.[11]

See your medical provider for tests that can detect low HCl levels in your stomach. Low stomach acid can be easily helped by taking supplements of betaine hydrochloride, a form of HCl available in capsules. Many digestive-enzyme supplements also contain some betaine hydrochloride.

A SIMPLE TEST FOR LOW HCL

One physician suggests the following simple test to determine if you have sufficient amounts of HCl. Mix one-quarter teaspoon of baking soda with 8 ounces of water. Drink this first thing in the morning, before eating or drinking. Note how long it takes until belching starts. If it takes longer than 2 or 3 minutes to produce a belch, this indicates low stomach acid. Immediate belching may indicate excess stomach acid. Children do not have to drink the entire 8 ounces.[12]

Another test for low stomach HCl is recommended by Dr. Mercola on his Web site, www.mercola.com. He gives instructions to locate the HCl reflex point—located on the lowest rib about 1 inch sideways from the center of the sternum. If this point is tender when pressed with a finger, it indicates an HCl deficiency. Mercola recommends taking 1 to 6 tablets of betaine HCl at the beginning of every meal and then adjusting the amount until the reflex point is no longer tender.[13]

LOW HCL LEVELS CAN PREVENT ABSORPTION OF FOLATE AND B VITAMINS

It is known that folate and vitamins B6 and B12 will not be absorbed without sufficient amounts of HCl.[14] Low levels of vitamin B12 can result in *depression, slower thinking, confusion, and memory lapses.* Other symptoms may include numbness or burning sensations in the feet.[15] One physician who specializes in treating patients with chronic fatigue syndrome gives injections of vitamin B12 and sees positive results in 80% of his patients.[16] Researchers point out that deficiencies of either vitamin B12 or folate may have a role in *depression[17], mood disorders[18], dementia, and psychiatric disturbances.[19]*

Nature's richest sources of vitamin B12 are clams, mussels, crabs,[20] meat, organ meats, fish, poultry, milk, and eggs.[21] Vitamin B complex supplements are popular and inexpensive. For more information on vitamin B and folate, refer to *Dr. Atkins' Vita-Nutrient Solution* (Simon & Schuster) and visit the Linus Pauling Institute Web site at www.lpi. oregonstate and select "micronutrients."

Folate is a B vitamin that is especially important for proper cell division and, therefore, is especially important for women before and during pregnancy.[22] One study showed that mothers who used multivitamins containing folic acid during the first 6 weeks of pregnancy had the lowest rates of brain and spinal cord defects in their babies.[23] Another study showed the risk of cleft lip in babies was lowest in mothers who ate plenty of fruits, vegetables, and other folate-containing foods and also took supplements of folic acid early in their pregnancy.[24] (Folic acid is a synthetic form of folate that is added to foods and is also available as supplements). Folate is also important for the production of HCl.[25] For more information and cautions about folate and folic acid supplements, visit the government-sponsored Web site for the Office of Dietary Supplements at ods.od.nih.gov/factsheets/folate.asp.[26]

Folate occurs naturally in many foods, including leafy green vegetables, especially spinach (which is very high in folate); broccoli; fruit; beans; peas; whole grains; and peanuts.[27] Be aware that cooking can destroy up to 90% of the folate in food.[28] Enriched breads, cereals, and other grain products such as pasta are often fortified with folic acid.[29]

Folate also helps remove homocysteine from the blood. Homocysteine is a blood protein that has been linked to increased risk of cardiovascular disease and stroke. Homocysteine levels in the blood are used as markers for the risk of cardiovascular disease and overclotting of blood.[30] High levels of homocysteine also increase the risk of diseases of the nervous system such as Alzheimer's and Parkinson's.[31] Animal studies show that too much homocysteine in the brain can damage the nerve cells that are involved in learning and memory.[32] Homocysteine slows the repair of DNA and induces oxidative stress, causing cells to dysfunction.[33]

Folate and folic acid may have other benefits. One interesting study showed folic acid supplements seemed to help reduce hearing loss in older adults.[34] Dr. Atkins writes, "Folic acid is the one vitamin we need more than any other." He recommends taking folic acid and vitamin B12 for treatment of acne and psoriasis.[35]

However, there are some cautions related to folate. Recent studies indicate that taking too much supplemental folic acid could promote the growth of certain cancer and precancer cells. It appears supplements of folic acid may do more harm than good later in life. The researchers also state, "There is absolutely no evidence that folate from foods alone is harmful."[36]

REFERENCES FOR CHAPTER 6

1. Le Veen HH, Hallinger L. "The role of pepsin, peptic inhibitory substances, and hydrochloric acid in normal subjects and in the production of peptic ulcers." Department of Surgery of the University of Chicago. July 23, 1946.

2. Atkins RC. *Dr. Atkin's Vita-Nutrient Solution.* Simon & Schuster, Inc. 1998. p.234.

3. Jonathan V. Wright, MD. "Theory of Aging Part II." Web site: Tahoma Clinic. Accessed 2/1/2008. <http://www.tahoma-clinc.com/afing2.shtml>.

4. Harrma k, Kamada T, Kawaguchi H, Okamoto S, Yoshihara M, Sumii K, Inoue M, Kishimoto S, Kajiyama G, Miyoshi A. "Effect of age and Helicobacter pylori infection on gastric acid secretion." *J Gastroenterol Hepatol.* 2000 Mar;15(3):277-83.

5. Thompson EH, Wolf ID, Allen CE. "GINGER RHIZOME: A NEW SOURCE OF PROTEOLYTIC ENZYME." *Journal of Food Science* -Volume 38 (1973). 652-6550

6.   Kalpana Platel & K. Srinivasan." Digestive stimulant action of spices: A myth or
      reality?" *Indian J Med Res.* 119, May 2004, pp 167-179.
7.   Atkins RC. *Dr. Atkin's Vita-Nutrient Solution.* Simon & Schuster, Inc. 1998. p.234.
8.   Atkins RC. *Dr. Atkin's Vita-Nutrient Solution.* Simon & Schuster, Inc. 1998. p.234.
9.   Atkins RC. *Dr. Atkin's Vita-Nutrient Solution.* Simon & Schuster, Inc. 1998. p.67,
      71.
10.   Leung LH. "Pantothenic acid deficiency as the pathogenesis of acne vulgaris,"
      Med Hypotheses. 1995 Jun;44(6):490-2.
11.   Davis A. *Lets Get Well.* Signet, Signet Classics, Signette, Mentor and Plume
      Books. New York, New York. November, 1972 p.142. (Authorized reprint of
      original by Harcourt Brace Jovanovich, Inc., 1965).
12.   "Autism Treatment Options". "Digestion Aids". Web site: Child-Autism-Parent-
      Cafe.com. Accessed 2/8/2008. <www.http://www.child-autism-parent-cafe.com/
      autism-treatment.html>.
13.   "Mercury Detoxification Protocol" Web site: mercola.com. Accessed 4/12/2008.
      <http://www.mercola.com/article/mercury/detox_protocol.htm>.
14a. Cichoke A, Dr. *The Complete Book of Enzyme Therapy* 1999, Avery Publishing,
      New York, NY 10014 p.264.
14b. Atkins RC. *Dr. Atkin's Vita-Nutrient Solution.* Simon & Schuster, Inc. 1998. p.234.
15.   Atkins RC. *Dr. Atkin's Vita-Nutrient Solution.* Simon & Schuster, Inc. 1998. p.74.
16.   Dr. Charles W. Lapp. "THE TREATMENT OF CHRONIC FATIGUE
      SYNDROME (CFS) THE PERSPECTIVE OF A PRIVATE SPECIALTY
      PRACTICE IN CHARLOTTE, NC." Lecture given in Nashville, TN, April
      1997 (translated by Angela). Accessed 2/13/2008. <http://www.co-cure.org/
      Lapp.htm>.
17.   Coppen A, Bolander-Gouaille C. "Treatment of depression: time to consider
      folic acid and vitamin B12." J Psychopharmacol. 2005 Jan;19(1):59-65.
18.   Reynolds E. "Vitamin B12, folic acid, and the nervous system." *Lancet Neurol.*
      2006 Nov;5(11):949-60.
19a. Reynolds E. "Vitamin B12, folic acid, and the nervous system." *Lancet Neurol.*
      2006 Nov;5(11):949-60.
19b. Bottiglieri T. "Folate, vitamin B12, and neuropsychiatric disorders." *Nutr Rev.*
      1996 Dec;54(12):382-90.
20.   "Vitamin B12" Web site: Linus Pauling Institute at Oregon State University.
      Accessed 2/13/2008. <http://lpi.oregonstate.edu/infocenter/vitamins/
      vitaminB12/>.
21.   Cichoke A, Dr. *The Complete Book of Enzyme Therapy.*1999, Avery Publishing,
      New York, NY 10014 p.57.
22.   "Dietary Supplement Fact Sheet: Folate." Web site: National Institutes of
      Health, Office of Dietary Supplements. Accessed 10/1/2008. <http://ods.od.nih.
      gov/factsheets/folate.asp>.
23.   Milunsky A, Jick H, Jick SS, Bruell CL, MacLaughlin DS, Rothman KJ, Willett

W. "Multivitamin/folic acid supplementation in early pregnancy reduces the prevalence of neural tube defects." JAMA. 1989 Nov 24;262(20):2847-52.

24. Wilcox AJ, Lie RT, Solvoll K, Taylor J, McConnaughey DR, Abyholm F, Vindenes H, Vollset SE, Drevon CA. "Folic acid supplements and risk of facial clefts: national population based case-control study." *BMJ*, 2007 Mar 3;334(7591):464. Epub 2007 Jan 26.

25a. Cichoke A, Dr. *The Complete Book of Enzyme Therapy* 1999, Avery Publishing, New York, NY 10014 p.57.

25b. "Nutrients in Spinach, Boiled." the world's healthiest foods. George Mateljan Foundation. Accessed 1/2/2008. <http://www.whfoods.com>.

26. "Dietary Supplement Fact Sheet: Folate." Web site: National Institutes of Health, Office of Dietary Supplements. Accessed 10/1/2008. <http://ods.od.nih.gov/factsheets/folate.asp>.

27. "Dietary Supplement Fact Sheet: Folate." Web site: National Institutes of Health, Office of Dietary Supplements. Accessed 10/1/2008. <http://ods.od.nih.gov/factsheets/folate.asp>.

28. Atkins RC. *Dr. Atkin's Vita-Nutrient Solution*. Simon & Schuster, Inc. 1998. p.72.

29. "Dietary Supplement Fact Sheet: Folate." Web site: National Institutes of Health, Office of Dietary Supplements. Accessed 10/1/2008. <http://ods.od.nih.gov/factsheets/folate.asp>.

30. Vermeulen EG, Stehouwer CD, Twisk JW, van den Berg M, de Jong SC, Mackaay AJ, van Campen CM, Visser FC, Jakobs CA, Bulterjis EJ, Rauwerda JA. "Effect of homocysteine-lowering treatment with folic acid plus vitamin B6 on progression of subclinical atherosclerosis: a randomized, placebo-controlled trial." *Lancet*. 2000 Feb 12;355(9023):517-22.

31. Mattson MP, Haberman F. "Folate and homocysteine metabolism: therapeutic targets in cardiovascular and neurodegenerative disorders." *Curr Med Chem*. 2003 Oct;10(19):1923-9.

32. "Folic Acid Possibly A Key Factor In Alzheimer's Disease Prevention." Web site: National Institutes of Health. NIH News Release. Friday, March 1, 2002. Accessed 1/29/2008. <http://www.nih.gov/news/pr/mar2002/nia-01.htm>.

33. Mattson MP, Haberman F. "Folate and homocysteine metabolism: therapeutic targets in cardiovascular and neurodegenerative disorders." *Curr Med Chem*. 2003 Oct;10(19):1923-9.

34. Durga J, Verhoef P, Anteunis LJC, Schouten E, Kok FJ. "Effects of folic acid supplementation on hearing in older adults. A randomized, controlled trial." Annals of Internal Medicine. 2 January 2007, Vol. 146, pages1-9.

35. Atkins RC. *Dr. Atkin's Vita-Nutrient Solution*. Simon & Schuster, Inc. 1998. p.67, 71.

36. Dr. Joel Mason, Dr. Young-In Kim. "Folate's Boost May Change with Age" American Institute for Cancer Research NEWSLETTER, Summer 20099, Issue 104.

CHAPTER 7

Heavy Metal Toxicity

CLUE #7: Consider the need to decrease toxic heavy metals in your body. Certain heavy metals can accumulate in body tissues, organs, and bones and can weaken the immune system, allowing for the recurrence of various infections and autoimmune reactions such as inflammation.[1] Heavy metals also produce large amounts of free radicals, which cause oxidative damage to our bodies' cells.[2] High levels of toxic metals can also cause *learning difficulties*[3], *impair hearing and speech, cause mental disturbances,*[4] *and reduce our quality of life.*[5] Chronic, long-term exposure to heavy metals has been linked to certain allergies. Long-term exposure to certain metals can also mimic various diseases such as Alzheimer's, Parkinson's, muscular dystrophy, and multiple sclerosis and can also result in cancer.[6] One researcher reports that mercury exists in cancer and precancer cells.[7]

Symptoms of metal toxicity develop slowly and may come and go, resulting in delaying the seeking of treatment.[8] In addition, it is known that antibiotic treatment for various infections is less effective if mercury is present in the body.[9]

In Danbury, Connecticut—the hat capital of the world during the 1800s—it was observed that some hat makers experienced various nervous disorders and certain mad behaviors. This disorder resulted from the frequent use of a mercury solution, which the hat makers used to remove hair from furs and produce a better quality of hats made from felt. The saying "mad as a hatter" became popularized during that era after the realization that high levels of mercury had poisoned these craftsmen.[10]

Researchers point out that the presence of mercury in our environment is widespread. It is known that mercury enters streams, rivers, lakes, and oceans, where naturally occurring microorganisms in the sediment transform it into a very toxic form called methylmercury. Methylmercury is readily absorbed by plants and fish and becomes many times more magnified as it works its way up the food chain.[11] Refer to the Web site www.americanpregnancy.org/pregnancyhealth/ sushimercury.htm for estimated mercury levels in various types of fish.

Dietrich Klinghardt, MD, PhD, and world-renowned expert in heavy metal detoxification with over thirty years of medical experience, states that symptoms of mercury toxicity may include: *anxiety, irritability, fearfulness, shyness, nervousness, impaired concentration, loss of self-confidence, learning disabilities, memory loss, emotional instability, insomnia, chronic fatigue, cancer* and hypoglycemia (low blood sugar).[12] Low blood sugar can also give a *spacey or foggy feeling* in the head.[13]

Exposure to mercury begins early—it can be passed to a developing baby through the umbilical cord,[14] breast milk, and formula.[15] Mercury has been a suspected link to autism[16] and various other neurological abnormalities such as *lack of social interaction, impaired communication,* and *repetitive behaviors.*[17] Childhood vaccinations in the United States prior to 2002 probably contained a mercury-based preservative called thimerosal which also has been a suspected link to autism. However, after thimerosal was removed from vaccinations (its removal was accelerated from 1999 to 2001) and surprisingly, levels of autism failed to decline, according to a California study.[18] This remains an intensely debated issue as other studies also cannot confirm a direct link between autism and thimerosal.[19] The incidence of autism-related behaviors for boys is believed to be about 4 times higher than for girls but could be as high as 15 boys for each girl. On the other hand, girls are less diagnosed because they are believed to be better at masking their behaviors than boys.[20] One study showed that girls are able to release more mercury into their urine than boys.[21] Other factors that can contribute to development of autism are parasite and fungal infections and genetics. Perhaps, still other considerations might be *Candida* overgrowth, low levels of selenium, exposure to mercury and other environmental toxins and methylation factors of both mother and child. Refer to the Web site www.hpakids.org and www.autism.org.uk for more information on autism.

Heavy metals in our bodies can promote the growth of Candida.[22] Dr. Klinghardt states that mercury "suffocates" our body's cells and causes cells to die. He suspects that the immune system's last resort to protect the body from mercury is to allow bacteria and fungi, such as *Candida*, to increase because these microbes can readily attach to mercury. This last-resort response allows our bodies' cells to breathe again.[23] This progression can take a strange and scary twist: it appears that *Candida* and certain bacteria in the mouth and digestive tract can change mercury into its most toxic form, methylmercury,[24] in a similar way that occurs in streams, rivers, lakes, and oceans. Researchers conclude that methyl-mercury "mimics" essential nutrients and is readily absorbed into the blood and brain.[25] Klinghardt estimates that methylmercury is more than 50 times more toxic than metallic forms of mercury.[26]

Mercury-based dental fillings (called amalgams) could be a source of mercury for some people[27] and could be a possible cause of *chronic fatigue syndrome,* as documented by numerous individuals on the Web site www.cfspages.com[28] and several other Web sites.

In addition to mercury, other potentially harmful metals include aluminum, arsenic, and lead. Sources of toxic metals may include the following: lead paint, lead-glazed ceramics, old water pipes, eating fish that contains mercury, broken thermometers, broken fluorescent light bulbs, pesticides, cigarette smoke, occupational exposure, coal power plants, and the possible presence of these metals in our food, water and air.[29]

It is thought that high levels of aluminum in the brain may be a possible link to Alzheimer's disease; however, a direct relationship has not yet been firmly established.[30] Illnesses having a direct link to aluminum toxicity include *dementia* (forgetfulness, decreased mental abilities) and anemia (low red blood cell count).[31]

Aluminum is all around us. It is the most common metal in the earth's crust.[32] Low levels of aluminum in our bodies generally do not pose an immediate threat; however, it is a good idea to reduce your exposure as practical. Sources of aluminum include certain antacid medications, some buffered aspirins, aluminum-containing baking powder, aluminum beverage cans, and antiperspirants. Uncoated aluminum cookware should be avoided, especially when cooking acidic foods such as tomatoes, which causes aluminum to leach into the food.[33]

The potential harm from these metals will be debated for a long time. Other factors come into play, such as genetic differences between people, the degree of absorption and methylation by each person, the amount of toxic metals received before birth, and deficiencies of vitamins and other nutrients. It is known that deficiencies of certain essential nutrients can allow the increased absorption of certain heavy metals.[34]

It appears that heavy metals are all around us, and, therefore, it is a good idea to eat foods that can help get toxic metals out of our bodies. Obviously, acute poisoning requires immediate medical attention and may require intravenous therapy. If you suspect toxic metals are diminishing your abilities, consult your medical practitioner for testing and an appropriate detoxification program.

Toxic metals can accumulate inside us unless steps are taken to remove them. The good news is that certain foods and supplements are very good at removing toxic metals from our body.

CHLORELLA—THE HEAVY METAL GRABBER

Chlorella is an algae supplement that can grab, or chelate to, heavy metals and move them out of the body. (Chelate, or chelation, means to grab or claw.) Chlorella supplements are a major part of many detoxification programs. Dr. Klinghardt writes that chlorella has at least 20 known actions involved in heavy metal detoxification[35] and that high doses of chlorella and cilantro are used in Germany for mercury detoxi-fication.[36] (Cilantro will be discussed shortly). *Caution is advised since about 30% of people cannot digest chlorella.* An enzyme supplement that contains the enzyme cellulase may help with digestion of chlorella. Dr. Klinghardt recommends starting out with one 500-mg tablet of chlorella (one-quarter teaspoon if using powder) once a day and, if experiencing no problems, then increasing up to five to ten tablets per day before meal time. These doses are for a 150-pound adult and should be reduced for children according to weight. (For example, a 30 pound child would only take one-fifth as much as a 150-pound adult.)[37]

Important: Dr. Klinghardt recommends taking chlorella 30 minutes *before* eating a meal to ensure the chlorella is present in the digestive tract. As bile is secreted into the small intestine upon eating, it contains some mercury. The mercury will be absorbed by the chlorella in the digestive tract and will be transported out of the body.[38] After a week or two of taking chlorella, eat some leaves of fresh cilantro with your meal to increase the release of mercury into the bile. Be sure to drink plenty of fresh water and eat fresh fruits and vegetables and other sources of fiber in order to speed the transit of mercury out of the body.

A broken portion of a chlorella tablet can be placed in the mouth next to a tooth that has a mercury filling or a root canal to absorb mercury from the gums.

I once had a major toothache for several weeks in a tooth that had a crown on it. It ached and throbbed, especially when exercising or in cold weather. In fact, the pain went all the way up the side of my face and into my head and interfered with my work and sleep. I hated the thought of having another root canal; however, my dentist did not feel a root canal was needed from his expert observation of the X-ray. I tried placing a portion of chlorella tablet next to the gum at bedtime and rinsed the tablet out of my mouth the next morning with water. Within a couple days, the pain went away, like a switch had been turned off. I am a firm believer in chlorella's ability to remove mercury from our bodies.

CILANTRO—THE HEAVY
METAL RELEASER

Cilantro is a very special herb that causes our bodies' cells to release mercury, lead, and aluminum. This amazing action was discovered by surprise in 1995 during a study of some people who happened to have eaten a Vietnamese soup containing cilantro. The researcher discovered that large amounts of mercury were being released into their urine. Amazingly, it was shown that cilantro can also help remove lead and aluminum from the body.[39] A further study showed that taking a 100-mg tablet of cilantro 4 times a day significantly reduced the absorption of mercury following the removal of a dental filling. Cilantro tablets (which were produced just for that study) were taken before the removal of the filling and were continued for two weeks after. *These amazing actions make cilantro one of the few known substances that can remove mercury from the brain and central nervous system.*[40]

The same researcher also discovered that the treatment of *Chlamydia* bacteria and the herpes family of viral infections was most effective when conventional medications were combined with cilantro. He concluded that these infectious microorganisms somehow use mercury or lead to protect themselves or that the heavy metals somehow reduced the effectiveness of the antibiotics and other medications.[41]

Remember to take chlorella 30 minutes before eating to ensure the chlorella is present in the digestive tract. Next, eat some fresh cilantro with your meal. As bile is secreted into the small intestine to aid digestion, it will contain even greater amounts of mercury released by the central nervous system. The mercury will be absorbed by the chlorella in the digestive tract and will be transported out of the body.[42]

Fresh cilantro is easy to grow and is available in grocery stores. You can eat the fresh leaves alone, in salads, or in recipes with other foods. You can also make a tea from the leaves. Other names for cilantro are coriander and Chinese parsley. Note: Dried cilantro is not effective at removing mercury from the central nervous system.[43]

Caution: Sudden detoxification can sometimes be dangerous and should be carried out under the supervision of a qualified practitioner.[44] Since *Candida* and bacterial infections can coexist with mercury,[45] it is important that these infections are brought under control prior to starting a heavy metal detoxification program. Consult your health care professional in regard to a detoxification program that is right for you. Refer to the following Web sites by Klinghardt and Mercola, two leading experts in metal detoxification, at www.neuraltherapy.com and www. mercola.com. Another term for heavy metal detoxification is chelation therapy.

GARLIC, MSM, AND THE SULFUR CONNECTION

Mercury and other heavy metals love to attach to sulfur, which is in every cell in our bodies but is most abundant in red blood cells. Garlic and MSM contain organic sources of sulfur and are used in detoxification programs because the sulfur readily combines with toxic metals and transports them out of the body.[46] (MSM is an abbreviation for methylsulfonylmethane). MSM supplements are inexpensive, harmless, odorless, and readily available. Some readers may know that MSM is also recommended to help build up the cartilage that cushions our joints.[47] An extra bonus: one study showed MSM to be helpful for reducing stuffy nose (seasonal allergic rhinitis). This study used 2.6 grams per day for 30 days.[48]

Dr. Mercola recommends starting out with one capsule of MSM twice a day. You can gradually increase to 3 capsules twice a day. For people with root canals who are also chronically sick, he recommends taking 5 capsules three times a day.[49]

Garlic's various sulfur compounds have been shown to have anti-cancer actions as well.[50] Garlic also contains significant amounts of selenium, which is probably the most helpful mineral for protecting against heavy metal toxicity. In addition, the selenium in garlic is easily absorbed by our bodies.[51] When using garlic, remember to crush it using a garlic press then let it set for 10 minutes so the phytochemicals have time to mix and reach their full effectiveness. Also, remember that cooking (and microwaving) garlic destroys many of its beneficial properties.[52] Refer to chapter 22 for recipe suggestions.

REMOVAL OF MERCURY-BASED DENTAL FILLINGS

Dr. Klinghardt's Web site, www.neuraltherapy.com, gives a protocol to be used when a mercury dental filling is removed. He recommends taking chlorella, MSM, cilantro, selenium, and vitamin E for two months prior to removal of the filling and continuing detoxification until symptoms disappear, which can be as long as three to four years for some people. [53] Experts also recommend having two or three bowel movements per day during detoxification, which reduces the chance of mercury being absorbed back into the body.

OTHER HELPFUL FOODS AND SUPPLEMENTS FOR HEAVY METAL DETOXIFICATION

Omega-3 essential fatty acids (EFAs): Dr. Klinghardt recommends we include sufficient omega-3 EFAs in our diet. He strongly recommends eating ground flaxseeds and taking supplements of evening primrose oil.[54] Remember that the omega-3 EFAs in flaxseeds deteriorate after grinding (when left exposed to air, light or heat) so be sure to mix the freshly ground flaxseeds (or flaxseed oil) with cottage cheese or yogurt for maximum absorption by our body. This is in accordance with Dr. Johanna Budwig's many years of research[55] and is discussed in chapter 13.

Vitamins C and E: These antioxidants aid the process of detoxification. Dr. Mercola recommends taking 500 mg of vitamin C three times a day and 400 mg of vitamin E once a day during detoxification.[56]

Selenium and zinc: Mercola and Klinghardt write that the body
will let go of toxic metals much easier when certain minerals
are present. Adequate amounts of selenium and zinc are
especially important for mercury detoxification. People with
mercury toxicity are often deficient in zinc.[57] Another study
confirms that adequate amounts of these and other micronutrients such as calcium and zinc can help the body resist heavy
metal toxicity.[58]

Selenium is an antioxidant that acts like a metal in the body;
however, selenium is not a metal. One study concluded that
workers in a mine in former Yugoslavia were exposed to high
levels of mercury; however, the men were protected from
mercury poisoning because of the high amounts of selenium in
their diets as a result of their selenium-rich soil.[59] It is known
that some parts of the world have high concentrations of selenium in the soil, while other locations have very low levels.
Brazil nuts are a natural source of selenium. One average Brazil
nut has about 70 micrograms of selenium, a bit more than the
recommended daily value.[60]

Dr. Atkins writes that multiple sclerosis may be a result of the
accumulation of toxic metals and notes that the disease occurs
more frequently in areas of the country where soils are low in
selenium.[61] Selenium supplements are readily available and
can be taken as directed on the bottle or by your health practitioner. Taking too much selenium can be toxic. Refer to the
following Web site for more information on recommended
amounts of selenium: ods.od.nih.gov/factsheets/selenium.asp.

Hydrochloric acid (HCl): HCl is required in the stomach in
adequate amounts for proper digestion of proteins and absorption of minerals. If you suspect your stomach does not secrete
enough HCl, you can take betaine hydrochloride supplements.

Mercola recommends taking 1 to 6 tablets just before a meal.[62] Refer to clue #6 in chapter 6 for more information.

Enzyme supplements and probiotics: These foods and supplements are also recommended by Klinghardt and Mercola and their importance is discussed in later chapters.

Humifulvate: A supplement derived from peat moss, humifulvate is another excellent chelating agent recommended by some experts for detoxification.[63]

Green leafy vegetables: One reason chlorella is effective as a chelating agent is its extremely high chlorophyll content—more than any other plant. Deep green leafy vegetables are rich in chlorophyll, which helps remove toxins from the body.[64] Some other ways chlorophyll and fiber protect us are by breaking down toxins[65] and helping our cells reproduce accurately rather than mutating into harmful forms.[66] The fiber in fresh, uncooked vegetables helps transport toxins out of the digestive tract quickly. Kale, spinach, and other dark green vegetables are good sources of chlorophyll and can help remove toxins from the body and prevent disease.[67] The highest amounts of chlorophyll are in various algae. Chlorella algae has about 13 times more chlorophyll than kale. Kale has about 3 times more chlorophyll than spinach.[68] Some amazing phytochemicals in kale and other foods are discussed in chapter 15.

Fresh ginger: How does fresh ginger fit into all this? Ginger helps detoxify the liver,[69] helps kill *Candida*, aids in the healing of leaky gut syndrome, and helps fight inflammation. I got my life back simply by eating small slices of fresh ginger. I only wish I had known about the many actions of ginger and these other foods twenty-five years ago; however, much of this

knowledge is fairly recent and has been researched by experts
all around the world.

One more interesting point: studies show that a common
Streptococcus bacteria in the mouth can convert mercury from
dental fillings into methylmercury,[70] which is readily absorbed
into the digestive tract.[71] Since fresh ginger's antibacterial
action can reduce the amount of this bacteria in the mouth, I
suspect the conversion of metallic mercury to methylmercury
is also reduced. This explanation is the opinion of this author
and has not been researched or proven. An interesting study
also showed that *Streptococcus* bacteria in the mouth speeds
the release of mercury out of mercury-based dental fillings.
The study also showed that mercury was no longer released
after the dental filling had aged two years due to the presence of a tarnish layer.[72] I also suspect having a slice of fresh
ginger in the mouth can help reduce tooth decay by reducing
the bacteria that causes dental plaque as further discussed in
chapter 18.

Water filter: Add a water filter to your kitchen spigot to reduce
metals in your drinking water. Be sure the water filter contains
charcoal, which absorbs and removes heavy metals, chlorine,
and many harmful chemicals.

PUTTING THE PIECES TOGETHER

As you may suspect, Clue #7 gives us an understanding into a string
of complex events and illness: heavy metal toxicity can promote *Candida*
overgrowth, *Candida* overgrowth and its many toxins can lead to leaky
gut syndrome, inflammation, and all sorts of problems in various parts
of the body. The remaining chapters give many details how the E-F-G
approach can help you have a clear head and improve your health and
your quality of life.

REFERENCES FOR CHAPTER 7

1a.   Joseph Mercola, D.O., Dietrich Klinghardt, M.D., Ph.D. "Mercury Toxicity and Systemic Elimination Agents." *Journal of Nutritional & Environmental Medicine.* (2001) 11, 53-62. Obtained from web site. Accessed 4/14/2008. <http://www.klinghardt.org/library.htm>.

1b.   Marth E, Jelovcan S, Kleinhappl B, Gutschi A, Barth S. "The effect of heavy metals on the immune system at low concentrations." *Int J Occup Med Environ Health.* 2001;14(4):375-86.

1c.   Bigazzi PE. "Metals and Kidney Autoimmunity." *Environmental Health Perspectives Supplements.* Volume 107, Number S5, October 1999.

1d.   Bernier J, Brousseau P, Krzystyniak K, Tryphonas H, Fournier M. "Immunotoxicity of Heavy Metals in Relation to Great Lakes." *Environmental Health Perspectives.* Vol 103, Supplement 9, December 1995.

1e.   Koller LD. "In Vitro Assessment of Humoral Immunity Following Exposure to Heavy Metals." *Environmental Health Perspectives.* Vol. 43, pp.37-39, 1982.

2a.   Houston MC. "The role of mercury and cadmium heavy metals in vascular disease, hypertension, coronary heart disease, and myocardial infarction." *Altern Ther Health Med.* 2007 Mar-Apr;13(2):S128-33.

2b.   Jie XL, Jin GW, Cheng JP, Wang WH, Lu J, Qu LY. "Consumption of mercury-contaminated rice induces oxidative stress and free radical aggravation in rats." *Biomed Environ Sci.* 2007 Feb;20(1):84-9.

2c.   Valko M, Morris H, Cronin MT. "Metals, toxicity and oxidative stress." *Curr Med Chem.* 2005;12(10):1161-208.

2d.   Schurz F, Sabater-Vilar M, Fink-Gremmels J. "Mutagenicity of mercury chloride and mechanisms of cellular defense: the role of metal-binding proteins." Mutagenesis, Vol. 15, No. 6, 525-530, November 2000.

3a.   Atkins RC. *Dr. Atkin's Vita-Nutrient Solution.* Simon & Schuster, Inc. 1998. pp.55,56,154. Citing Blakely, B.R., et al.. *Journal of Applied Toxicology.* 1990;10(2): 93-97.

3b.   Jim O'Brien. "Mercury Amalgam Toxicity." Web site: LifeExtension, LE Magazine. May 2001. Accessed 3/28/2008. <http://www.lef.org>.

4.   Murata K, Grandjean P, Dakeishi M. "Neurophysiological evidence of methyl mercury neurotoxicity." *Am J Ind Med.* 2007 Oct;50(10):765-71.

5.   Jim O'Brien. "Heavy Metal Toxicity." Web site: LifeExtension, LE Magazine. Updated: 06/12/2003. Citing (Ferner 2001). Accessed 3/28/2008. <http://www.lef.org>.

6.   Jim O'Brien. "Heavy Metal Toxicity." Web site: LifeExtension, LE Magazine. Updated: 06/12/2003. Citing (International Occupational Safety and Health Information Centre 1999). Accessed 3/28/2008. <http://www.lef.org/LEFCMS/aspx/PrintVersionMagic.aspx?CmsID=104400>.

7.   Omura Y, Shimotsuura Y, Fukuoka H, Nomoto T. "Significant mercury

deposits in internal organs following the removal of dental amalgam, & development of pre-cancer on the gingiva and the sides of the tongue and their represented organs as a result of inadvertent exposure to strong curing light (used to solidify synthetic dental filling material) & effective treatment: a clinical case report, along with organ representation areas for each tooth." *Acupunct Electrother Res.* 1996 Apr-Jun;21(2):133-60.

8.   Jim O'Brien. "Heavy Metal Toxicity." Web site: LifeExtension, LE Magazine. Updated 06/12/2003. Accessed 3/28/2008. <http://www.lef.org/LEFCMS/ aspx/PrintVersionMagic.aspx?CmsID=104400>.

9a.   Omura Y, Shimotsuura Y, Fukuoka H, Nomoto T. "Significant mercury deposits in internal organs following the removal of dental amalgam, & development of pre-cancer on the gingiva and the sides of the tongue and their represented organs as a result of inadvertent exposure to strong curing light (used to solidify synthetic dental filling material) & effective treatment: a clinical case report, along with organ representation areas for each tooth." *Acupunct Electrother Res.* 1996 Apr-Jun;21(2):133-60.

9b.   Omura Y, Beckman SL. "Role of mercury (Hg) in resistant infections & effective treatment of Chlamydia trachomatis and Herpes family viral infections (and potential treatment for cancer) by removing localized Hg deposits with Chinese parsley and delivering effective antibiotics using various drug uptake enhancement methods." *Acupunct Electrother Res.* 1995 Aug-Dec;20(3-4):195-229.

10.   Peg Van Patten. "The Mad Hatter Mercury Mystery" Communications Director, Connecticut Sea Grant. Accessed 3/31/2008. <http://www.seagrant. ucom.edu/HATTER.HTML."

11a.   "Mercury Health Hazards." Web site: U.S. Office of Research Facilities, Development and Operations. Accessed 4/25/2008. <http://orf.od.nih.gov/ factsheets/thimerosal.htm>.

11b.   Watras CJ, Back RC, Halvorsen S, Hudson RJ, Morrison KA, Wente SP. "Bioaccumulation of mercury in pelagic freshwater food webs." *Sci Total Environ.* 1998 Aug 28;219(2-3):183-208.

11c.   Cynthia C. Gilmour, David P. Krabbenhoft. "Appendix 7-4: Status of Methylmercury Production Studies." 2001 Everglades Consolidated Report.

11d.   Anwar M, Ando T, Maaz A, Ghani S, Munir M, Qureshi IU, Naeem S, Tsuji M, Wakamiya J, Nakano A, Akiba S. "Scalp hair mercury concentrations in Pakistan." *Environ Sci.* 2007;14(4):167-75.

11e.   "NIAID Research on Thimerosal." Web site: National Institute of Allergy and Infectious Diseases, National Institutes of Health, U./S. Department of Health and Human Services. Accessed 4/22/2008. <http://www.niaid.nih.gov/fact- sheets/thimerosal.htm>.

12.   Joseph Mercola, D.O., Dietrich Klinghardt, M.D., Ph.D. "Mercury Toxicity

and Systemic Elimination Agent." *Journal of Nutritional & Environmental Medicine.* (2001) p.4. Accessed 4/14/2008. <http://www.neuraltherapy.com>.

13. "Control" "Low Blood Sugars (Hypoglycemia)" "Low blood Sugar Symptoms" Web site: DiabetesNet.com. Accessed 3/26/2010. <http://www.diabetesnet. com/diabetes_control_tips/hypoglycemia_symptoms.php>

14. Murata K, Dakeishi M, Shimada M, Satoh H. "Assessment of intrauterine methylmercury exposure affecting child development: messages from the newborn." *Tohoku J Exp Med.* 2007 Nov;213(3):187-202.

15a. Drasch G, Aigner S, Roider G, Staiger F, Lipowski G. "Mercury in human colostrum and early breast milk. Its dependence on dental amalgam and other factors." *J Trace Elem Med Biol.* 1998 Mar;12(1):23-7.

15b. Vimy MJ, Hooper DE, King WW, Lorscheider FL. "Mercury from maternal "silver" tooth fillings in sheep and human breast milk. A source of neonatal exposure." *Biol Trace Elem Res.* 1997 Feb;56(2):143-52.

16. Geier DA, Geier MR. "A case series of children with apparent mercury toxic encephalopathies manifesting with clinical symptoms of regressive autistic disorders." *J Toxicol Environ Health A.* 2007 May 15;70(10):837-51.

17. Bernard S, Enayati A, Redwood L, Roger H, Binstock T. "Autism: a novel form of mercury poisoning." *Med Hypotheses.* 2001 Apr;56(4):462-71.

18. Schechter R, Grether JK. "Continuing increases in autism reported to California's development services system: mercury in retrograde." *Arch Gen Psychiatry.* 2008 Jan;65(1):19-24.

19a. Fombonne E. "Thimerosal disappears but autism remains." *Arch Gen Psydhiatry.* 2008 Jan;65(1):15-6.

19b. Stehr-Green P, Tull P, Stellfeld M, Mortenson PB, Simpson D. "Autism and thimerosal-containing vaccines: lack of consistent evidence for an association." *Am J Prev Med.* 2003 Aug;25(2):101-6.

20. "Autism: why do more boys than girls develop it?" Web site: The National Autistic Society. Accessed 6/3/2009. <http://www.autism.org.uk/nas/jsp/polo-poly.jsp?d=1049&a=3370&view=print>

21. Woods JS, Martin MD, Leroux BG, DeRouen TA, Leitao JG, Bernardo MF, Luis HS, Simmonds PL, Kushleika JV, Huang Y. "The contribution of dental amalgam to urinary mercury excretion in children." *Environ Health Perspect.* 2007 Oct;115(10):1527-31.

22a. "Heavy Metal Toxicity." Web site: The Modern Herbalist. Accessed 3/26/2008. <http://www.modernherbalist.com/heavymetal.html>.

22b. Harrison JJ, Ceri H, Yerly J, Rabiei M, Hu Y, Martinuzzi R, Turner RJ. "Metal ions may suppress or enhance cellular differentiation in Candida albicans and Candida tropicalis biofilms." *Appl Environ Microbiol.* 2007 Aug;73(15):4940-9. Epub 2007 Jun 8.

22c. Harrison JJ, Rabiei M, Turner RJ, Badry EA, Sproule KM, Ceri H.

"Metal resistance in Candida biofilms." *FEMS Microbiol Ecol.* 2006 Mar;55(3):479-91.

23. Joseph Mercola, D.O., Dietrich Klinghardt, M.D., Ph.D. "Mercury Toxicity and Systemic Elimination Agents." *Journal of Nutritional & Environmental Medicine.* (2001) 11, 53-62. Accessed 4/14/2008. <http://www.klinghardt. org/library.htm>.

24a. Yannai S, Berdicevsky I, Duek L. "Transformations of Inorganic Mercury by Candida albicans and Saccharomyces cerevisiae." *Applied and Environmental Microbiology.* 1991 Jan;57(1): 245-7.

24b. Rowland IR, Grasso P, Davies MJ. "The methylation of mercuric chloride by human intestinal bacteria. *Experientia.* 1975 Sep 15;31(9):1064-5.

25. Simmons-Willis, TA, Koh AS, Clarkson TW, Ballatori N. "Transport of a neurotoxicant by molecular mimicry: the methylmercury-L-cysteine complex is a substrate for human L-type large neutral amino acid transporter (LAT) 1 and LAT2." *Biochem. J.* (2002) 367, 239-246.

26. Dietrich Klinghardt, MD, PhD. "A Comprehensive Review of Heavy Metal Detoxification and Clinical Pearls from 30 Years of Medical Practice." Accessed 4/14/2008. < http://www.neuraltherapy.com/articlesProtocols.asp>

27. Lorsheider FL, Vimy MJ, Summers AO. "Mercury exposure from "silver" tooth fillings: emerging evidence questions a traditional dental paradigm. *FASEB J.* 1995 Apr;9(7):504-8.

28. "Chronic Fatigue Syndrome? or Chronic Mercury Poisoning?" Health Update. Web site for chronic fatigue syndrome testimonials. Accessed 4/21/2008. <http://www.cfspages.com/update.html>.

29a. "Mercury Levels in Sushi." Web site: American Pregnancy Association. Accessed 4/2/2008. <http://www.americanpregnancy.org/pregnancyhealth/ sushimercury.htm>.

29b. "Heavy Metal Toxicity." Updated: 06/12/2003. Web site: LifeExtension, LE Magazine. Accessed 3/28/2008. <http://www.lef.org/LEFCMS/aspx/ PrintVersionMagic.aspx?CmsID=104400>.

29c. "Secondhand Smoke: Questions and Answers" Web site: National Cancer Institute. U.S. National Institutes of Health. Accessed 3/26/2008. <http:// www.nci.nih.gov/cancertopics/factsheet/Tobacco/ETS...>

30. Web Site: Alzheimer's Society. "Aluminum and Alzheimer's disease - Alzheimer's Society". Accessed 3/25/2008. <www.alzheimers.org.uk>.

31. "Definition of Aluminum" Web site: MedicineNet.com. Accessed 4/3/2008. <http://www.medterms.com/script/main/art.asp?articlekey=39609>.

32. "Definition of Aluminum" Web site: MedicineNet.com. Accessed 4/3/2008. <http://www.medterms.com/script/main/art.asp?articlekey=39609>.

33. Linda Paul, Guest Author. "Dangers of Aluminum Toxicity Part II." Web site: BellaOnline The Voice of Women. Accessed 4/3/2008. <http://www.bellaon-line.com/articles/art12624.asp>.

34. Peraza MA, Ayala-Fierro F, Barber DS, Casarez E, Rael LT. "Effects of Micronutrients on Metal Toxicity." *Environmental Health Perspectives.* Vol 106, Supplement 1, February 1998.

35. Dietrich Klinghardt, MD, PhD. "A Comprehensive Review of Heavy Metal Detoxification and Clinical Pearls from 30 Years of Medical Practice. Web site accessed 4/14/2008. <http://www.neuraltherapy.com/articlesProtocols.asp>

36. Joseph Mercola, D.O., Dietrich Klinghardt, M.D., Ph.D. "Mercury Toxicity and Systemic Elimination Agents." *Journal of Nutritional & Environmental Medicine* (2001) p.10. Article obtained from web site. Accessed 4/14/2008. <http://www.klinghardt.org/library.htm>.

37. Joseph Mercola, D.O. "Mercury Detoxification Protocol." Web site: Mercola. com. Accessed 4/12/2008. <http://mercola.com/article/detox_protocol.htm>.

38. Dietrich Klinghardt M.D., Ph.D. "The Klinghardt Neurotoxin Elimination Protocol" Article from Web site. Accessed 4/28/2009. <http://www.kling hardtacademy.com/Protocols/>.

39. Omura Y, Beckman SL. "Role of mercury (Hg) in resistant infections & effective treatment of Chlamydia trachomatis and Herpes family viral infections (and potential treatment for cancer) by removing localized Hg deposits with Chinese parsley and delivering effective antibiotics using various drug uptake enhancement methods." *Acupunct Electrother Res.* 1995 Aug-Dec;20(3-4):195-229.

40. Omura Y, Shimotsuura Y, Fukuoka H, Nomoto T. "Significant mercury deposits in internal organs following the removal of dental amalgam, & development of pre-cancer on the gingiva and the sides of the tongue and their represented organs as a result of inadvertent exposure to strong curing light (used to solidify synthetic dental filling material) & effective treatment: a clinical case report, along with organ representation areas for each tooth." *Acupunct Electrother Res.* 1996 Apr-Jun;21(2):133-60.

41. Omura Y, Beckman SL. "Role of mercury (Hg) in resistant infections & effective treatment of Chlamydia trachomatis and Herpes family viral infections (and potential treatment for cancer) by removing localized Hg deposits with Chinese parsley and delivering effective antibiotics using various drug uptake enhancement methods." *Acupunct Electrother Res.* 1995 Aug-Dec;20(3-4):195-229.

42. Dietrich Klinghardt M.D., Ph.D. "The Klinghardt Neurotoxin Elimination Protocol" Article from Web site. Accessed 4/28/2009. <http://www.klinghard-tacademy.com/Protocols/>.

43. Joseph Mercola, D.O., Dietrich Klinghardt, M.D., Ph.D. "Mercury Toxicity and Systemic Elimination Agents." *Journal of Nutritional & Environmental Medicine.* (2001) p.8. Obtained from web site. Accessed 4/14/2008. <http://www.klinghardt.org/library.htm>.

44a. Dietrich Klinghardt, MD, PhD. "A Comprehensive Review of Heavy

Metal Detoxification and Clinical Pearls from 30 Years of Medical Practice"
Obtained from web site. Accessed 4/14/2008. <http://.klinghardt.org/library.
htm>.

44b.   Joseph Mercola, D.O., Dietrich Klinghardt, M.D., Ph.D. "Mercury Toxicity
        and Systemic Elimination Agents." *Journal of Nutritional & Environmental
        Medicine* (2001) 11, 53-62. Obtained from web site: Accessed 4/14/2008.
        <http://www.klinghardt.org/library.htm>.

45a.   Shmuel Yannai, Israela Berdicevsky, and Lea Duek. "Transformations of
        Inorganic Mercury by *Candida albicans* and *Saccharomyces cerevisiae*" Applied
        and Environmental Microbiology, Jan 1991, Vol. 57, No. 1, pp.245-247.

45b.   Rowland IR, Grasso P, Davies MJ. "The methylation of mercuric chloride by
        human intestinal bacteria. *Experientia*. 1975 Sep 15;31(9):1064-5.

46a.   Joseph Mercola, D.O., Dietrich Klinghardt, M.D., Ph.D. "Mercury Toxicity
        and Systemic Elimination Agents." *Journal of Nutritional & Environmental
        Medicine* (2001) pp.6,9. Obtained from web site. Accessed 4/14/2008.
        <http://www.neuraltherapy.com>.

46b.   Cha CW. "A study on the effect of garlic to the heavy metal poisoning of rat."
        J Korean Med Sci. 1987 Dec;2(4):213-24.

47.   Lipski E. *Digestive Wellness*. McGraw-Hill, New York, NY. 2004. p.296.

48.   Barrager E, Veltmann JR Jr, Schauss AG, Schiller RN. "A multicentered, open-
        label trial on the safety and efficacy of methylsufonylmethane in the treatment
        of seasonal allergic rhinitis." *J Altern Complement Med*. 2002 Apr;8(2):167-73.

49.   Joseph Mercola, D.O. "Mercury Detoxification Protocol." Web site: Mercola.
        com. Accessed 4/12/2008. <http://mercola.com/article/detox_protocol.htm>.

50a.   Ariga T, Seki T. "Antithrombotic and anticancer effects of garlic-derived sulfur
        compounds: a review." *Biofactors*. 2006;26(2):93-103.

50b.   Milner JA. "A historical perspective on garlic and cancer." *J Nutr*. 2001
        Mar;131(3s):1027S-31S.

50c.   Lea MA. "Organosulfur compounds and cancer." *Adv Exp Med Biol*.
        1996;401:147-54.

51.   Dietrich Klinghardt M.D., Ph.D. "The Klinghardt Neurotoxin Elimination
        Protocol" Article fom web site. Accessed 4/28/2009. <http://www.klinghard-
        tacademy.com/Protocols/>.

52.   "Garlic and Organosulfur Compounds" Web site: Linus Pauling Institute at
        Oregon State University. Accessed 4/15/2008. <http://lpi.oregonstate.edu/
        infocenter/phytochemicals/garlic/>.

53.   Joseph Mercola, D.O., Dietrich Klinghardt, M.D., Ph.D. "Mercury Toxicity
        and Systemic Elimination Agents." *Journal of Nutritional & Environmental
        Medicine* (2001) 11, 53-62. Obtained from web site. Accessed 4/14/2008.
        <http://www.klinghardt.org/library.htm>.

54.   Joseph Mercola, D.O., Dietrich Klinghardt, M.D., Ph.D. "Mercury Toxicity
        and Systemic Elimination Agents." *Journal of Nutritional & Environmental*

Medicine (2001) p.9. Obtained from web site. Accessed 4/14/2008. <http://www.klinghardt.org/library.htm>.

55. Budwig, Johanna. *Flax Oil as a True Aid Against Arthritis, Heart Infarction, Cancer and Other Diseases.* Apple Publishing Co. Ltd. 1994 p.22.

56a. Joseph Mercola, D.O., Dietrich Klinghardt, M.D., Ph.D. "Mercury Toxicity and Systemic Elimination Agents." *Journal of Nutritional & Environmental Medicine* (2001) p.9. Obtained from web site. Accessed 4/14/2008. <http://www.klinghardt.org/library.htm>.

56b. Peraza MA, Ayala-Fierro F, Barber DS, Casarez E, Rael LT. "Effects of Micronutrients on Metal Toxicity." *Environmental Health Perspectives.* Vol 106, Supplement 1, February 1998.

57. Joseph Mercola, D.O., Dietrich Klinghardt, M.D., Ph.D. "Mercury Toxicity and Systemic Elimination Agents." *Journal of Nutritional & Environmental Medicine* (2001). p.8. Obtained from web site. Accessed 4/14/2008. <http://www.klinghardt.org/library.htm>.

58. Peraza MA, Ayala-Fierro F, Barber DS, Casarez E, Rael LT. "Effects of Micronutrients on Metal Toxicity." *Environmental Health Perspectives.* Vol 106, Supplement 1, February 1998.

59. Atkins RC. *Dr. Atkin's Vita-Nutrient Solution.* Simon & Schuster, Inc. 1998. pp.154-5. Citing Hu Y. *Biological Trace Element Research.* 1997;56:331-42.

60. Duke JA. *The Green Pharmacy.* Rodale Press, Emmaus, PA. 1997 pp.24-25.

61. Atkins RC. *Dr. Atkin's Vita-Nutrient Solution.* Simon & Schuster, Inc. 1998. p.154. Citing Mai J., et al., *Biological Trace Element Research.* 1990; 24: 109-17.

62. Joseph Mercola, D.O., Dietrich Klinghardt, M.D., Ph.D. "Mercury Toxicity and Systemic Elimination Agents." *Journal of Nutritional & Environmental Medicine* (2001) p.8. Obtained from web site. Accessed 4/14/2008. <http://www.klinghardt.org/library.htm>.

63. "Humifulvate Product Range Raw Materials Licenses for Scientists & Experts The Inventor" Web site: Humet. Accessed 10/16/2008. <http://www.humet.hu/index>.

64a. "Chlorophyll and Chlorophyllin." Web site: Linus Pauling Institute at Oregon State University. Accessed 4/4/2008. <http://lpi.oregonstate.edu/infocenter/phytochemicals/chlorophylls/index.html>.

64b. Harttig U, Baily GS. "Chemoprotection by natural chlorophylls in vivo: inhibition of dibenzo[a,l]pyrene-DNA adducts in rainbow trout liver." *Carcinogenesis.* vol 19, no. 7 pp.1323-1326, 1998.

65a. Tachino N, Guo D, Dashwood WM, Tamane S, Larsen R, Dashwood R. "Mechanism of the in vitro antimutagenic action of chlorophyllin against benzo[a] pyrene: studies of enzyme inhibition, molecular complex formation and degradation of the ultimate carcinogen." *Mutat Res.* 1994 Jul 16;308(2):191-203.

65b.   Wu ZL, Chen JK, Ong T, Brockman HE, Whong WZ. "Antitransforming activity of chlorophyllin against selected carcinogens and complex mixtures." *Teratog Carcinog Mutagen.* 1994;14(2):75-81.

66a.   Ghosh AK, Sen S, Sharma A, Talukder G. "Effect of chlorophyllin on mercuric chloride-induced clastogenicity in mice." *Food Chem Toxicol.* 1991 Nov;29(11):777-9.

66b.   Ong TM, Whong WZ, Stewart J, Brockman HE. "Chlorophyllin: a potent antimutagen against environmental and dietary complex mixtures." *Mutat Res.* 1986 Feb;173(2):111-5.

67.   "Chlorophyll and Chlorophyllin." Web site: Linus Pauling Institute at Oregon State University. Accessed 4/4/2008. <http://lpi.oregonstate.edu/infocenter/phytochemicals/chlorophylls/index.html>.

68a.   "Composition of Chlorella". Web site:chlorella-africa.com. Accessed 10/18/2008. <http://www.chlorella-africa.com/chlorellacomp.html>.

68b.   Mark Lefsrud, Dean Kopsell, Adam Wenzel, Joseph Sheehan. "Changes in kale (*Brassica oleracea* L. var. *acephala*) carotenoid and chlorophyll pigment concentrations during leaf ontogeny" *Scientia Horticulturae.* 112 (2007) 136-141.

68c.   T. Bohn, T. Walczyk, S. Leisibach, R.F. Hurrell. "Chlorophyll-bound Magnesium in Commonly Consumed Vegetables and Fruits: Relevance to Magnesium Nutrition" *Journal of Food Science.* Volume 69, Issue 9, Pages S347-S350. Published Online: 31 May 2006.

69.   Hikino H, Kiso Y, Kato N, Hamada Y, Shioiri T, Aiyama R, Itokawa H, Kiuchi F, Sankawa U. "Antihepatotoxic actions of gingerols and diarylheptanoids." *J Ethnopharmacol.* 1985 Sep;14(1):31-9.

70.   Heintze U, Edwardsson S, Derand T, Birkhed D. "Methylation of mercury from dental amalgam and mercuric chloride by oral streptococci in vitro." *Scand J Dent Res.* 1983 Apr;91(2):150-2.

71.   Gianpaolo Guzzi, Claudio Minoia, Paolo D. Pigatto, Gianluca Severi. "Methylmercury, Amalgams, and Children's Health." *Environ Health Perspect.* 2006 March; 114(3): A149.

72.   Lyttle HA, Bowden GH. "The level of mercury in human dental plaque and interaction in vitro between biofilms of Streptococcus mutans and dental amalgam." *J Dent Res.* 1993 Sep;72(9):1320-4.

PART II

Ginger

**SOME SIMPLE
GUIDELINES AND
INSTRUCTIONS**

CHAPTER 8

Using Ginger

GINGER'S botanical name is *Zingiber officinale,* and it is actually a rhizome, not a root. A rhizome is a stem that extends underground while the actual roots are tiny sprouts that extend from the rhizome. Ginger is known to most of us only as a flavoring for foods, ginger ale, and various Oriental and Indian dishes. Interestingly, the ginger rhizome is also consumed as a vegetable in several countries.[1]

It was Hippocrates (born 460 BC, died 377 BC) who declared, "Let food be your medicine and medicine be your food." Hippocrates is known as the "father of medicine" for his many important discoveries that are still in practice today. It is interesting to know that about 25% of all pharmaceutical medications involve substances that originate from plants.[2]

AN "INTERNAL SAUNA"

Stephen Fulder, PhD, author of *The Ginger Book,* sums it up well when he describes the working of ginger as an "internal sauna" that "brings body fluids to affected areas, warming them up. This mobilizes the body's defenses ... As a result, in the case of a cough, secretions are increased, so phlegm becomes thinner and can be coughed up. Sweating is increased, driving out toxins or viruses. Immune-system functioning is increased, more white blood cells are produced, and, above all, circulation to all those hard-to-reach places is improved." He further states that ginger "can help mobilize our immunity and our body's defenses, which in turn can mean faster recovery from a variety of infections, from the common cold to chronic bronchial problems. It can open vessels and bring healing fluids to places that have closed down and atrophied, thus helping rheumatic and arthritic problems in particular. It can keep the current of liquids moving properly in the body, helping problems such as menstrual irregularities. These are some of the more subtle and yet powerful effects of ginger which are well known in traditional medicine and will now, hopefully, come to be enjoyed by many more of us."[3]

One of the first things I noticed after I began eating slices of fresh ginger was that I no longer needed to frequently clear my throat. Ginger's warming and thinning effects help the sinuses to drain naturally, making it no longer necessary for all the throat-clearing and snorting and growling noises I used to make. (My wife is extremely grateful that this issue has been resolved.)

A Suggested Schedule for Taking Fresh Ginger

1.   Be like Confucius and eat a slice of fresh ginger with every meal—breakfast, lunch, and dinner.
2.   Feel free to take it throughout the day. I remember taking a slice every twenty or thirty minutes, which helped reduce congestion and pressure in my head.
3.   If you have a minor food sensitivity, it may help to take a slice of ginger before and after eating that food. If you are sensitive to cold weather, taking ginger may help you feel a bit warmer.
4.   I take a slice at bed time.
5.   Take ginger with you when you travel.

A Word about Taste and Effects

The taste of fresh ginger has been described many ways, such as warm, citrusy, peppery, sharp, strong, and distinct, and some people say fresh ginger is too strong for them to eat. I enjoy the lemony flavor most of the time. The flavor can vary widely with each rhizome, from rich and satisfying to bitter and undesirable. If your first experience is unpleasant, try purchasing ginger at another store or another time. You can also make fresh ginger tea, which may taste milder. It is easy to tell if ginger is fresh enough to use; the color should be bright yellow when cut open and it should not taste rancid or spoiled.

You can make fresh ginger tea by first heating water to less than 140°F (60°C). The delicate enzymes will remain active at these lower temperatures. Next, cut off a chunk of rhizome and place into a garlic press. Gently squeeze the rhizome so that juice comes out but do not completely crush it as you would garlic. Add honey for sweetness.

Some of ginger's compounds are absorbed into the body very quickly. One of the main reasons ginger is commonly used in Oriental and Indian traditional medicine is its ability to carry other medications into the body quickly and thoroughly. There seems to be a lot of wisdom behind that old famous folk rhyme: "Run, run, as fast as you can; you can't catch me, I'm the gingerbread man!"[4]

BUYING AND STORING FRESH GINGER

If your local grocery store keeps a supply of fresh ginger in the produce section, you're in luck. If not, go to one that does or order it by mail. Fresh ginger should be firm when squeezed with your fingers, and the skin should be smooth (not wrinkled) and have a slight shine. Before use, rinse it with water to remove any dirt and residue. I store fresh ginger in the refrigerator in a plastic sandwich bag, although it can also be stored in a dry place at room temperature without a plastic bag. You don't need to peel off the skin, but if you do, be certain to remove only a thin layer as valuable aromatic resin lies just beneath the skin.

If you slice the ginger and see a light blue ring near the outer edge, it has been scientifically confirmed that the rhizome packs a potent supply of enzymes.[5] Enzymes are desperately lacking in many of the foods we eat today.

TAKE DRY GINGER POWDER FOR HEALTH MAINTENANCE

Dried ginger powder is much more potent than fresh ginger and is commonly available as a spice but is also available in capsules that are easy to swallow. While dried ginger does not provide the throat-clearing and head-clearing effects of fresh ginger, it has many benefits that have been studied in great detail. Dried ginger has been used by many cultures throughout history for treating a variety of ailments.

A recommended amount for health maintenance is 1/2 to 2 grams of dried powder per day, taken with a meal. For dose measurement, 1 level teaspoon of dried powder is about 1.6 to 1.8 grams. Be sure to check the label on your bottle for the recommended daily amount.

Loose powder is inexpensive and can be mixed with a cup of water and drunk. Sometimes, I make a quick and soothing tea by adding 1/2 to 1 teaspoon of dry ginger powder to a cup of warm water. Add honey for sweetness.

FRESH GINGER VERSUS DRIED GINGER POWDER

One of ginger's astonishing natural characteristics is that new sets of chemicals are created when it is dried. Fresh ginger contains gingerols, which are responsible for its pungent taste, its many therapeutic properties, and its head-clearing effects.

Dried ginger is much more potent than fresh ginger. This is because water is removed and upon drying, the gingerols (abundant in fresh ginger) are transformed into a new group of chemicals called shogaols and zingerone. The shogaols have characteristics similar to aspirin and can have up to 10 times the concentration and potency of the gingerols in fresh ginger.[6] Shogaols have anti-inflammatory and other therapeutic properties as well.

Many people take capsules of dried ginger powder every day. Swallowing the capsules will not produce the head-clearing effect of fresh ginger. It is important to set limits on the amount of dried ginger powder consumed. The following chapter will provide some guidance based on past experience and studies.

REFERENCES FOR CHAPTER 8

1. Puri HS and Pandey G. "Glimpses into the crude drugs of Sikkim." *Bulletin Medical Ethnobotany Research* 1 (1980):55-71. (As cited by Schulick, P. *Ginger: Common Spice & Wonder Drug.* 3rd ed. Prescott, AZ. Hohm Press, 1996, p.11).

2. "Department of Health and Human Services Food and Drug Administration". Web site. Accessed 11/12/2006. <http://www.technology.gov/Reports/Compendium/dohhs.pdf>.

3. Fulder S, Ph.D. *The Ginger Book.* Avery Publishing Group, Garden City Park, New York. pp.46, 52.

4. Fulder S, Ph.D. *The Ginger Book.* Avery Publishing Group, Garden City Park, New York. pp.42-43.

5. Thompson EH, Wolf ID, Allen CE. "Ginger Rhizome: A New Source of Proteolytic Enzyme." Meat Science Lab, Dept. of Animal Science, University of Minnesota, St. Paul, MN 55101.

6. Schulick, P. *Ginger: Common Spice & Wonder Drug.* 3rd ed. Prescott, AZ. Hohm Press, 1996, pp.80-81.

CHAPTER 9

How Much Ginger Should You Take?

WHEN considering recommended amounts, the distinction needs to be made between low supplemental/maintenance amounts versus higher therapeutic/medicinal dosages. You should consult with your health expert before taking therapeutic/medicinal dosages if you are attempting to target a particular condition such as a chronic inflammatory condition or another suspected illness. Supplemental/maintenance amounts can also provide many health benefits.

FRESH GINGER

Because fresh ginger is a food, there is very little research data suggesting a daily limit. One thin slice about the size of a quarter is about 2 to 3 grams (1 gram is 1000 milligrams). One teaspoon of grated ginger is about 5 grams. I may consume as few as 3 slices a day or as many as 10 slices. It is hard to overdose on fresh ginger by taking one slice at a time unless you experience some negative side effects, sensitivities, or allergies. Paul Schulick, researcher and author of *Ginger: Common Spice and Wonder Drug*, writes, "One is most likely to err by taking too little or by selecting an improper or low quality form." His research shows that 7 grams of fresh ginger is considered a minimal daily amount for an adult in order to receive some health benefit.[1] In one study, a patient consumed as much as 50 grams of ginger root daily (lightly cooked with other vegetables and meat) for three months for increased relief of rheumatoid arthritis with no negative side effects.[2] I've found that just 1 or

2 slices are enough to help clear my throat. It should be noted that fresh ginger, like other herbs and crops, could contain some contaminants which, over a long period of time, could be a concern. An alternative would be to obtain a supply of certified organically grown ginger to eliminate this concern.

DRIED GINGER—IT'S POTENT STUFF!

Because dried ginger powder can have many times the potency of some compounds (mainly shogaols) compared to fresh, the amount of dried ginger consumed needs to be limited. For supplemental/main-tenance purposes, 1 or 2 capsules (1/2 to 2 grams) a day is generally recommended. I give my kids 1 capsule of dry ginger powder every other day. I alternate this with 1 capsule of turmeric in between the ginger days. An amount above 2 grams a day of dried ginger is considered a therapeutic/medicinal dosage, and you should consult your physician before taking these higher dosages. Be sure to check the label on the bottle for the recommended amount, as concentrations may vary.

For children, the above amounts need to be reduced according to the child's weight. Since most herbal dosages are for a 150-pound adult, a child weighing 50 pounds should take one-third the adult dosage. Ginger should not be used by children under two years old,[3] as there are no studies to assess ginger's safety with very young children.

GINGER IS SAFE

According to a past director of the World Health Organization (WHO), ginger is "one of the three most thoroughly studied plants in the history of the world." (The other two are garlic and ginseng.)[4] Ginger has been used throughout history for its healing properties with no side effects. It is one of the few herbs that is also a food. Historical evidence shows very few, if any, interactions with other medications. Refer to the next chapter for cautions.

The United States Food and Drug Administration (FDA) classifies fresh ginger as one of the safest herbs when used as a food additive. It is rated "generally recognized as safe" (GRAS) for its intended use by a consensus of scientific opinion. This is the same category as parsley, pepper, mustard, horseradish, garlic, and other common herbs, spices, and natural seasonings.[5] Ginger is consumed all over the world in many ways. Paul Schulick sums it up this way: "The historical literature contains virtually no mention of adverse effects and modern scientific literature supports this with a unanimous verdict of: *no side effects.*" Schulick also writes, "Animals have been given ginger on a daily basis in the amounts equivalent to a human's consumption of about 7 1/2 pounds without noticeable side effects. When animals are fed pure gingerol or shogaol, they can tolerate amounts equivalent to a human's consumption of about 4 1/2 pounds of dried ginger."[6]

REFERENCES FOR CHAPTER 9

1.   Schulick, P. *Ginger: Common Spice & Wonder Drug.* 3rd ed. Prescott, AZ. Hohm Press, 1996, pp.83-85.
2.   Srivastava KC, Mustafa T. "Ginger (Zingiber officinale) and rheumatic disorders." *Medical Hypotheses.* 29, no. 1 (May 1989): 25-28
3.   "Ginger" Web site: USADrug.com. Accessed 11/15/03. <http://www.usadrug.com/IMCAccess/ConsHerbs/Gingerch.shtml>.
4.   Schulick P. "The healing power of ginger." *Vegetarian Times.* May 1996. Quoting Norman Farnsworth, Ph.D. Director of the World Health Organization Collaborating Centre for Traditional Medicine and Research Professor of Pharmacognosy at the University of Chicago at Illinois
5.   United States Government Web Sites:
     Dr. Duke's Phytochemical and Ethnobotanical Databases. "Module 19. Botanicals Generally Recognized As Safe" Accessed 2/11/2003. <http://www.ars-grin.gov/duke/syllabus/gras.htm>
     21CFR582.1 "TITLE 21 – FOODS AND DRUGS, CHAPTER 1—FOOD AND DRUG ADMINISTRATION, DEPARTMENT OF HEALTH AND HUMAN SERVICES, PART 582—SUBSTANCES GENERALLY RECOGNIZED AS SAFE" Accessed 2/11/2003. <http://www.accessdata.fda.gov...>
6.   Schulick, P. *Ginger: Common Spice & Wonder Drug.* 3rd ed. Prescott, AZ. Hohm Press, 1996, pp.83, 104.

CHAPTER 10

Cautions When Taking Ginger

GINGER has a reputation down through history of being very safe, and several expert sources also affirm its safety.[1] However, some commonsense guidelines and limitations need to be followed, especially when taking dried ginger because of its high concentration of certain compounds. The FDA has not evaluated ginger for safety or effectiveness for treating any condition or illness. Guidelines for using ginger are largely based on its documented historical use for the past 2,500-plus years along with many studies regarding its therapeutic applications around the world.

The American Herbal Products Association (AHPA) gives *fresh* ginger a class 1 safety rating, meaning it "can be safely consumed when used appropriately."[2] Dried ginger is rated class 2b and 2d by the AHPA. The class 2b rating means it should not be used during pregnancy unless directed by a professional with expertise in the use of ginger during pregnancy. The class 2d rating means there are some other restrictions according to professional guidance. Persons with gallstones should consult with their physician before using ginger according to the AHPA *Botannical Safety Handbook*.[3] If you are pregnant or nursing, consult with your physician.

Other sources for reviewing the safety of vitamins, herbs, and medications are: The University of Maryland Medical Center Web site www.umm.edu/altmed and the Web site www.drugdigest.org.

Cautions

- Due to a lack of knowledge of its effects on infants, ginger should not be used during breast-feeding nor given to children under the age of two.[4]
- Do not take ginger during times of high fever or if you feel hot or are red and sweating.[5]
- Discontinue use in the cases of allergic reaction, development of rash, abnormal bleeding, or if any other adverse medical condition occurs.

Consult Your Physician

Consult your physician before taking dried ginger if any of the following apply to you:

- Are pregnant or planning to become pregnant
- Are breast-feeding
- Are prone to bleeding
- Have diabetes (ginger has a lowering effect on blood sugar)
- Have hypoglycemia (low blood sugar)
- Have hemophilia (improper clotting of blood) or hereditary clotting disorders
- Have gallstones or gallbladder problems (ginger increases the flow of bile, which may aggravate the problem)
- Are taking medications for diabetes, blood thinning, or any other condition
- Have any health conditions for which you are being monitored[6]

Nausea during Pregnancy

Even though ginger is one of the most widely used herbal remedies for nausea and vomiting, there have been no large, controlled trials to establish its safety for use during pregnancy. Yet, a 2001 survey among obstetricians and gynecologists in the United States found that 51.8% of physicians who responded to the survey had recommended ginger for treatment of moderate nausea during pregnancy.[7] After consulting with your physician, it would make sense to start with 1 or 2 cups of ginger tea unless there is a history of miscarriage, in which case ginger should be avoided during the first trimester, according to one ob/gyn physician.[8] One source states the amount used in tea is about 250 mg (about 1/4 teaspoon).[9] Alternatively, you could make tea from fresh ginger, but it would be a good idea to obtain some that is certified organic.

An interesting study completed in 2005 in the United States reported successful treatment of postoperative nausea using a 5% solution of essential oil of ginger by means of *aromatherapy before surgery*.[10] Another study indicated that *Helicobacter pylori* bacteria may be one possible cause of nausea and vomiting during pregnancy.[11] Ginger's effectiveness at inhibiting this common bacteria is covered in chapter 18.

Paul Schulick, author of *Ginger: Common Spice and Wonder Drug*, recommends not exceeding the following amounts each day during the first trimester:

- Dried ginger: 1 gram (1000 milligrams)
- Fresh ginger: 1 teaspoon, grated (about 5 to 7 grams)
- Liquid extract: 2 droppers (2 milliliters)
- Syrup: 2 teaspoons (10 milliliters)[12]

Here are the results of some studies about the use of ginger. More studies relating to nausea and pregnancy are given in chapter 20.

A 1991 landmark study of thirty pregnant women with morning sickness was conducted by the University of Copenhagen in Denmark. The women were given 250 milligrams of dried ginger powder 4 times a day (equal to 1 gram a day). Ginger was given for only 4 days. 70% of the women preferred the time period that ginger was given. No side effects on pregnancy outcome were observed as a result of using ginger in this short study.[13]

A later study of 70 pregnant women (at or before 17 weeks into pregnancy) who were experiencing nausea and vomiting was conducted in 2001 by the Chiang Mai University in Thailand. Women were given 250 milligrams of ginger, 4 times a day, for 4 days. 87% of the women reported improvement in nausea symptoms. No adverse effect on pregnancy outcome was detected. This study also showed that the greatest relief from nausea came 48 hours after the ginger was first taken.[14]

A small study conducted in 2002 by the University of South Florida involved women who were experiencing nausea and vomiting in their first trimester of pregnancy. Half of the woman were given 1 tablespoon of commercially prepared ginger syrup mixed with 4 to 8 ounces of water (divided into 4 doses) and given 4 times a day for 2 weeks. 67% of the women who received ginger syrup and water had stopped vomiting by day six. (The ginger syrup was equivalent to taking 1 gram of dried ginger powder per day.) The other group of women received a placebo (a supplement with no effect) and only 20% had stopped vomiting by day six. The study lasted 2 weeks.[15]

A systematic literature search of past studies was reported in 2005 in Italy and involved 675 pregnant women who were experiencing nausea and vomiting during pregnancy. Results of the studies showed ginger to be superior to a placebo. Also, ginger was just as effective as the reference drug vitamin B6. There were no significant side effects or adverse effects on pregnancy outcomes. The study concluded that ginger may be an effective treatment for nausea. However, more studies using larger groups are needed to further investigate the safety of ginger during pregnancy.[16] (Vitamin B6, also called pyridoxine, is one of the drugs of choice used in Canada for treatment of nausea during pregnancy.)[17]

Another study was reported in 2007 in Thailand and involved 123 women who were less than 16 weeks pregnant and were experiencing nausea and vomiting. The women were given daily doses of either 650 mg of ginger or 25 mg of vitamin B6 (divided into 3 doses per day) and given 3 times a day for four days. Both ginger and vitamin B6 were shown to significantly reduce nausea and vomiting. Ginger was more effective than vitamin B6. Some side effects from both groups were reported but were minor and did not require any treatment.[18]

INTERACTIONS WITH MEDICATIONS

In general, interactions between ginger and medications (or herbs) are rare, unknown, or have not been reported. The Web site EdrugDigest. org and other sources state that ginger can increase the effectiveness of certain medications while decreasing the effectiveness of others.[19] Another informative Web site is www.drugdigest.org, which contains a list of drugs and herbs that could interact with ginger.

Interactions with diabetes medications: Taking large amounts of ginger may have a lowering effect on blood sugar and could increase the effectiveness of medications used to treat diabetes. Persons with diabetes should not take large amounts of ginger (no more than 2 grams of dried powder or 3 grams of fresh ginger per day). Consult your physician or pharmacist before taking ginger if you are using insulin or other medications for diabetes.[20]

Interactions with stomach medications: Ginger may alter stomach acid and interfere with antacids and other medications for the stomach.[21]

Interactions with medications for the heart and circulatory system:

- Medications that lower blood pressure may be affected by taking over 4 grams of dried ginger per day or over 10 grams of fresh ginger per day.[22]
- High doses of ginger should not be taken at the same time as aspirin, as slower blood clotting could result.[23]
- One finding was reported of a seventy-six-year-old white

European woman who was using the blood-thinning medication phenprocoumon (used in Europe) who also began
eating various ginger products. She experienced overthin-
ning of blood but the condition was easily corrected after
she stopped eating ginger products. This was the first case of
a reported action between a blood-thinning medication and
ginger. Recommendations were issued to refrain from using
garlic, *Ginkgo biloba,* and other herbs when bleeding could
be critical.[24]

• There appears to be no evidence of interactions between
ginger, garlic, and warfarin.[25] There was one reported case
where using both *Ginkgo biloba* and warfarin resulted in
bleeding in the brain.[25] Warfarin is a popular blood thinning medication in the United States.

GINGER AND BLOOD-THINNING

Since ginger may have some slight blood-thinning actions, ginger
should not be taken two weeks prior to surgery as blood clotting times
after surgery could be affected. Refer to chapter 19 for additional guidelines and studies about the possible blood-thinning actions of the E-F-G
approach.

A 1994 study in the United Kingdom of eight healthy male volunteers showed that 2 grams of dried ginger had no detectable effect on
blood platelet function;[26] however, a 1991 study in India showed that
10 grams of dried ginger powder produced *significant* blood thinning in
patients with coronary artery disease. It is also interesting that 4 grams
of dry ginger powder given daily for three months did *not* produce blood
thinning in these same patients.[27]

Other foods and supplements that may also have blood-thinning
actions include the following: flax oil,[28] fish oil,[29] olive oil,[30] onions and
garlic,[31] curcumin (from turmeric),[32] *Ginkgo biloba,*[33] ginseng,[34] grape
skins and seeds,[35] soy sauce,[36] tomato,[37] quercetin (abundant in onions
and apples),[38] vitamin E,[39] and, although not a food, long-term moderate

exercise can also thin the blood while intense and strenuous exercise has the opposite effect of making blood thicker.[40] Ginger's potential blood-thinning actions are further reviewed in chapter 19.

REFERENCES FOR CHAPTER 10

1a.   Schulick, P. *Ginger: Common Spice & Wonder Drug*. 3rd ed. Prescott. AZ. Hohm Press. 1996. p.83.

1b.   Kaul PN, Joshi BS. "Alternative medicine: herbal drugs and their critical appraisal--partII." Prog Drug Res. 2001;57:1-75.

1c.   Weidner MS, Sigwart K. "Investigation of the teratogenic of a zingiber officinale extract in the rat." *Reprod Toxicol*. 2001 Jan-Feb;15(1):75-80.

2.   McGuffin M, Hobbs C, Upton R and Goldberg A. *Botannical Safety Handbook*. American Herbal Products Associations Botanical Safety Handbook, CRC Press, Boca Raton 1997. pp.125, introduction.

3.   McGuffin M, Hobbs C, Upton R and Goldberg A. *Botannical Safety Handbook*. American Herbal Products Associations Botanical Safety Handbook, CRC Press, Boca Raton 1997. pp.125, introduction.

4.   "Ginger - Drugs & Vitamins - Drug Library – DrugDigest" Web site: E DrugDigest. Accessed 11/19/03. <http://www.drugdigest.org/DD/ PrintablePages/herbMonograph/0,11475,4016,00.html>.

5.   Fulder S. *The Ginger Book: The Ultimate Home Remedy*. Avery Publishing Group. Garden City Park, New York. 1996. p.48.

6.   "Ginger - Drugs & Vitamins - Drug Library – EDrugDigest" Web site: E DrugDigest. Accessed 11/19/03. <http://www.drugdigest.org/DD/ PrintablePages/herbMonograph/0,11475,4016,00.html>.

7.   Chandra K, Einarson A, Koren G. "Taking ginger for nausea and vomiting during pregnancy." *Canadian Family Medicine* Vol.48:September 2002. College of Family Physicians of Canada www.cfpc.ca *The Motherrisk Newsletter* Accessed Nov. 2003. <http://www.motherrisk.org/prof/updatesDetail. jsp?content_id=354>.

8.   Kelly Shanahan, M.D. "Ginger & Miscarriage." Web site: iVilllage. Accessed 5/18/02. <http://www.ivillagehealth.com/experts/womens/ qas/0,11816,166315_151238,00.html>.

9.   "Morning Sickness." Web site: MotherNature.com. Accessed 11/16/03. <http://mothernature.com/Library/bookshelf/Books/41/85.cfm>.

10.   James L. Geiger. "The essential oil of ginger, Zingiber officinale, and anaesthesia." *The International Journal of Aromatherapy*. (2005) 15, 7-14.

11.   Quinla JD, Hill DA. "Nausea and vomiting of pregnancy." *Am Fam Physician*. 2003 Jul 1;68(1):121-8.

12. Schulick, P. *Ginger: Common Spice & Wonder Drug.* 3rd ed. Prescott. AZ. Hohm Press. 1996. pp.84, 88.

13. Fischer-Rasmussen W, Kjaer SK, Dahl C, and Asping, U. "Ginger treatment of hyperemesis gravidarum." *European Journal Obstetrics, Gynecology,and Reproductive Biology* 38, no. 1 (Jan. 1991): 19-24.

14. Vutyavanich T, Kraisarin T, Ruangsri R "Ginger for nausea and vomiting in pregnancy: randomized, double-masked, placebo-controlled trial." *Obstetrics and Gynecology* (Apr 2001) 97(4):577-82.

15. Keating A, Chez RA. "Ginger syrup as an antiemetic in early pregnancy." Altern Ther Health Med. 2002 Sep-Oct;8(5):89-91.

16. Borrelli F, Capasso R, Aviello G, Pittler MH, Izzo AA. "Effectiveness and safety of ginger in the treatment of pregnancy-induced nausea and vomiting." Obstet Gynecol. 2005 Apr;105(4):849-56.

17. Chandra K, Einarson A, Koren G. "Taking ginger for nausea and vomiting during pregnancy." *Canadian Family Medicine* Vol.48:September 2002. College of Family Physicians of Canada www.cfpc.ca *The Motherrisk Newsletter* Accessed Nov. 2003. <http://www.motherrisk.org/prof/updatesDetail. jsp?content_id=354>.

18. Chittumma P, Kaewkiattikum K, Wiriyasiriwach B. "Comparison of the effectiveness of ginger and vitamin B6 for treatment of nausea and vomiting in early pregnancy: a randomized double-blind controlled trial." *J Med Assoc Thai.* 2007 Jan;90(1):15-20.

19a. "Ginger - Drugs & Vitamins - Drug Library – DrugDigest" Web site: E DrugDigest. Accessed 11/19/03. <http://www.drugdigest.org/DD/ PrintablePages/herbMonograph/0,11475,4016,00.html>.

19b. Lala LG, D'Mello PM, Naik SR. "Pharmacokinetic and pharmacodynamic studies on interaction of "Trikatu" with diclofenac sodium." J Ethnopharmacol. 2004 Apr;91(2-3):277-80.

20. "Ginger - Drugs & Vitamins - Drug Library – DrugDigest" Web site: E DrugDigest. Accessed 11/19/03. <http://www.drugdigest.org/DD/ PrintablePages/herbMonograph/0,11475,4016,00.html>.

21. "Ginger - Drugs & Vitamins - Drug Library – DrugDigest" Web site: E DrugDigest. Accessed 11/19/03. <http://www.drugdigest.org/DD/ PrintablePages/herbMonograph/0,11475,4016,00.html>.

22. "Ginger - Drugs & Vitamins - Drug Library – DrugDigest" Web site: E DrugDigest. Accessed 11/19/03. <http://www.drugdigest.org/DD/ PrintablePages/herbMonograph/0,11475,4016,00.html>.

23. "Ginger - Drugs & Vitamins - Drug Library – DrugDigest" Web site: E DrugDigest. Accessed 11/19/03. <http://www.drugdigest.org/DD/ PrintablePages/herbMonograph/0,11475,4016,00.html>.

24. Kruth P, Brosi E, Fux R, Morike K, Gleiter CH. "Ginger-associated overanti-

coagulation by phenprocoumon." *Ann Pharmacother.* 2004 Feb;38(2):257-60. Epub 2003 Dec 19.

25a.   Jiang X, Blair EY, McLachlan AJ. "Investigation of the effects of herbal medicines on warfarin response in healthy subjects: a population pharmacokinetic-pharmacodynamic modeling approach." *J Clin Pharmacol.* 2006 Nov;46(11):1370-8.

25b.   Vaes LP Chyka PA. "Interactions of warfarin with garlic, ginger, ginkgo, or ginseng: nature of the evidence." *Ann Pharmacother.* 2000 Dec;37(12):1478-82.

26.   Lumb AB. "Effect of dried ginger on human platelet function." *Thromb Haemost.* 1994 Jan;71(1):110-1.

27.   Bordia A, Verma SK, Srivastava KC. "Effect of ginger (Zingiber officinale Rosc.) and fenugreek (Trigonella foenumgraecum L.) on blood lipids, blood sugar and platelet aggregation in patients with coronary artery disease." *Prostaglandins Leukot Essent Faty Acids.* 1997 May;56(5):379-84.

28.   Allman MA, Pena MM, Pang D. "Supplementation with flaxseed oil versus sunflowerseed oil in healthy young men consuming a low fat diet: effects on platelet composition and function." *Eur J Clin Nutr.* 1995 Mar;49(3):169-78.

29a.   Agren JJ, Vaisanen S, Hanninen O, Muller AD, Hornstra G. "Hemostatic factors and platelet aggregation after a fish-enriched diet or fish oil or docosahexaenoic acid supplementation." *Prostaglandins Leukot Essent Fatty Acids.* 1997 Oct;57(4-5):419-21.

29b.   Mori TA, Beilin LJ, Burke V, Morris J, Ritchie J. "Interactions between dietary fat, fish, and fish oils and their effects on platelet function in men at risk of cardiovascular disease." *Arterioscler Thromb Vasc Biol.* 1997 Feb; 17(2):279-86.

29c.   Oosthuizen W, Vorster HH, Jerling JC, Barnard HC, Smuts CM, Silvis N, Kruger A, Venter CS. "Both fish oil and olive oil lowered plasma fibrinogen in women with high baseline fibrinogen levels." *Thromb Haemost.* 1994 Oct;72(4):557-62.

30a.   Larsen LF, Jaspersen J, Marckmann P. "Are olive oil diets antithrombotic? Diets enriched with olive, rapeseed, or sunflower oil affect postprandial factor VII differently." *The American Journal of Clinical Nutrition.* 70(6), 1999, pages 976-982. Obtained from web site: Atkins.com Accessed 2/5/2004. <http://atkins.com/Archive/20026/20-65315.html>.

30b.   Oosthuizen W, Vorster HH, Jerling JC, Barnard HC, Smuts CM, Silvis N, Kruger A, Venter CS. "Both fish oil and olive oil lowered plasma fibrinogen in women with high baseline fibrinogen levels." *Thromb Haemost.* 1994 Oct;72(4):557-62.

31.   Srivastava KC. "Aqueous extracts of onion, garlic and ginger inhibit platelet aggregation and alter arachidonic acid metabolism." *Biomed Biochim Acta.* 1984;43(8-9):S335-46.

32a.   Shah BH, Nawaz Z, Pertani SA, Roomi A, Mahmood H, Saeed SA, Gilani

AH. "Inhibitory effect of Curcumin, a food spice from turmeric, on platelet-activating factor- and arachidonic acid-mediated platelet aggregation through inhibition of thromboxane formation and Ca2+ signaling." *Biochem Pharmacol.* 1999 Oct 1;58(7):1167-72.

32b.   Srivastava KC, Bordia A, Verma SK. "Curcumin, a major component of food spice turmeric (Curcuma longa) inhibits aggregation and alters eicosanoid metabolism in human blood platelets." *Prostaglandins Leukot Essent Fatty Acids.* 1995 Apr;52(4):223-7.

33.   Bent S, Goldberg H, Padula A, Avins A. "Spontaneous Bleeding Associated with Ginkgo biloba." *J Gen Intern Med.* 2005 July; 20(7):657-661.

34.   Teng CM, Kuo SC, Ko FN, Lee JC, Lee LG, Chen SC, Huang TF. "Antiplatelet actions of panaxynol and ginsenosides isolated from ginseng." *Biochim Biophys Acta.* 1989 Mar 24;990(3):315-20.

35.   Shanmuganayagam D, Beahm MR, Osman HE, Krueger CG, Reed JD, Folts JD. "Grape Seed and Grape Skin Extracts Elicit a Greater Antiplatelet Effect When Used in Combination than When Used Individually in Dogs and Humans." *J. Nutr.* 132:3592-3598, December 2002.

36.   Tsuchiya H, Sato M, Watanabe I. "Antiplatelet activity of soy sauce as functional seasoning." *J Agric Food Chem.* 1999 Oct;47(10):4167-74.

37.   O'kennedy N, Crosbie L, Whelan S, Luther V, Horgan G, Broom JI, Webb DJ, Duttaroy AK. "Effects of tomato extract on platelet function: a double-blinded crossover study in healthy humans." *Am J Clin Nutr.* 2006 Sep;84(3):561-9.

38a.   Hubbard GP, Wolffram S, de Vos R, Bovy A, Gibbins JM, Lovegrove JA. "Investigation of onion soup high in quercetin inhibits platelet aggregation and essential components of the collagen-stimulated platelet activation pathway in man: a pilot study." *Br J Nutr.* 2006 Sep;96(3):482-8.

38b.   Hubbard GP, Wolffram S, Lovegrove JA, Gibbons JM. "Ingestion of quercetin inhibits platelet aggregation and essential components of the collagen-stimulated platelet activation pathway in humans." *J Thromb Haemost.* 2004 Dec;2(12):2138-45.

39a.   Stuart MJ, Oski FA. "Vitamin E and platelet function." *Am J Pediatr Hematol Oncol.* 1979 Spring;1(1):77-82.

39b.   Freedman JE, Keaney JF Jr. "Vitamin E Inhibition of Platelet Aggregation Is Independent of Antioxidant Activity." *Journal of Nutrition.* 2001;131:374S-377S.

40a.   Imhof A, Koenig W. "Exercise and thrombosis." *Cardiol Clin.* 2001 Aug;19(3):389-400.

40b.   Koenig W, Ernst E. "Exercise and thrombosis." *Coron Artery Dis.* 2000 Mar;11(2):123-7.

CHAPTER 11

The History of Ginger and the Spice Trade

L ET'S take a break from the technical stuff and enjoy a brief review of the importance of spices throughout history. To study the history of ginger and the spice trade is really a lesson in ancient cultures, dynasties, and world empires. Spices have been used for thousands of years to spice up a regular diet of bland staple foods, to help preserve meats, and as fragrances and medicines.

The use of ginger dates back more than five thousand years, originating in the subtropical regions of China and India.[1] Spices from Sri Lanka and China made their way to the Middle East as early as 2000 BC.[2] For several thousand years, until about 200 BC, the Arabs led the spice trade in and out of Asia and were known to travel these long journeys in large caravans with as many as 4,000 camels.[3] The book of Genesis tells of Joseph being sold as a slave to a passing Ishmaelite caravan carrying spices on the way to Egypt around 1500 BC. About 1000 BC, the Queen of Sheba traveled over twelve hundred miles to test King Solomon's wisdom and presented him with expensive gifts of gold, precious stones, and large quantities of spices.[4] It was the Arabs who brought spices to the Greeks and Romans. Traders often told tales exaggerating the dangers of obtaining spices to keep prices high and hide the origins of the spices.[5]

As the Roman Empire expanded, and likewise its vast maritime capabilities, the Romans began sailing to India and other countries in the first century AD.[6] The Romans were able to increase their wealth by trading directly with India and Asia and dominated the spice trade until the empire's decline between 400 and 500 AD. After the fall of the Roman empire, spices became scarce and were available only to the wealthy. History then repeated itself as the Arabs regained dominance of the spice trade for about another thousand years.[7]

In 1298, Marco Polo returned from China, bringing with him new knowledge of the origins of many spices. His influence rekindled interest in direct trade with the spice-producing countries of the Orient.[8] Over the next one hundred years, huge profits were made by Italian, Portuguese, and Spanish explorers in an effort to satisfy Europe's desire and taste for spices.[9] Having exotic and expensive spices became a status symbol and a means to impress dinner guests.[10]

In 1492, Christopher Columbus sailed westward, hoping to find a new route to India, but instead he sailed into the Americas, ushering in another era of exploration and trade. He brought back knowledge of new peoples and places and also some new spices, including red pepper (chilies), allspice, and vanilla.[11] Several years later, in 1498, Vasco de Gama's newly discovered trade route around Africa allowed tiny Portugal to become a center for world commerce and, in turn, become one of the wealthiest countries in Europe.[12] The demand for spices, gold, and other goods motivated traders and explorers to brave long and often dangerous journeys to distant lands. Also important was the exploration of new peoples and their cultures, skills, goods, technologies, and art forms. The ports became centers for the exchange of information as well as for the trading of food, spices, and other goods.[13]

The various sea routes linking the East to the West became known as the "Spice Routes." These routes spanned from Japan, China, and India in the East, down around Africa, and continued westward to the Middle East and Europe. The network of sea routes covered some 93,000 miles and included stops at ports in many other countries as well.[14]

American-born Elihu Yale spent his childhood in England and later was employed as a young clerk for the British East India Trading Company, which had a monopoly on the spice trade. In 1672, he set up his own spice trade business in India and earned his fortune. He provided the largest gift of financial backing to start a new university in his hometown of Boston, and, in his honor, the new learning institution was named Yale University.[15]

America had entered the lucrative spice trade in the early 1800s, but it later became too risky and dangerous because of pirate attacks on the Java and China seas.[16] The young nation could not defend international shipping, and, as a result, direct exchange with the native spice cultures of the world ceased. However, spices still entered America by way of Europe and other countries.

Valued throughout history for its complex flavor and therapeutic properties, ginger was second only to pepper in the spice trade.[17] Ginger is often mentioned in the historical literature and folklore of many cultures. Spices were used as currency for the payment of taxes, rents, bribes, and ransoms and were even valued as highly as gold by some traders.[18]

Ginger is now widely grown in warm, moist climates in many countries, including China, India, Africa, the West Indies, Australia, Jamaica, Brazil, and Hawaii. The spread of ginger to many cultures and its historical staying power makes a very important statement—it was highly prized and useful to many people for thousands of years.

REFERENCES FOR CHAPTER 11

1.   "History of Ginger" Web site: National Importers, Inc. Accessed 3/2/2004. <http://www.nationalimporters.com/history>.

2.   Reid, S. *East Meets West - Exploration by Sea*. Thameside Press. 2002. p.6. Distributed in the U.S. by Smart Apple Media, 1980 Lookout Drive, North Mankato, MN 56003.

3.   V. Krishna Moorthy, Bhaskar Karnick. "Indian Spices - Tastes of Paradise" Web site. Accessed 4/3/04. <http://www.vigyanprasar.com/comcom/reature66. htm>.

4.   The Bible. Genesis Chapter 37, verse 25. I Kings Chapter 10. II Chronicles Chapter 9.

5.   "The Enspicelopedia - The History of Spices" Web site: McCormick & Company, Inc. Accessed 4/3/2004. <http://www.mccormick.com>.

6.   "Ginger - Introduction." Web site: National Importers. Accessed 3/2/2004.
     <http://www.nationalimporters.com.history>.
7.   "History of Ginger" Web site: National Importers, Inc. Accessed 3/2/2004.
     <http://www.nationalimporters.com/history/history.asp?articleid=14>.
8.   "A Timeline of Spice History..." Web site: The American Spice Trade
     Association. 20025 M Street, NW Suite 800, Washington, DC 20036.
     Accessed 4/3/2004. <http:www.astaspice.org/history/timeline.htm>.
9.   "History of Ginger." Web site: National Importers, Inc. Accessed 3/2/2004.
     <http://www.nationalimporters.com/history>.
10. V. Krishna Moorthy, Bhaskar Karnick. "Indian Spices - Tastes of Paradise"
     Accessed 4/3/04. <http://www.vigyanprasar.com/comcom/reature66.htm>.
11. "The Enspicelopedia - The History of Spices." Web site: McCormick &
     Company, Inc. Accessed 4/3/2004. <http://www.mccormick.com>.
12. V. Krishna Moorthy, Bhaskar Karnick. "Indian Spices - Tastes of Paradise"
     Accessed 4/3/04. <http://www.vigyanprasar.com/comcom/reature66.htm>.
13. Reid, S. East Meets West - Exploration by Sea. Thameside Press. 2002. p.7.
     Distributed in the U.S. by Smart Apple Media, 1980 Lookout Drive, North
     Mankato, MN 56003.
14. Reid, S. East Meets West - Exploration by Sea. Thameside Press. 2002. p.6.
     Distributed in the U.S. by Smart Apple Media, 1980 Lookout Drive, North
     Mankato, MN 56003.
15a. V. Krishna Moorthy, Bhaskar Karnick. "Indian Spices - Tastes of Paradise"
     Accessed 4/3/04. <http://www.vigyanprasar.com/comcom/reature66.htm>.
15b. "The Enspicelopedia - The History of Spices." Web site: McCormick &
     Company, Inc. Accessed 4/3/2004. <http://www.mccormick.com>.
16. "The Enspicelopedia - The History of Spices." Web site: McCormick &
     Company, Inc. Accessed 4/3/2004. <http://www.mccormick.com>.
17. "Ginger - Your Food is Your Medicine." Web site: Steven Foster Group.
     Accessed 1/29/2004. <http://www.stevenfoster.com/education/monograph/
     ginger.html>.
18. V. Krishna Moorthy, Bhaskar Karnick. "Indian Spices - Tastes of Paradise"
     Accessed 4/3/04. <http://www.vigyanprasar.com/comcom/reature66.htm>.

PART III

Answers to Clues

A Look Under the Hood

CHAPTER 12

Digestion and Leaky Gut Syndrome

HOW important are digestion and diet? A 1996 study by the U.S. Department of Health estimates that *one-third to one-half of all adults in America are affected in some way by a digestive illness.* This startling study suggests an epidemic in the United States with a huge cost—estimated to be over 41 billion dollars per year.[1] The National Cancer Institute estimates at least 35% of cancers are related to diet, but that number could be as high as 60%.[2]

Ginger is best known throughout history for treating problems with digestion and nausea. Confucius, one of history's great teachers and administrators (551–479 BC), was known to eat ginger with every meal.[3] What did Confucius know? Besides composing many wise sayings about life, he was very much aware of ginger's use for improving digestion and helping with many ailments.

When taken with food during a meal, fresh ginger's enzymes jump-start the digestion process by breaking down food proteins in the stomach. Fresh ginger provides one of nature's richest sources of proteolytic (protein-digesting) enzymes.[4] It was first proposed in 1935 that undigested food proteins that are absorbed into the blood can trigger food allergies,[5] and this was confirmed by later studies and enzyme-treatment programs.[6]

Ginger promotes healthy digestion several other ways:

- Antinausea and antivomiting actions (see chapter 20)

- Antiulcer actions[7]: Gingerols (most abundant in fresh ginger) were shown to be effective at inhibiting the growth of all 19 strains of *Helicobacter pylori*, the bacteria most responsible for dyspepsia, peptic ulcer disease, and the development of gastric and colon cancer[8]
- Anti-inflammatory actions (see chapter 16)
- Antifungal actions[9]
- Increases the flow of bile into the small intestine in animal studies[10] (bile is produced by the liver, is stored in the gall bladder, and is released into the small intestine after eating; it has strong detergent properties that act to break down fats into fatty acids, helps neutralize toxins, and has potent antibiotic actions)[11]

Ginger also helps detoxify the liver, the body's largest internal organ. The liver has the important job of removing toxins from the blood by breaking down harmful substances like ammonia, drugs, alcohol, and other toxins so they can be excreted out of the body. The liver also plays a large role in removing inflammatory toxins from the body. One interesting animal study showed that gingerols (most abundant in fresh ginger) exerted stronger activity in removing a test toxin from the liver than did shogaols (which are most abundant in dried ginger).[12] Gingerols are the compounds in fresh ginger most responsible for its pungent flavor and its many therapeutic actions. Gingerols are transformed into shogaols when ginger is dried.

Our digestive system has a huge job. It must break down our food into very tiny particles that can be absorbed by the millions of microscopic finger-like projections (called "villi") that cover the inside wall of the small intestine. It is estimated that 10–15 percent of our bodies' energy is used for digestion.[13] When you eat a slice of fresh ginger with your meal, as Confucius did, its potent proteolytic enzymes start the digestion process by breaking down proteins, resulting in better digestion and freeing up enzymes and energy that would otherwise be spent on digestion.

The digestive tract is the largest component of our immune system. For an average adult, the total surface area of the intestines, with its many folds and millions of microscopic villi, is about the size of a tennis court! Even more amazing is that this huge area must be highly selective in allowing tiny, microscopic nutrients to be absorbed into the bloodstream while keeping out toxins and waste products meant to be excreted out of the body. The inside wall of the intestines has a protective mucosa coating that is home to trillions of bacteria that protect us in many ways.

A healthy digestive tract is home to over 500 kinds of good bacteria, which are often called "friendly flora" or "beneficial bacteria." These beneficial bacteria perform many functions, such as the following:

- Inhibiting growth of yeasts such as *Candida albicans*[14] and harmful bacteria such as *Escherichia coli* (*E. coli*)[15]
- Manufacturing antibiotics and producing vitamins A, B1, B2, B3, B5, B6, B12, K, and folic acid
- Increasing absorption of calcium and other minerals[16]
- Fighting against tumors[17]
- Neutralizing the detergent-like properties of bile into a harmless form that will not harm the large intestine[18] (this is extremely important because un-neutralized bile is actually a carcinogen and may play a role in colon cancer and other related cancers;[19] some experts believe the destruction of beneficial bacteria from antibiotic use may play a role in causing colon cancer,[20] the third most common cancer in the United States)[21]

When beneficial bacteria are disturbed or destroyed, the protective mucosa barrier can no longer keep harmful toxins out—our body reacts, our health suffers, and our energy declines—setting the stage for sickness and disease.

You can help the beneficial bacteria become re-established in your body by eating yogurt and taking probiotic supplements, which contain active bacteria cultures, and taking other important steps for healing the digestive tract.

Leaky Gut Syndrome
(also called increased intestinal permeability)

Leaky gut syndrome (LGS) occurs when the wall of the intestine becomes inflamed, disturbed, or damaged, allowing undigested food particles, harmful bacteria, toxins, and waste products to leak into the bloodstream. Normally, toxins and waste products are contained within the intestinal wall and then excreted out of the body, but with LGS, the waste products can pass into the bloodstream. An inflamed intestine has enlarged spaces between the cells of the intestinal wall, allowing leakage of these potentially harmful products into the bloodstream.[22]

When undigested food particles, toxins, and waste products enter the bloodstream, the immune system attacks them and releases antibodies, which can cause inflammatory reactions in other parts of the body. If too many of these undigested food particles and toxins leak into the bloodstream, the liver can become overloaded and unable to detoxify the blood. A chronic condition of discomfort, fatigue, and illness can set in, making life very difficult for some people with LGS.

Symptoms associated with LGS include the following: abdominal pain, *aggressive behavior, anxiety,* asthma, bed-wetting, bloating, chronic joint pain, chronic muscle pain, *confusion,* constipation, diarrhea, *fatigue and malaise,* fevers of unknown origin, *fuzzy thinking,* gas, indigestion, *mood swings, nervousness,* poor exercise tolerance, poor immunity, *poor memory,* recurring bladder infections, recurring vaginal infections, shortness of breath, and skin rashes.[23]

A list of these and other symptoms and conditions associated with LGS can be found at the Web site www.leakygut.co.uk/symptoms.htm.

A big problem is that LGS and inflammation appear to build on each other, setting up a vicious cycle. Consider these two important findings:

- Undigested proteins that are absorbed into the bloodstream (from LGS) can trigger food-related allergic reactions. This was proposed as early as 1935.[24]
- In 1991, it was observed that allergic reactions by the intestine can cause temporary increases in gut leakiness.[25]
- Allergic reactions in the intestines can hinder absorption of nutrients, even when we eat nutritious food.[26]

It is logical that these reactions can make our health spiral downward unless corrective action is taken.

- LGS also seems related to the way our bodies respond to odors, chemicals, and environmental pollutants. One medical practitioner believes that 70% of her patients who have multiple chemical sensitivities also have LGS.[27]
- Studies during the 1980s showed how LGS in infants can trigger allergic-type responses.[28] It is also known that many substances in human breast milk (such as antibodies) help protect premature newborns from allergic reactions until their intestinal barriers are developed.[29]
- LGS is associated with multiple illnesses and diseases, which are discussed at the end of this chapter. Dr. Jake Paul Fratkin, OMD, a leading expert and practitioner in treating LGS, states that "LGS is a major cause of disease and dysfunction in modern society, and in my practice accounts for at least 50% of chronic complaints, as confirmed by laboratory tests," and he firmly believes "LGS is reaching epidemic proportions within our population."[30] Dr. Fratkin's article is available at the Web site www.hpakids.org (select "Articles," then "Leaky Gut Syndrome"). Dr. Fratkin uses holistic and Chinese medicine in his practice.

What Causes LGS?

LGS is a modern, twentieth-century illness. How does it happen? The exact cause of LGS is not fully understood, although research suggests it may be triggered by many factors. Some of these factors may include the use of broad-spectrum (broad-acting) antibiotics;[31] frequent use of NSAIDs (nonsteroidal anti-inflammatory drugs);[32] aspirin (the most well-known NSAID);[33] alcoholism;[34] aging;[35] bacterial, viral, and yeast/*Candida* infections in the intestine;[36] food allergies;[37] poor food choices;[38] pancreatic insufficiency;[39] heredity;[40] immune overload; environmental toxins; chronic stress; trauma; or complications from chemotherapy, radiation therapy, or disease (such as AIDS).[41]

LGS appears to be initiated by a decrease in the population of beneficial bacteria and an increase in harmful bacteria, yeast over-growth, or other infections. This condition is called "dysbiosis." It is known that the overuse of antibiotics is a leading cause of dysbiosis.[42] Another cause of dysbiosis and LGS is the frequent use of NSAIDs such as aspirin, ibuprofen, and indomethacin. It is known that NSAIDs disrupt the mucosa lining of the intestine, interfere with its healing, and increase intestinal permeability (leakiness).[43] It is known that the overuse of NSAIDs can damage this protective mucosa lining and lead to "ulcerations, hemorrhage, perforation, stricture formation, and the exacerbation of inflammatory bowel disease."[44]

Other factors that can contribute to dysbiosis include bad diet, chronic stress, and environmental chemicals such as chlorine and fluoride added to our drinking water, which also can harm beneficial bacteria.[45]

When large amounts of beneficial bacteria and its protective proper-ties are destroyed, a condition is created that allows bad bacteria, yeast, and other infections to grow more quickly than the beneficial bacteria, especially when the immune system is already weakened. The most common yeast to take over is *Candida albicans,* which can change into an aggressive fungal infection that can invade the digestive tract and cause reactions in other parts of the body. *A pattern of antibiotic use followed by Candida overgrowth is probably the leading cause of LGS.*[46] *Candida* overgrowth is discussed in chapter 14.

Parasite infections can also cause LGS.[47] It is interesting that the Japanese have a long tradition of serving slices of pickled ginger with sushi (raw fish), probably because of ginger's effectiveness at killing certain parasites and their larvae. Research backs this up.[48]

Pancreatic insufficiency (the pancreas not producing enough digestive enzymes) can also contribute to LGS. It is the job of the pancreas to produce digestive enzymes that break down our food. When food is not completely broken down, additional stress is placed on the body. Taking digestive enzyme supplements orally (by mouth) has been shown to reduce allergy symptoms by breaking down undigested foods into pieces too small to cause allergic reactions.[49] Remember that fresh ginger's proteolytic enzymes also help break down food proteins and fight inflammation, helping to reduce stress on the body. It is logical that fresh ginger's anti-inflammatory actions can help reduce inflammation of the digestive tract.

Diagnosing and Healing LGS

By now, you should have a pretty good idea if LGS is a condition you need to explore further. Elizabeth Lipski MS, CCN, in her books *Leaky Gut Syndrome* (Keats Publishing, Inc.) and *Digestive Wellness* (McGraw-Hill), has provided a questionnaire to help assess the functioning of the small intestine. Also, your health care provider can request a test for LGS, known as the Intestinal Permeability Assessment, as described on the Web at www.genovadiagnostics.com. The test is simple and involves drinking two types of sugar water and then comparing sugar levels in the urine several hours later. Consult your health care provider for this and other helpful diagnostic tests.

Healing a leaky gut requires multiple strategies and a lot of discipline. While the methods of treatment vary among practitioners, the steps below will provide a good start. You may need to try various strategies to determine which are best for you or your loved one. Some symptoms should improve after a few weeks of implementing various strategies. Substantial healing may take from four to nine months or even longer. Some cases of LGS may require careful and specific antibiotic treatment, according to Dr. Leo Galland, LGS medical expert and practitioner.[50] Dr. Galland has authored many informative articles that are available on his Web site at www.mdheal.org.

You can take the following steps right away to get the healing process started.

1. **Reduce** and **rotate** **foods that stress the immune system.**
   To rotate a food means to eat it once every four to seven days and substitute other foods in between. Foods that can stress the immune system and prevent healing include the following:

   Sugar-loaded foods and snacks: Since sugar has very little nutritional value (except for carbohydrates), it requires nutrients from elsewhere in our body to metabolize it.[51] (Metabolize means to break down into simpler substances that our body can use or get rid of as waste.)

   Try to reduce foods with refined sugar as much as you can. At the same time, don't feel guilty about treating yourself from time to time for good behavior. If *Candida* overgrowth is suspected, avoid all forms of sugar since *Candida* thrives on sugar and can cause an aggressive fungal infection in the digestive tract. More on this in chapter 14.

   Be aware that fruit juices usually contain a lot of sugar unless they are freshly squeezed. Other forms of sugar include dextrose, sucrose, fructose, and other food items such as corn syrup, pancake syrup, pastries, candy, soft drinks, high-sugar breakfast cereals, snacks, and desserts.

I enjoy using a powdered sweetener called stevia, which is produced from the leaves of the stevia plant, one of the sweetest plants known to man. Stevia powder is available at grocery stores and vitamin and health food stores. Stevia has been recently approved by the FDA as a sweetener and has long been approved as a supplement. (1/2 teaspoon of stevia has about the same sweetness as 1 cup of sugar.)

Yeasts, vinegar, and fermented foods: If you suspect *Candida*, it is important to eliminate yeast-containing foods for a period of time because yeast fosters the growth of *Candida*. Vinegar and many fermented foods also foster the growth of *Candida*. Yeast foods include bread, bagels, rolls, and pastries. Vinegar foods include mayonnaise and salad dressings. Fermented foods include sauerkraut, tofu, and sourdough bread.

Note: There is some disagreement among experts whether yeast-containing foods contribute to *Candida* or not. Some yeasts can actually fight against *Candida*.

Foods with refined white flour and corn: Wheat and corn rank high in causing allergic reactions. Wheat foods include bread, bagels, pasta, and pastry. Try to rotate with other grains such as white and brown rice, wild rice, oats, barley, millet, and other whole grains. If you do not have allergies to wheat, try to include whole wheat foods into your diet. Most wheat foods are made from white flour that is stripped of bran, fiber, and wheat germ, which contain the nutrients our bodies need.

Dairy: Milk and milk products are known to cause allergic reactions in many people. The late Dr. Frank Oski at John Hopkins School of Medicine described the condition "allergic tension-fatigue syndrome" as a cause of recurring abdominal pain, repeated headaches, aching muscles and joints, and even bed-wetting. He cites milk as the food most responsible for allergic symptoms in adults and children.[52] The pasteurizing process involves heating, which destroys harmful bacteria but also destroys enzymes that would have aided in the digestion of the milk. An interesting study involving 87 healthy teenagers showed that approximately 50% of adolescents had some difficulty in digesting the milk sugar lactose. (This condition is called lactose intolerance.) The study further analyzed lactose intolerance by ethnic group: 81% of African American teenagers, 80% of Asian American teenagers, and 36% of white adolescents experienced symptoms of lactose intolerance.[53] Milk with added probiotic bacteria *L. acidophilus* or *L. bulgaricus* has shown improved digestion of milk lactose.[54] Taking a lactase enzyme supplement with milk is also helpful. Enzymes are discussed in chapter 15.

It is known that many people who cannot tolerate milk can safely eat yogurt and other fermented milk products that contain active probiotic bacteria and natural enzymes that help digest the milk. Many people groups around the world have traditionally used foods made from fermented milk because refrigeration is not available. Probiotic bacteria such as *L. acidophilus, L. bulgaricus,* and others are available as supplements and will help recolonize beneficial bacteria in the digestive tract.

Chlorinated drinking water: Chlorine and fluoride added to drinking water may disrupt beneficial bacteria.[55] Water purifiers that mount on your spigot are fairly easy to install and do a good job of removing chlorine and other chemicals.

Foods that trigger migraine headaches: If you experience frequent headaches, you may want to reduce and rotate the following foods: alcohol, citrus fruits (oranges, grapefruit, lemon), chocolate, smoked or processed meats (such as hot dogs, bacon, ham, and salami), excessive caffeine, and food additives such as MSG (monosodium glutamate).[56] Smoked meats and processed meats usually contain nitrates or nitrites, which are added to maintain a fresh red color, otherwise the meat would turn pale gray. Reduce and rotate these nitrate-containing foods. Other factors that can trigger migraines include low blood sugar, cigarette smoke, changes in weather, barometric changes, and altitude changes.[57]

Dr. Seymour Diamond, MD, author of *Conquering Your Migraine*, lists many warning symptoms of migraine headaches that provide us with some more clues:[58]

- Difficulty in focusing, distorted perception, impaired concentration, and confusion
- Difficulty with speech—such as difficulty in finding the right word or using wrong words in speaking or writing—or slurred speech
- Word deafness—the inability to understand what has been said
- Changes in personality, becoming withdrawn or irritable

- Restlessness, agitation, frequent urination, thirst, and general muscle weakness

Dr. John A. Allocca, a leading authority on migraines, states that LGS, *Candida*, congestive bowel toxicity, and other factors can trigger migraine headaches and depression.[59] His Web site, www.allocca.com, includes a self-evaluation questionnaire.

At least two studies show ginger to be helpful for some relief of migraine headaches.[60]

2. Consider an elimination diet.

The goal of an elimination diet is to avoid potentially allergenic foods for five to ten days or longer; then each food is introduced one at a time while you carefully watch for signs of allergy or intolerance. Several sources recommend you do this under the care of a physician when there is the possibility of allergic reactions. Allow at least two days after eating each new food to check for any discomfort or reactions. Several books with information on elimination diets are listed at the end of this section.

Elizabeth Lipski, in her book *Leaky Gut Syndrome*, has had success putting her patients on the following foods during an elimination diet:[61]

- Rice
- Fish
- Fruit (except citrus)
- Vegetables (except potatoes, tomatoes, eggplant, and peppers)
- Olive oil

For people with *Candida* overgrowth, she eliminates all fruit and substitutes poultry. For people with Crohn's disease or ulcerative colitis, she eliminates rice and adds poultry. Be aware that some ready-to-eat fish fillets (breaded or batter dipped) may contain MSG (monosodium glutamate), which can trigger headaches and other reactions in some people. The late William G. Crook, MD, and Marjorie Hurt Jones, RN, authors of *The Yeast Connection Cookbook,* recommend that oats, brown rice, and millet be used during the elimination diet but should be alternated with grain substitutes such as amaranth or quinoa (pronounced keen'wa). These practitioners advise against eating wheat and corn during the elimination diet because these rank high in causing allergies.[62]

3. **Avoid foods that cause allergic reactions. Reduce and rotate foods that cause sensitivities.**

According to the American Academy of Allergy, Asthma, & Immunology, these six foods cause 90% of food allergy reactions in children: milk, egg, wheat, soy, peanuts, and tree nuts (such as pecans and walnuts).

The four foods that cause 90% of food allergy reactions in adults are: peanuts, tree nuts, fish, and shellfish.[63]

Real food allergies often produce an immediate, inflammatory response (from the rapid release of histamine) and may cause damage to the body and, in some cases, life-threatening reactions. Allergic reactions include closing of the throat and other breathing problems, itching of the skin, rashes, hives, or other severe reactions. Generally, food allergies are repeatable every time the offending food is eaten.

Unlike allergic reactions, which often occur immediately, food sensitivities are generally delayed and occur several hours or days later. Food sensitivities often produce some type of discomfort and may irritate or damage the digestive tract. Delayed reactions may be a result of undigested food particles entering the bloodstream. Elizabeth Lipski, in her book *Digestive Wellness,* states that food sensitivities and environmental sensitivities are often a result of LGS. Food sensitivities and environmental sensitivities have been known to disappear after the offending food or environmental allergen has been avoided for a period of time and the digestive tract has healed. She states that 80% of food sensitivities are from beef, citrus, dairy products, egg, pork, and wheat.[64]

4. *Do* **eat foods that are easy on the digestive tract and are least likely to cause sensitivities or allergic reactions.**
This usually means eating more foods in their natural forms, like fresh, uncooked fruits and vegetables; whole grains; and home-cooked, unprocessed meats. Try to include fresh, uncooked fruits and vegetables as often as possible. Also, be sure to chew your food thoroughly to aid digestion as much as possible.
If you suspect sensitivities to wheat, try other grains such as corn, oats, rice, barley, millet, or rye.

If you are allergic to gluten (a protein abundant in wheat, barley, rye, and, to a lesser extent, oats), then you must use gluten-free grains such as rice, corn, millet, buckwheat, amaranth, and quinoa. Teff is a grain substitute that has very little gluten. Some of these other grains can be relatively expensive. Rice cakes can be substituted for bread. Rice noodles can be substituted for pasta.
Gluten reacts with yeast to give dough its stretchiness and a loaf of bread its sponginess. However, gluten can damage the intestinal wall and cause severe reactions in people with gluten allergies. Individuals with gluten allergies must avoid it at all costs and be sure that other foods and grains are not contaminated with gluten from processing or cooking. An enzyme supplement made from ginger can help with gluten allergies and is available at www.biohawk.com.au.

5. *Do* eat foods and supplements that help heal the digestive tract.

> **Ginger** and **turmeric** have strong anti-inflammatory actions that can help heal the digestive tract. Be like Confucius and eat a slice of fresh ginger with every meal as well as 1 to 2 grams of dried ginger powder every day. Reducing inflammation of the digestive tract will help stop the leaks.

> **Yogurt** is a wonderful probiotic food because it contains active bacteria cultures, which promote recolonization of beneficial bacteria in the digestive tract. Make sure the label reads "contains live or active cultures." Avoid yogurt that has been heat treated because it has *no* active bacteria cultures.
> The active bacteria in yogurt can provide amazing health benefits:
> - *Lactobacillus acidophilus* (also called *acidophilus*) is added to many yogurts and is also a beneficial bacteria in the digestive tract. *Acidophilus* inhibits the growth of *Candida albicans* yeast, *E. coli* and other harmful bacteria,[65] and has cholesterol-lowering actions.[66] The name *Lactobacillus* means this beneficial bacteria produces lactic acid as it breaks down lactose (the sugar in milk). This lactic acid gives yogurt its sour taste.
> - *Bifidus* (also called *Bifidobacterium*) is another bacteria added to yogurt and is also the most abundant beneficial bacteria in the digestive tract. *Bifidus* provides many benefits, such as helping lower cholesterol,[67] potentially helping prevent food poisoning by fighting *Salmonella* (an infec-

tion from eating contaminated food),[68] and helping break down lactose, the sugar in milk.[69]

- *Lactobacillus casei* (*L. casei*) is another bacteria added to yogurt, and it also provides many benefits to the intestine such as decreasing ammonia levels,[70] reducing intestinal permeability (leaky gut),[71] reducing *Candida albicans*,[72] fighting against *H. pylori* (a common bacteria linked to stomach ulcers),[73] fighting against *E. coli* (another foodborne infection),[74] shortening the duration of "winter infections" in elderly persons,[75] and, in two studies, significantly decreasing recurrence of bladder cancer.[76]

The amazing benefits of yogurt were scientifically documented in 1908 by Nobel Prize–winner Dr. Elie Metchnikoff, an immunologist and close friend of Louis Pasteur. Dr. Metchnikoff studied a people group in Bulgaria who were very healthy and lived exceptionally long lives. He concluded this was due to their high consumption of yogurt and other foods made from fermented milk. Even the type of bacteria required to be present in yogurt is named after these people: *bulgaricus*. The National Yogurt Association requires that yogurt must contain the active bacteria *Lactobacillus bulgaricus* and *Streptococcus thermophilus* in order to be sold as yogurt.[77]

Other health benefits of yogurt are:

- Helps decrease diarrhea[78]
- Stimulates the immune system[79] and may help decrease allergic symptoms[80]
- Can produce some natural antibiotics and some

B vitamins (think of B vitamins as the "brain vitamins")[81]

- Contains anti-tumor properties,[82] fights against colon cancer,[83] and may help fight breast cancer[84]
- Increases absorption of calcium[85]
- Is a source of milk for lactase-deficient individuals[86] (lactase is the enzyme that breaks down the milk sugar lactose); it is also important to note that lactose intolerance is a frequent condition in older adults[87]
- Can help promote weight loss[89]
- Stimulates physical growth in animal studies[90]
- Is an excellent source of enzymes[91]
- Significantly lowers ammonia levels in the colon in animal studies[92] (ammonia is produced by *H. pylori* bacteria,[93] is damaging to the digestive tract,[94] and also can interfere with normal brain function[95]); remember that ginger can help fight against *H. pylori*[96], and garlic, turmeric, and some other herbs have antibiotic actions to fight against some of these harmful bacteria, as discussed in chapter 18.

At least one company adds the bacteria *Lactobacillus reuteri* to its yogurt. This bacteria can help inhibit *Salmonella, E. coli, Staphylococcus, Listeria,* and *Candida albicans.*[97] See the Web sites www.stonyfield.com and www.askdrsears.com for additional information.

Although other studies may discount some of the claims of yogurt's benefits, I believe many of us would benefit by eating it frequently. In addition, *if you are taking antibiotic medications, remember to eat yogurt and take probiotic supplements, which will help recolonize the beneficial bacteria of the digestive tract.*

Probiotic supplements contain active bacteria cultures
that promote the recolonization of beneficial bacteria
in the digestive tract. In addition to eating yogurt,
taking probiotic supplements offers another way to
increase beneficial bacteria and add new ones that are
not in yogurt. Probiotics can help stabilize the protective mucosal barrier of the digestive tract, strengthen
the immune system, crowd out bad bacteria, and
decrease inflammation of the intestine.[98] Additional
research confirms that probiotics help reduce the level
of ammonia in the blood and colon[99] and can help
reduce the risk of colon cancer by deactivating toxic
chemicals in the colon.[100] These are just a few of the
many advantages of eating yogurt and taking probiotic
supplements.

Oats have been shown to be effective in healing leaky gut
and preventing liver injury in alcohol-fed rats.[101] For
an economical breakfast, I like to sprinkle cinnamon
over finely rolled oats, then I add water. I prefer to eat
oatmeal uncooked because it tastes kind of like cookie
dough. I like to add fruit such as bananas, fresh pineapple, kiwi, applesauce, or whatever fruit or topping
happens to be on hand.

Psyllium seeds and husks provide water-soluble fiber and
contain short-chain fatty acids and other nutrients that
aid the growth of beneficial bacteria. Other benefits
include inhibiting the growth of harmful organisms and
decreasing inflammation of the intestine.[102] Psyllium
is available in capsules, tablets, and powder. Psyllium
seeds and husks are the active ingredient in popular
fiber supplements and laxatives. (People with asthma

or allergies to psyllium must avoid psyllium until it is proven safe for them.)

Bananas contain a sugar called fructooligosaccharides (abbreviated FOS), which is also available as a supplement. FOS is amazing in that it is sweet like sugar; however, it is not absorbed by the body. FOS actually aids the growth of beneficial bacteria and may reduce inflammation of the digestive tract.[103] Another important property of FOS is that it decreases the pH in the digestive tract (increases acidity), which supports the growth of beneficial bacteria and discourages the growth of harmful bacteria.[104] FOS is also found in garlic, onion, asparagus, tomatoes, barley, oats, wheat, wheat bran, wheat germ, and honey.

If you suspect *Candida* overgrowth, remember to avoid fruits and reduce starchy vegetables (such as potatoes and yams) until healing is well under way, after which you can begin eating these foods in small amounts. *Candida* overgrowth is discussed in chapter 14.

Omega-3 essential fatty acids also decrease inflammation of the digestive tract. Fish oil, a popular omega-3 supplement, was shown to help reduce symptoms of Crohn's disease for patients who were in remission. (The fish oil capsules in this study had an enteric coating, which dissolves and releases the fish oil after entering the small intestine.)[105] Omega-3s are discussed in chapter 13.

Quercetin is a natural antihistamine[106] found in apples, berries, pears, kale, broccoli, onions, tea,[107] and is also available in capsules. (Antihistamines help prevent inflammatory reactions.) James Duke, PhD, author of

The Green Pharmacy, writes that onion skins are a rich source of quercetin; he recommends cooking the onion skins in soups and removing them just before eating.[108] A recent animal study showed that quercetin can slow down a tumor's ability to form blood vessels and also can help block a type of protein needed by a tumor to divide and grow.[109] Another animal study showed that quercetin has some actions against colon cancer.[110]

Zinc aids in healing a leaky gut,[111] is important in maintaining a healthy immune system,[112] and also helps resist *Candida*.[113] Dr. Duke recommends eating spinach because of its high zinc content. Other natural sources listed in order of decreasing potency of zinc content are parsley, collard greens, Brussels sprouts, cucumbers, string beans, endive, asparagus, and prunes.[114]

Gelatin was shown to help protect the mucosal lining of the digestive tract against alcohol damage in animal studies. Its effectiveness was a result of increased blood circulation to the digestive tract by its blood-thinning effect.[115] The best source of gelatin is from soups and slow-cooked meats that have been cooked with the cartilage. Cartilage and gelatin supplements are also available in capsules. You may even reap other benefits from cartilage, such as a healthier immune system, heart, muscles, and skin, according to some sources. An entire book could be written about the amazing benefits of gelatin and cartilage.

Other supplements used by medical practitioners include folate (folic acid is the synthetic form used in supplements), the amino acids glutamine and L-arginine, and enteric-coated mint oil (the enteric coating keeps the mint oil intact until it reaches the intestine).

6. *Do* **eat foods that are rich in enzymes.**

Since it is known that food rests in the upper stomach 1/2 to 1 hour before being acted on by the protein-digesting enzyme pepsin in the lower stomach,[116] it is logical that fresh ginger's enzymes will go to work and jump-start the digestion of food proteins. It has been shown that plant enzymes are active even in highly acidic conditions such as in the stomach.[117] Fresh pineapple, kiwi, papaya, and figs are also good sources of protein-digesting enzymes. Fresh, raw fruits and vegetables have their own natural enzymes that aid in their digestion. You should eat lots of fresh produce if possible. Yogurt and other fermented foods also contain enzymes.[118]

Sprouted seeds are also a good source of enzymes. In the wintertime, I like to sprout mung beans because they sprout very quickly. In his book *Enzyme Nutrition*, Dr. Howell points out that seeds have their highest enzyme content when their sprouts measure 1/4 inch long.[119] Small sprouting kits are inexpensive. A good Web site for buying seeds for sprouting is www.wheatgrasskits.com.

7. *Do* **take enzyme supplements.**

Some people do not produce enough enzymes for proper digestion. This is called pancreatic insufficiency. Dr. Howell cites several human studies showing that as we age, our body's digestive enzymes become weaker and weaker, and in some cases are only a fraction of the strength of younger people.[120] Worse yet, animal studies show that the intestinal barrier becomes less efficient at blocking out harmful environmental substances with increasing age.[121] Enzyme supplements can help with digestion and also have healing and anti-inflammatory properties. Enzymes are discussed in chapter 15.

8. **Eat foods that fight against parasites, worms, and other microbe infections of the digestive tract.**

   Dr. Leo Galland, medical expert in treating gastrointestinal illnesses, believes most of the world's population is infected by intestinal parasites, even in the Unite States. He also reported that many cases of chronic fatigue syndrome and irritable bowel syndrome were linked to parasite infections within the intestine.[122] Many physicians recommend parasite testing. Common foods that help fight against intestinal infections include ginger, garlic, turmeric, papaya, pineapple, and cloves.[123] Ginger's anti-worm and antimicrobial actions are discussed in chapter 18. You may visit Dr. Galland's Web site at mdheal.org.

9. *Avoid* **smoke, dust, mold, mildew, and other environmental pollutants.**

   Environmental pollutants stress the immune system. If your immune system has been overloaded, it will need a chance to rest and recover. If possible, reduce or avoid using harsh household cleaners and chemicals. Construction materials, new furniture, fabrics, and rugs can release chemicals such as formaldehyde, which can further stress our immune system. Avoid mold and mildew, but be aware that they are often present in basements and houseplants. For more information, refer to Dr. Galland's Web site at mdheal.org and locate his article on "A Healthy Home."[124]

10. **Remember, as your digestive tract heals, you may gradually add foods that once caused some discomfort.**

11. **Consider reading the following books:**

Leaky Gut Syndrome, by Elizabeth Lipski, MS, CCN (New Canaan, CT: Keats Publishing).

Digestive Wellness, by Elizabeth Lipski, MS, CCN (New York: McGraw-Hill).

The Yeast Connection Handbook, by William Crook, MD (Jackson, TN: Professional Books).

The Yeast Connection Cookbook, by William Crook, MD, and Marjorie Jones (Jackson, TN: Professional Books).

The Allergy Self-Help Cookbook, by Marge Jones (Emmaus, PA: Rodale Press).

Allergy and Candida Cooking Made Easy, by Sondra Lewis (Coralville, IA: Canary Connect Publications).

Allergy Cooking with Ease, by Nicolette Dumke (Lancaster, PA: Starburst Publishers).

LGS AND OTHER ILLNESSES

LGS appears to be closely related to many inflammatory-type conditions, including the following:

- **Food allergies**[125]
- **Asthma**[126]
- **Eczema (also called atopic dermatitis):**[127] An inflammatory skin disorder characterized by a patch rash that is dry, slightly reddened, and itchy. Patches may also feel leathery.
- **Celiac disease:**[128] A condition of chronic inflammation of the digestive tract caused by allergic reactions to gluten-containing foods such as wheat, rye, barley, and other foods. Allergic reactions to gluten can damage the small intestine. Celiac disease appears to be a genetic disease and can result in an increased rate of osteoporosis and other conditions. (Osteoporosis is the weakening and deterioration of bones.)
- **Crohn's disease:**[129] A condition of chronic inflammation of the

digestive tract causing intestinal permeability that can be six times greater than normal.

- **Vasculitis:** Blood vessels become inflamed and narrowed and can weaken and stretch, increasing the chance of an aneurysm (a balloon-like bulge of a blood vessel). An aneurysm is a life-threatening condition if the blood vessel bursts. (My father passed away from a burst aneurysm in his brain at the relatively young age of fifty-one. This underscores the importance of getting inflammation under control.) Vasculitis can also cause blood vessels to become blocked—another dangerous condition. Vasculitis can also cause inflammation of the digestive tract leading to LGS and other harmful conditions.[130] *Ginger has many benefits for the heart and blood vessels* as discussed in chapter 19.

LGS also appears to be related to the following inflammatory joint diseases:

- **Rheumatoid arthritis:**[131] Inflammation of the joints that may even result in crippled and deformed joints. As early as 1947, the link between rheumatic diseases and the incomplete digestion of proteins was suggested.[132]
- **Ankylosing spondylitis:**[133] A form of arthritis and inflammation of the spinal column resulting in back pain and stiffness.
- **Fibromyalgia:**[134] A condition resulting in fatigue; anxiety; depression; and pain, stiffness, and tenderness of the muscles, tendons, and joints. It is characterized by restless sleep, waking up tired, and disturbances in bowel function.

REFERENCES FOR CHAPTER 12

1.   "Digestive Diseases in the United States." US Department of Health. 1996
2.   "Cancer Rates and Risks." National Cancer Institute, Washington DC: 1985 and Doll R, Peto R. *Journal of the National Cancer Institute.* 1981; 66(6):1191-1308.

3. Confucius. *Confucian Analects*. 500 BC. (The *Analects* are a collection of sayings of Confucius and stories about his life).

4. Thompson EH, Wolf ID, Allen CE. "Ginger rhizome: A new source of proteolytic enzyme." *Journal of Food Science* 38, no. 4 (1973): pp.652-55.

5. Oelgoetz AW, Oelgoetz PA, Wittenkind J. "The treatment of food allergy and indigestion of pancreatic origin with pancreatic enzymes." *Am. J. Dig. Dis. Nutr.* 1935; 2:422-6.

6a. Cichoke AJ. The Complete Book of Enzyme Therapy. Avery Publishing, New York, NY 1999. pp.110-113.

6b. McCann M. "Pancreatic enzyme supplement for treatment of multiple food allergies." *Ann. Allergy.* 1993; 71:269 [abstract #17].

6c. Howell E. Dr. *Enzyme Nutrition*. Avery Publishing, 1985. pp.143-144.

7a. Yoshikawa M, Hatakeyama S, Taniguchi K, Matuda H, Yamahara J. "6-Gingesulfonic acid, a new anti-ulcer principal, and ginger-glycolipids A, B, and C, three new monoacyldigalactosylglycerols from Zingiberis rhizoma originating in Taiwan." *Chemical and Pharmaceutical Bulletin* 40, no. 8 (1992): 2239-41.

7b. Yamahara J, Hatakeyama S, Taniguchi K, Kawamura M, Yoshikawa M. "Stomachic principles in ginger. II. Pungent and anti-ulcer effects of low polar constituents isolated from ginger, the dried rhizoma of Zingiber officinale Roscoe cultivated in Taiwan. The absolute stereostructure of a new diarylheptanoid." *Yakugaku Zasshi.* 1992 Sep;112(9):645-55.

7c. al-Yahya MA, Rafatullah S, Mossa JS, Ageel AM, Parmer NS, Tariq M. "Gastroprotective activity of ginger, zingiber officinale rosc., in albino rats." *American Journal of Chinese Medicine* 1989;17,(1-2): 51-6.

7d. Wu H, Ye D, Bai Y, Zhao Y. "Effect of dry ginger and roasted ginger on experimental gastric ulcers in rats." *Zhongguo Zhong Yao Za Zhi.* 1990 May;15(5):278-80, 317-18.

7e. Yamahara J, Mochizuki M, Rong HQ, Matsuda H, Fujimura H. "The anti-ulcer effect in rats of ginger constituents." *Journal of Ethnopharmacology.* 1988 July-Aug; 23(2-3):299-304.

8. Mahady GB, Pendland SL, Yun GS, Lu ZZ, Stoia A. "Ginger (Zingier officinale Roscoe) and the gingerols inhibit the growth of Cag A+ strains of Helicobacter pylori. *Anticancer Res.* 2003 Sep-Oct;23(5A):3699-702.

9. Ficker CE, Amason JT, Vindas PS, Alvarez LP, Akpagana K, Gbéassor M, De Souza C and Smith ML. "Inhibition of human pathogenic fungi by ethnobotanically selected plant extracts." Mycoses Feb. 2003;46:p.29.

10. Yamahara J, Miki K, Chisaka T, Sawada T, Fugimura H, Tomimatsu T, Nakano K, Nohara T. "Cholagogic effect of ginger and its active constituents." *Journal of Ethnopharmacology.* 1985 May;13(2):217-25.

11a. Begley M, Gahan CG, Hill C. "The interaction between bacteria and bile." *FEMS Microbiol.* 2005 Sep;29(4):625-51.

11b.   Gunn JS. "Mechanisms of bacterial resistance and response to bile." *Microbes Infect.* 2000 Jul;2(8):907-13.

12.   Hikino H, Kiso Y, Kato N, Hamada Y, Shioiri T, Aiyama R, Itokawa H, Kiuchi F, Sankawa U. "Antihepatotoxic actions of gingerols and diarylheptanoids." *Journal of Ethnopharmacology* 1985 Sep;14(1): 31-9.

13.   Calles-Escandon J, Horton ES. "The thermogenic role of exercise in the treatment of morbid obesity: a critical evaluation." *Am J Clin Nutr.* 1992;55:533S-7S.

14.   Kennedy MJ, Volz PA. "Ecology of *Candida albicans* Gut Colonization: Inhibition of *Candida* Adhesion, Colonization, and Dissemination from the Gastrointestinal Tract by Bacterial Antagonism." *Infect Immun.* Sept. 1985 pp.654-663.

15a.   Itoh K, Freter R. "Control of Escherichia coli populations by a combination of indigenous clostridia and lactobacilli in gnotobiotic mice and continuous-flow cultures." *Infect Immun.* 1989 Feb;57(2):559-65.

15b.   Freter R. Stauffer E, Cleven D, Holdeman LV, Moore WE. "Continuous-flow cultures as in vitro models of the ecology of large intestinal flora." *Infect Immun.* 1983 Feb;36(2):666-75.

16.   Lipski, E. *Leaky Gut Syndrome.* Keats Publishing, Inc., New Canaan, CT 06840. 1998 pp.36-37.

17a.   Sakamoto K, Konishi K. "Antitumor effect of normal intestinal microflora on Ehrlich ascites tumor." *Jpn J Cancer Res.* 1988 Jan;79(1):109-16.

17b.   Morinaga S, Sakamoto K, Konishi K. "Antitumor activity and its properties of Eubacterium lentum." *Jpn J Cancer Res.* 1988 Jan;79(1):117-24.

18a.   Liong MT, Shah NP. "Bile salt diconjugation ability, bile salt hydrolase activity and cholesterol co-precipitation ability of lactobacilli strains." Int. Dairy J. 2005 1;15:391-8.

18b.   McAuliffe O, Cano RJ, Klaenhammer TR. "Genetic analysis of two bile salt hydrolase activities in Lactobacillus acidophilus NCFM." *Appl. Environ. Microbiol.* 2005 Aug; 71(8):4925-9.

18c.   Corzo G, Gilliland SE. "Bile salt hydrolase activity of three strains of Lactobacillus acidophilus." *J. Dairy Sci.* 1999 Mar; 82(3):472-80.

18d.   Brashears MM, Gilliland SE, Buck LM. "Bile salt deconjugation and cholesterol removal from media by Lactobacillus casei." *J Dairy Sci.* 1998 Aug;81(8):2103-10.

18e.   Gilliland SE, Speck ML. "Deconjugation of bile acids by intestinal lactobacilli." *Appl Environ Microbiol.* 21977 Jan;33(1):15-8.

19.   Bernstein H, Bernstein C, Payne CM, Dvorakova K, Garewal H. "Bile acids as carcinogens in human gastrointestinal cancers." *Mutat Res.* 2005 Jan;589(1):47-65.

20.   Fratkin, JP. "Leaky Gut Syndrome." Published 07/28/2004. Article available

at Holistic Pediatric Association web site. Accessed 12/1/2006. <http://www.hpakids.org/holistic-health/articles/149/1/Leaky-Gut-Syndrome>.

21. "Colorectal Cancer: Early Detection." Web site: American Cancer Society web site. Accessed 1/18/2007. <http://www.cancer.org/docroot/CRI_2_6X_Colorectal_Cancer_Eatly_Detecti...>.

22a. Mielants H, De Vos M, Goemaere S, Schelstraete K, Cuvelier C, Goethals K, Maertens M, Ackerman C, Veys EM. "Intestinal mucosal permeability in inflammatory rheumatic diseases. II. Role of disease." *J Rheumatol.* 1991 Mar;18(3):394-400.

22b. Madara JL, Nash S, Moore R, Atisook K. "Structure and function of the intestinal epithelial barrier in health and disease." *Monogr Pathol.* 1990;(31):306-24.

22c. Isolauri E, Juntunen M, Wiren S, Vuorinen P, Koivula T. "Intestinal permeability changes in acute gastroenteritis: effects of clinical factors and nutritional management." *J Pediatr Gastroenterol Nutr.* 1989 May;8(4):466-73.

22d. Olaison G, Sjodahl R, Tahesson C. "Abnormal intestinal permeability in Crohn's disease. A possible factor." *Scand J Gastroenterol.* 1990 Apr; 25(4):321-28.

23. Galland L. "Solving the Digestive Puzzle." (conference manual), Great Smokies Diagnostic Laboratory / HealthComm International, Inc., San Francisco, May 1995, p.10. Cited by Elizabeth Lipski, M.S., C.C.N., *Leaky Gut Syndrome*, Keats Publishing, Inc. 1998, p.9.

24a. Oelgoetz AW, Oelgoetz PA, Wittenkind J. "The treatment of food allergy and indigestion of pancreatic origin with pancreatic enzymes." *Am. J. Dig. Dis. Nutr.* 1935; 2:422-6.

24b. McCann M. "Pancreatic enzyme supplement for treatment of multiple food allergies". *Ann. Allergy.* 1993; 71:269 [abstract #17].

25a. Andre F, Andre C, Feknous M, et al. "Digestive permeability to different-sized molecules and to sodium cromoglycate in food allergy." *Allergy Proc.* 1991; 12:293-8.

25b. Jalonen T. "Identical intestinal permeability changes in children with different clinical manifestations of cow's milk allergy." *J. Allergy Clin. Immunol.* 1991; 88:737-42.

26. Doe WF. "An overview of intestinal immunity and malabsorption." *Am J Med.* 1979;67(6):1077-84.

27. Munroe J., M.D. "Medical Causes and Treatment of Leaky Gut Syndrome." (audiotape), Asherville, N.C.: Great Smokies Diagnostic Laboratory. Cited by Elizabeth Lipski, M.S., C.C.N., *Leaky Gut Syndrome*, Keats Publishing, Inc. 1998, p.31.

28. Reinhardt M. "Macromolecular absorption of food antigens in health and disease." *Ann Allergy* 1984;53:597-601 [review].

29.   Walker WA. "Pathophysiology of intestinal uptake and absorption of antigens in food-allergy." Ann Allergy. 1987 Nov;59(5 Pt 2):7-16.

30.   Fratkin, JP. "Leaky Gut Syndrome." Published 07/28/2004. Article available at Holistic Pediatric Association web site. Accessed 12/1/2006. <http://www. hpakids.org/holistic-health/articles/149/1/Leaky-Gut-Syndrome>.

31a. Atkins, R. *Dr. Atkins' Vita-Nutrient Solution.* Simon & Schuster, 1998, p.230.

31b. Fratkin, JP. "Leaky Gut Syndrome." Published 07/28/2004. Article available at Holistic Pediatric Association web site. Web site. Accessed 12/1/2006. <http:// www.hpakids.org/holistic-health/articles/149/1/Leaky-Gut-Syndrome>.

31c. Berg RD, Wommack E, Deitch EA. "Immunosuppression and intestinal bacterial overgrowth synergistically promote bacterial translocation." *Arch Surg.* 1988 Nov;123(11):1359-64.

31d. Berg RD. "Promotion of the translocation of enteric bacteria from the gastro-intestinal tracts of mice by oral treatment with penicillin, clindamycin, or metronidazole." *Infect Immun.* 1981 Sep;33(3):854-61.

31e. Heimdahl A, Nord CE. "Effect of phenoxymethylpenicillin and clinda-mycin on the oral, throat and fecal microflora of man." *Scand J Infect Dis.* 1979;11(3):233-42.

32a. Davies GR, Wilkie ME, Rampton DS. "Effects of metronidazole and misopro-stol on indomethacin-induced changes in intestinal permeability." *Dig Dis Sci.* 1993 Mar;38(3):417-25.

32b. Babb RR. "Gastrointestinal complications of nonsteroidal anti-inflammatory drugs." *West J Med.* 1992 October; 157(4):444-447.

32c. Jenkins AP, Trew DR, Crump BJ, Nukajam WS, Foley JA, Menzies IS, Creamer B. "Do non-steroidal anti-inflammatory drugs increase colonic permeability?" *Gut.* 1991 Jan;32(1):66-9.

32d. Rooney PJ, Jenkins RT. "Nonsteroidal antiinflammatory drugs (NSAID"s) and the bowel mucosa: changes in intestinal permeability may not be due to changes in prostaglandins." *Clin Exp Rheumatol.* 1990 May-Jun;8(3):328-9.

32e. Bjarnason I, Zanelli G, Smith T, Smethurst P, Price AB, Gumpel MJ, Levi AJ. "Nonsteroidal anti-inflammatory drug-induced intestinal inflammation in humans." *Scand J Rheumatol Suppl.*1987;64:55-62.

32f. Jenkins RT, Rooney PJ, Jones DB, Bienenstock J, Goodacre RL. "Increased intestinal permeability in patients with rheumatoid arthritis: a side-effect of oral nonsteroidal anti-inflammatory drug therapy?" *Br J Rheumatol.* 1987 Apr;26(2):13-7.

32g. Bjarnason I, Williams P, Smethurst P, Peters TJ, Levi AJ. "Effect of non-steroidal anti-inflammatory drugs and prostaglandins on the permeability of the human small intestine." *Gut.* 1986 Nov;27(11):1292-7.

33.   Hochain P, Capet C, Colin R. "[Digestive complications of aspirin]". *Rev Med Interne.* 2000 Mar;21 Suppl 1:50s-59s.

34.   Bjarnason I, Peters TJ, Wise RJ. "The leaky gut of alcoholism: Possible route of entry for toxic compounds." *Lancet.* 1984 Jan 28;1(8370):179-82.

35a.   Katz D, Hollander D, Said HM, Dadufalza V. "Aging-associated increase in intestinal permeability to polyethylene glycol 900." *Dig Dis Sci.* 1987 Mar;32(3):285-88.

35b.   Hollander D, Tarnawski H. "Aging-associated increase in intestinal absorption of macromolecules." *Gerontology.* 1985;31(3):133-37.

36a.   Isolauri E, Juntunen M, Wiren S, Vuorinen P, Koivula T. "Intestinal permeability changes in acute gastroenteritis: effects of clinical factors and nutritional management." *J Pediatr Gastroenterol Nutr.* 1989;8(4):466-73.

36b.   Serrander R, Magnusson KE, Kihlstrom E, Sundqvist T. "Acute yersinia infections in man increase intestinal permeability for low-molecular weight polyethylene glycols (PEG 400)." *Scand J Infec Dis.* 1986;18(5):409-13.

36c.   Fratkin, JP. "Leaky Gut Syndrome." Published 07/28/2004. Article available at Holistic Pediatric Association web site. Accessed 12/1/2006. <http://www.hpakids.org/holistic-health/articles/149/1/Leaky-Gut-Syndrome>.

37.   Andre C, Andre F, Colin L, Cavagna S. "Measurement of intestinal permeability to mannitol and lactulose as a means of diagnosing food allergy and evaluating therapeutic effectiveness of disodium cromoglycate." *Ann Allergy.* 1987 Nov;59(5 Pt 2):127-30.

38.   Lipski, E. *Leaky Gut Syndrome.* Keats Publishing, Inc., New Canaan, CT 06840. 1998. pp.23-24.

39a.   Mack DR, Flick JA, Durie PR, Rosenstein BJ, Ellis LE, Perman JA. "Correlation of intestinal lactulose permeability with exocrine pancreatic dysfunction." *J Pediatrics.* 1992 May;120(5):696-701.

39b.   Murphy MS, Sheldon W, Brunetto A, Pearson AD, Laker MF, Eastham EJ, Nelson R. "Active and passive sugar absorption in pancreatic insufficiency." *J Pediatr Gastroenterol Nutr.* 1989 Feb;8(2):189-94.

40a.   Soderholm JD, Olaison G, Lindberg E, Hannestad U, Vindels A, Tysk C, Jarnerot G, Sjodahl R. "Different intestinal permeability patterns in relatives and spouses of patients with Crohn's disease: an inherited defect in mucosal defense?" *Gut.* 1999 Jan;44(1):96-100.

40b.   Butkus SN, Mahan LK. "Food allergies: immunological reactions to food." *J Am Diet Assoc.* 1986 May;86(5):601-8.

41a.   Kryger-Baggesen N, Moldow B, Rasmussen G, Dissing I, Moller EH, Ladefoged K, Jarnum S. "[Chronic radiation enterotheropathy. A retrospective study]." *Ugeskr Laeger.* 1993 Dec 20;155(51):4180-4.

41b.   Jaffe R, MD. "Gut hyperpermeability." *Serammune Physicians Laboratory Newsletter* 2(1), Jan. 1992. [Reference cited in *Leaky Gut Syndrome* by Elizabeth Lipski, Keats Publishing]. p.17.

41c.   Coltart RS, Howard GC, Wraight EP, Bleehen NM. "The effect of hyperthermia and radiation on small bowel permeability using 51Cr EDTA and 14C mannitol in man." *Int J Hyperthermia.* 1988 Sep-Oct;4(5):467-77.

41d. Deitch EA, Bridges RM. "Effect of stress and trauma on bacterial translocation from the gut." *J Surg Res.* 1987 May;42(5):536-42.

41e. Ruppin H, Hotze A, During A, Reichert M, Baur J, Stoll R, Herbst M, Mahlstedt J. "[Reversible functional disorders of the intestinal tract caused by abdominal radiotherapy]." *Z Gastroenterol.* 1987 May;25(5):261-9.

42a. Johnston BC, Supina AL, Vohra S. "Probiotics for pediatric antibiotic-associated diarrhea: a meta-analysis of randomized placebo-controlled trials." *CMAJ.* 2006 Aug 15;175(4):377-83.

42b. Kelly CP, LaMont JT. "Clostridium difficile infection." *Annu Rev Med.* 1998;49:375-90.

42c. Heimdahl A, Nord CE. "Effect of phenoxymethylpenicillin and clindamycin on the oral, throat and fecal microflora of man." *Scand J Infect Dis.* 1979;11(3):233-42.

42d. Atkins, R. *Dr. Atkins' Vita-Nutrient Solution.* Simon & Schuster, 1998, p.230.

42e. van der Waaij D, Hofstra H, Wiegersma N. "Effect of beta-lactam antibiotics of the resistance of the digestive trat of mice to colonization." J Infect Dis. 1982 Sep;146(3):417-22.

43a. Babb RR. "Gastrointestinal complications of nonsteroidal anti-inflammatory drugs." *West J Med.* 1992 October; 157(4):444-447.

43b. Jenkins AP, Trew DR, Crump BJ, Nukajam WS, Foley JA, Menzies IS, Creamer B. "Do non-steroidal anti-inflammatory drugs increase colonic permeability?" *Gut.* 1991 Jan;32(1):66-9.

43c. Rooney PJ, Jenkins RT. "Nonsteroidal antiinflammatory drugs (NSAID"s) and the bowel mucosa: changes in intestinal permeability may not be due to changes in prostaglandins." *Clin Exp Rheumatol.* 1990 May-Jun;8(3):328-9.

43d. Bjarnason I, Zanelli G, Smith T, Smethurst P, Price AB, Gumpel MJ, Levi AJ. "Nonsteroidal anti-inflammatory drug-induced intestinal inflammation in humans." *Scand J Rheumatol Suppl.*1987;64:55-62.

43e. Jenkins RT, Rooney PJ, Jones DB, Bienenstock J, Goodacre RL. "Increased intestinal permeability in patients with rheumatoid arthritis: a side-effect of oral nonsteroidal anti-inflammatory drug therapy?" *Br J Rheumatol.* 1987 Apr;26(2):13-7.

43f. Bjarnason I, Williams P, Smethurst P, Peters TJ, Levi AJ. "Effect of non-steroidal anti-inflammatory drugs and prostaglandins on the permeability of the human small intestine." *Gut.* 1986 Nov;27(11):1292-7.

43g. Lanza FL. "A double-blind study of prophylactic effect of misoprostol on lesions of gastric and duodenal mucosa induced by oral administration of tolmetin in health subjects." Dig Dis Sci. 1986 Feb;31(2 Suppl):131S-136S.

44. Babb RR. "Gastrointestinal complications of nonsteroidal anti-inflammatory drugs." *West J Med.* 1992 Oct;157(4):444-7.

45. Atkins, R. *Dr. Atkins' Vita-Nutrient Solution.* Simon & Schuster, 1998, pp.28-30, 230.

46. Fratkin, JP. "Leaky Gut Syndrome." Published 07/28/2004. Article available at Holistic Pediatric Association web site. Accessed 12/1/2006. <http://www.hpakids.org/holistic-health/articles/149/1/Leaky-Gut-Syndrome>.

47. Lipski E. *Leaky Gut Syndrome.* Keats Publishing, New Canaan, CT. 1998. pp.29-31.

48. Goto C, Kasuya S, Koga K, Ohtomo H, Kagei N. "Lethal efficacy of extract from Zingiber officinale (traditional Chinese medicine) or [6]-shogaol and [6]-gingerol in Anisakis larvae in vitro." *Parasitol Res.* 1990;76(8):653-6.

49. McCann M. "Pancreatic enzyme supplement for treatment of multiple food allergies." *Ann. Allergy.* 1993; 71:269 [abstract #17].

50. Galland L. "Leaky Gut Syndromes: Breaking the Vicious Cycle." Foundation for Integrated Medicine. Accessed 11/30/2006. <http://www.mdheal.org/leakygut.htm>.

51. Atkins, R. *Dr. Atkins' Vita-Nutrient Solution.* Simon & Schuster, 1998, p.30.

52. Oski FA, M.D. *Don't Drink Your Milk.* Teach Services, Brushton N.Y. 1993 ninth edition.

53. Kwon PH Jr, Rorick MH, Scrimshaw NS. "Comparative tolerance of adolescents of differing ethnic backgrounds to lactose-containing and lactose-free dairy drinks. II. Improvement of a double-blind test." *Am J Clin Nutr.* 1980 Jan;33(1):22-6.

54. Lin MY, Yen CL, Chen SH. "Management of lactose maldigestion by consuming milk containing lactobacilli." *Dig. Dis. Sci.* 1998;43(1):133-137.

55. Atkins, R. *Dr. Atkins' Vita-Nutrient Solution.* Simon & Schuster, 1998, p.230.

56. Diamond S. *Conquering Your Migraine.* Fireside/Simon & Schuster. New York, NY 2001 pp.35-37.

57. Diamond S. *Conquering Your Migraine.* Fireside/Simon & Schuster. New York, NY 2001 pp.36-37.

58. Diamond S. *Conquering Your Migraine.* Fireside/Simon & Schuster. New York, NY 2001 pp.38-40, 43-45.

59. Dr. John A. Allocca. "Migraine, Depression, and other Serotonin and Norepinephrine Disorders." Web site: Allocca Biotechnology, LLC. Accessed 3/14/2008. <http://www.allocca.com/migraine.htm>.

60a. Cady RK, Schreiber CP, Beach ME, Hart CC. "Gelstat Migraine (sublingually administered feverfew and ginger compound) for acute treatment of migraine when administered during the mild pain phase." *Med Sci Monit.* 2005 Sep;11(9):PI65-9.

60b. Mustafa T, Srivastava KC. "Ginger (Zingiber officinale) in migraine headache." *J Ethnopharmacol.* 1990 Jul;29(3):267-73.

61. Lipski, E. *Leaky Gut Syndrome.* Keats Publishing, Inc., New Canaan, CT. 1998 p.31.

62. Crook WG MD, Jones MH RN. *The Yeast Connection Cookbook*. Professional Books, Jackson, TN 1997 p.61.

63. "Food Reactions" Web site: American Academy of Allergy, Asthma & Immunology. Accessed 1/12/2005. <http://www.aaaai.org/ar/working_vol3/069.asp>.

64. Lipski E. *Digestive Wellness*. McGraw-Hill. 2004, pp.89-90, 95, 337.

65a. Hilton E, Isenberg HD, Alperstein P, France K, Borenstein MT. "Ingestion of yogurt containing Lactobacillus acidophilus as prophylaxis for candidal vaginitis." *Ann Intern Med*. 1992 Mar 1;116(5):353-7.

65b. Burkitt D. *PCRM Update*. May-June, 1990; 1-9.

65c. Gorbach SL. "Lactic acid bacteria and human health." *Ann Med*. 1990 Feb;22(1):37-41.

65d. Kennedy MJ, Volz PA. "Ecology of Candida albicans gut colonization: inhibition of Candida adhesion, colonization, and dissemination from the gastrointestinal tract by bacterial antagonism." *Infect Immun*. 1985 Sep;49(3):654-63.

66a. Akalin AS, Gonc S, Duzel S. "Influence of yogurt and acidophilus yogurt on serum cholesterol levels in mice." *J Dairy Sci*. 1997 Nov;80(11):2721-5.

66b. Anderson JW, Gilliland SE. "Effect of fermented milk (yogurt) containing Lactobacillus acidophilus L1 on serum cholesterol in hypercholesterolemic humans." *J Am Coll Nutr*. 1999 Feb;18(1):43-50.

66c. Mital BK, Garg SK. "Anticarcinogenic, hypocholesterolemic, and antagonistic activities of Lactobacillus acidophilus." *Crit Rev Microbiol*. 1995;21(3):175-214.

66d. Gilliland SE, Nelson CR, Maxwell C. "Assimilation of Cholesterol by Lactobacillus acidophilus." *Applied and Environmental Microbiology*. 1985 Feb;49(2):377-381.

66e. Mann GV. "A factor in yogurt which lowers cholesteremia in man." *Atherosclerosis*. 1977 Mar;26(3):335-40.

67. Beena A, Prasad V. "Effect of yogurt and bifidus yogurt fortified with skim milk powder, condensed whey and lactose-hydrolysed condensed whey on serum cholesterol and triacylglycerol levels in rats." *J Dairy Res*. 1997 Aug;64(3):453-7.

68. Silva AM, Bambirra EA, Oliveira AL, Souza PP, Gomes DA, Vieira EC, Nicoli JR. "Protective effect of bifidus milk on the experimental infection with *Salmonella enteritidis* subsp. *typhimurium* in conventional and gnotobiotic mice." J Applied Micribiolgy. 1999;86:331-6.

69. Jiang T, Savaiano DA. "Modification of colonic fermentation by bifidobacteria and pH in vitro. Impact on lactose metabolism, short-chain fatty acid, and lactate production." *Dig Dis Sci*. 1997 Nov;42(11):2370-7.

70. Yaeshima T, Takahashi S, Matsumoto N, Ishibashi N, Hayasawa H, Iino H. "Effect of Yogurt Containing Bifidobacterium longum BB536 on the

Intestinal Environment, Fecal Characteristics and Defecation Frequency: A Comparison with Standard Yogurt." *Bioscience Microflora.* 1997 Vol.16;(2):73-77.

71. Isolauri E, Majamaa H, Arvola T, Rantala I, Virtanen E. Arvilommi H. "Lactobacillus casei strain GG reverses increased intestinal permeability induced by cow milk in suckling rats." *Gastroenterology.* 1993;105: 1643-1650.

72. Wagner RD, Pierson C, Warner T, Dohnalek M, Farmer J, Roberts L, Hilty M, Balish E. "Biotherapeutic effects of probiotic bacteria on candidiasis in immunodeficient mice." *Infect Immun.* 1997 October; 65(10):4165-4172.

73. Sykora J, Valeckova K, Amlerova J, Siala K, Dedek P, Watkins S, Varvarovska J, Stozicky F, Pazdiora P, Schwarz J. "Effects of a specially designed fermented milk product containing probiotic Lactobacillus casei DN-114 001 and the eradication of H. pylori in children: a prospective randomized double-blind study." *J Clin Gastroenterol.* 2005 Sep;39(8):692-8.

74. Ingrassia I, Leplingard A, Darfeuille-Michaud A. "Lactobacillus casei DN-114 001 Inhibits the Ability of Adherent-Invasive Escherichia coli Isolated from Crohn's Disease Patients To Adhere to and To Invade Intestinal Epithelial Cells." *Appl Environ Microbiol.* 2005 June;71(6):2880-7.

75. Turchet P, Laurenzano M, Auboiron S, Antoine JM. "Effect of fermented milk containing the probiotic Lactobacillus casei DN-114001 on winter infections in free-living elderly subjects: a randomized, controlled pilot study." *Journal of Nutrition, Health and Aging.* 2003;7:75-7.

76a. Aso Y, Akaza H, Kotake T, Tsukamoto T, Imai K, Naito S. "Preventive effect of a Lactobacillus casei preparation on the recurrence of superficial bladder cancer in a double-blind trial. The BLP Study Group." *Eur Urol.* 1995;27:104-9.

76b. Aso Y, Akaza H. "Prophylactic effect of a Lactobacillus casei preparation on the recurrence of superficial bladder cancer. BLP Study Group." *Urol Int.* 1992;49(3):125-9.

77. "Live and Active Culture (LAC) Yogurt Facts." The Official Web Site of the National Yogurt Association. Accessed 12/7/2006. <http://www.aboutyogurt. com/lacYogurt/facts.asp>.

78a. Boudraa G, Benbouabdellah M, Hachelaf W, Boisset M, Desjeux JF, Touhami M. "Effect of feeding yogurt versus milk in children with acute diarrhea and carbohydrate malabsorption." *J Pediatr Gastroenterol Nutr.* 2001 Sep;33(3):307-13.

78b. Pedone CA, Arnaud CC, Postaire ER, Bouley CF, Reinert P. "Multicentric study of the effect of milk fermented by Lactobacillus casei on the incidence of diarrhoea." *Int J Clin Pract.* 2000 Nov;54(9):568-71.

78c. Salminen S, Salminen E. "Lactulose, lactic acid bacteria, intestinal microecology and mucosal protection." *Scand J Gastroenterol Suppl.* 1997;222:45-8.

78d. Salminen E, Elomaa I, Minkkinen J, Vapaatalo H, Salminen S. "Preservation of intestinal integrity during radiotherapy using live Lactobacillus acidophilus cultures." *Clin Radiol.* 1988 Jul;39(4):435-7.

78e.   Niv M, Levy W, Greenstein NM. "Yogurt in the treatment of infantile diarrhea." *Clin Pediatr.* 1963;2:407-11.

79a.   Perdigon G, Vintini E, Alvarez S, Medina M, Medici M. "Study of the possible mechanisms involved in the mucosal immune system activation by lactic aid bacteria." *J Dair Sci.* 1999 Jun;82(6):1108-14.

79b.   Perdigon G, Alvarez S, Rachid M, Aguero G, Gobbato N. "Immune system stimulation by probiotics." *J Dairy Sci.* 1995 Jul;78(7):1597-606.

79c.   De Simone C, Vesely R, Negri R, Bianchi SB, Zanzoglu S, Cille A, Lucci L. "Enhancement of immune response of murine Peyer's patches by a diet supplemented with yogurt." *Immunopharmacol Immunotoxicol.* 1987;9(1):87-100.

80.   Van de Water J, Keen CL, Gershwin ME. "The influence of chronic yogurt consumption on immunity." *J Nutr.* 1999 Jul;129(7 Suppl):1492S-5S.

81.   Shahani KM, Chandan RC. "Nutritional and healthful aspects of cultured and culture-containing dairy foods." *J Dairy Sci.* 1979 Oct;62(10):1685:94.

82.   de Moreno de Leblanc A, Perdigon G. "Yogurt feeding inhibits promotion and progression of experimental colorectal cancer." *Med Sci Monit.* 2004 Apr;10(4):BR96-104.

83.   de Moreno de Leblanc A, Perdigon G. "Yogurt feeding inhibits promotion and progression of experimental colorectal cancer." *Med Sci Monit.* 2004 Apr;10(4):BR96-104.

84.   van't Veer P, Dekker JM, Lamers JW, Kok FJ, Schouten EG, Brants HA, Sturmans F, Hermus RJ. "Consumption of fermented milk products and breast cancer: a case-control study in The Netherlands." *Cancer Res.* 1989 Jul 15;49(14):4020-3.

85.   Wynckel A, Jaisser F, Wong T, Drueke T, Chanard J. "Intestinal absorption of calcium from yogurt in lactase-deficient subjects." *Reprod Nutr Dev.* 1991;31(4):411-8.

86a.   Marteau P, Flourie B, Pochart P, Chastang C, Desjeux JF, Rambaud JC. "Effect of the microbial lactase (EC 3.2.1.23) activity in yogurt on the intestinal absorption of lactose: an in vivo study in lactase-deficient humans." *Br J Nutr.* 1990 Jul;64(1):71-9.

86b.   Kolars JC, Levitt MD, Aouji M, Savaiano DA. "Yogurt-an autodigesting source of lactose." *N Engl J Med.* 1984 Jan 5;310(1):1-3.

87.   Saltzman JR, Russell RM. "The aging gut. Nutritional issues." *Gastroenterol Clin North Am.* 1998;27(2):309-24.

88.   Not used.

89.   Zemel MB, Richards J, Mathis S, Milstead A, Gebhardt L, Silva E. "Dairy augmentation of total and central fat loss in obese subjects." *Int J Obes (Lond).* 2005 Apr;29(4):391-7.

90.   Wong NP, McDonough FE, Hitchins AD. "Contribution of Streptococcus

thermophilus to growth-stimulating effect of yogurt on rats." *J Dairy Sci.* 1983 Mar;66(3):444-9.

91. Cichoke AJ. The Complete Book of Enzyme Therapy. Avery Publishing, New York, NY 1999. pp.30-31.

92. Kim K, Lee W, Benevenga NJ. "Feeding Diets Containing High Levels of Milk Products or Cellulose Decrease Urease Activity and Ammonia Production in Rat Intestine." *J Nutr.* 1998 Jul;128(7):1186-91.

93. Triebling AT, Korsten MA, Dlugosz JW, Paronetto F, Lieber CS. "Severity of Helicobacter-induced gastric injury correlates with gastric juice ammonia." *Dig Dis Sci.* 1991 Aug;36(8):1089-96.

94a. Triebling AT, Korsten MA, Dlugosz JW, Paronetto F, Lieber CS. "Severity of Helicobacter-induced gastric injury correlates with gastric juice ammonia." *Dig Dis Sci.* 1991 Aug;36(8):1089-96.

94b. Lin HC, Visek WJ. "Colon mucosal cell damage by ammonia in rats." *J Nutr.* 1991 Jun;121(6):887-93.

95. Galland L. "Intestinal Parasites, Bacterial Dysbiosis and Leaky Gut." Foundation for Integrated Medicine. Accessed 3/14/2008. <http://www.mdheal.org/parasites.htm>.

96a. Nostro A, Cellini L, Di Bartolomeo S, Cannatelli MA, Di Campli E, Procopio F, Grande R, Marzio L, Alonzo V. "Effects of combining extracts (from propolis or Zingiber officinale) with clarithromycin on Helicobacter pylori." *Phytither Res.* 2006 Mar;20(3):187-90.

96b. Mahady GB, Pendland SL, Yun GS, Lu ZZ, Stoia A. "Ginger (Zingiber officinale Roscoe) and the gingerols inhibit the growth of Cag A+ strains of Helicobacter pylori." *Anticancer Res.* 2003 Sep-Oct;23(5A):3699-702.

97. "Probiotics: For Life!" Stonyfield Farms web site. Accessed 12/7/2006. <www.stonyfield.com>.

98a. Saxelin M, Tynkkynen S, Mattila-Sandholm T, de Vos WM. "Probiotic and other functional microbes: from markets to mechanisms." *Curr Opin Biotechnol.* 2005 Apr;16(2):204-11.

98b. Viljanen M, Kuitunen M, Haahtela T, Juntunen-Backman K, Korpela R, Savilahti E. "Probiotic effects on faecal inflammatory markers and on faecal IgA in food allergic atopic eczema/dermatitis syndrome infants." *Pediatr Allergy Immunol.* 2005 Feb;16(1):65-71.

98c. Rosenfeldt V, Benfeldt E, Valerius NH, Paerregaard A, Michaelsen KF. "Effect of probiotics on gastrointestinal symptoms and small intestinal permeability in children with atopic dermatitis." *J Pediatr.* 2004 Nov;145(5):612-6.

98d. Elmer GW. "Probiotics: "living drugs." *Am J Health Syst Pharm.* 2001 Jun 15;58(12):1101-9.

98e. Kailasapathy K, Chin J. "Survival and therapeutic potential of probiotic organisms with reference to Lactobacillus acidophilus and Bifidobacterium spp." *Immunol Cell Biol.* 2000 Feb;78(1):80-8.

98f. von Wright A, Salminen S. "Probiotics: established effects and open questions." *Eur J Gastroenterol Hepatol.* 1999 Nov;11(11):1195-8.

98g. Dunne C, Murphy L, Flynn S, O'Mahony L, O'Halloran S, Feeney M, Morrissey D, Thornton G, Fitzgerald G, Daly C, Kiely B, Quigley EM, O'Sullivan GC, Shanahan F, Collins JK. "Probiotics: from myth to reality. Demonstration of functionality in animal models of disease and in human clinical trials." *Antonie Van Leeuwenhoek.* 1999 Jul-Nov;76(1-4):279-92.

98h. Salminen S, Salminen E. "Lactulose, lactic acid bacteria, intestinal microecology and mucosal protection." *Scand J Gastroenterol Suppl.* 1997;222:45-8.

98i. Majamaa H, Isolauri E. "Probiotics: a novel approach in the management of food allergy." *J Allergy Clin Immunol.* 1997 Feb;99(2):179-85.

98j. Salminen S, Isolauri E, Salminen E. "Clinical uses of probiotics for stabilizing the gut mucosal barrier: successful strains and future challenges." *Antonie Van Leeuwenhoek.* 1996 Oct;70(2-4):347-58.

98k. Salminen E, Elomaa I, Minkkinen J, Vapaatalo H, Salminen S. "Preservation of intestinal integrity during radiotherapy using live Lactobacillus acidophilus cultures." *Clin Radiol.* 1988 Jul;39(4):435-7.

99. Zhao HY, Wang HJ, Lu Z, Xu SZ. "Intestinal microflora in patients with liver cirrhosis." *Chinese Journal of Digestive Diseases.* 2004 Apr;5(2):64-7.

100. Wollowski I, Rechkemmer G, Pool-Zobel BL. "Protective role of probiotics and prebiotics in colon cancer." *Am J Clin Nutr.* 2001 Feb;73(2 Suppl):451S-455S.

101. Keshavarzian A, Choudhary S, Holmes EW, Yong S, Banan A, Jakate S, Fields JZ. "Preventing gut leakiness by oats supplementation ameliorates alcohol-induced liver damage in rats." *J Pharmacol Exp Ther.* 2001 Nov;299(2):442-8.

102a. Rodriguez-Cabezas ME, Galvez J, Camuesco D, Lorente MD, Concha A, Martinez-Augustin O, Redondo L, Zarauelo A. "Intestinal anti-inflammatory activity of dietary fiber (Plantago ovata seeds) in HLA-B27 transgenic mice." *Clin Nutr.* 2003 Oct;22(5):43-71.

102b. Fernandez-Banares F, Hinojosa J, Sanchez-Lombrana JL, Navarro E, Martinez-Salmeron JF, Garcia-Puges A, Gonzalez-Huix F, Riera J, Gonzalez-Lara V, Dominguez-Abascal F, Gine JJ, Moles J, Gomollon F, Gassull MA. "Randomized clinical trial of Plantago ovata seeds (dietary fiber) as compared with mesalamine in mainaining remission in ulcerative colitis. Spanish Group for the study of Crohn's Disease and Ulcerative Colitis (GETECCU). *Am J Gastroenterol.* 1999 Feb;94(2):427-33.

102c. Nordgaard I, Hove H, Clausen MR, Mortensen PB. "Colonic production of butyrate in patients with previous colonic cancer during long-term treatment with dietary fibre (Plantago ovata seeds)." *Scand J Gastroenterol.* 1996;31:1011-1020.

102d. Ward PB, Young GP. "Dynamics of Clostridium difficile infection. Control using diet." *Adv Exp Med Biol.* 1997;412:63-75.

103. Cherbut C, Michel C, Lecannu G. "The prebiotic characteristics of fructooligosaccharides are necessary for reduction of TNBS-induced colitis in rats." *J Nutr.* 2003 Jan;133(1):21-7.

104a. Bounik Y, Raskine L, Simoneau G, Paineau D, Bornet F. "The capacity of short-chain fructo-oligosaccharides to stimulate faecal bifidobacteria: a dose-response relationship study in healthy humans." *Nutr J.* 2006 Mar 28;5:8.

104b. Barrangou R, Altermann E, Hutkins R, Cano R, Klaenhammer TR. "Functional and comparative genomic analyses of an operon involved in fructooligsaccharide utilization by Lactobacillus acidophilus." *Proc Natl Acad Sci U S A.* 2003 Jul 22;100(15):8957-62. Epub 2003 Jul 7.

104c. Bouhnik Y, Flourie B, Riottot M, Bisetti N, Gailing MF, Guibert A, Bornet F, Rambaud JC. "Effects of fructo-oligosaccharides ingestion on fecal bifidobacteria and selected metabolic indexes of colon carcinogenesis in healthy humans." *Nutr Cancer.* 1996;26(1):21-9.

104d. May T, Mackie RI, Fahey GC Jr, Cremin JC, Garleb KA. "Effect of fiber source on short-chain fatty acid production and on the growth and toxin production by Clostridium difficile." *Scand J Gastroenterol.* 1994 Oct;29:916-922.

104e. Mitsuoka T, Hidaka H, Eida T. "Effect of fructo-oligosaccharides on intestinal microflora." *Nahrung.* 1987;31(5-6):427-36.

105. Belluzi A, Brignola C, Campieri M, Pera A, Boschi S, Miglioli M. "Effect of an enteric-coated fish-oil preparation on relapses in Crohn's disease." *N Engl J Med.* 1996 Jun 13;334(24):1557-1560.

106a. Bronner C, Landry Y. "Kinetics of the inhibitory effect of flavonoids on histamine secretion from mast cells." *Agents Actions.* 1985 Apr;16(3-4):147-51.

106b. Middleton E Jr, Drzewiecki G. "Flavanoid inhibition of human basophil histamine release stimulated by various agents." *Biochem Pharmacol.* 1984 Nov 1;33(21):3333-8.

106c. Pearce FL, Befus AD, Bienenstock J. "Mucosal mast cells. III. Effect of quercetin and other flavonoids on antigen-induced histamine secretion from rat intestinal mast cells." *J Allergy Clin Immunol.* 1984 Jun;73(6):819-23.

106d. Fewtrell CM, Gomperts BD. "Quecetin: a novel inhibitor of Ca2+ influx and exocutosis in rat peritoneal mast cells." *Biochim Biophys Acta.* 1977 Aug 15;469(1): 52-60.

107. "Flavanoids" Linus Pauling Institute at Oregon State University. Web site accessed 11/25/2009. <http://lpi.oregonstate.edu/infocenter/phytochemicals/flavanoids/.

108. Duke JA, Ph.D. *The Green Pharmacy.* Rodale Press, Emmaus, PA 1997 pp.283-4.

109. Jackson SJ, Venema RC. "Quercetin inhibits eNOS, microtubule polymerization, and miotic progression in bovine aortic endothelial cells." *J Nutr.* 2006 May;136(5):1178-84.

136   Lynn Smith

110. Dihal AA, de Boer VC, van der Woude H, Tilburgs c, Bruijntjes JP, Alink GM, Rietjens IM, Woutersen RA, Stierum RH. "Quercetin, but not its glycosidated conjugate rutin, inhibits azoxymethane-induced colorectal carcinogenesis in F344 rats." J Nutr. 2006 Nov;136(11):2862-7.

111a. Sturniolo GC, Di Leo V, Ferronato A, D'Odorico A, D'Inca R. "Zinc Supplementation Tightens "Leaky Gut" in Crohn's Disease." *Inflammatory Bowel Diseases*. 7(2):94-98, May 2001.

111b. Roy SK, Behrens RH, Haider R, Akramuzzaman SM, Mahalanabis D, Wahed MA, Tomkins AM. "Impact of zinc supplementation on intestinal permeability in Bangladeshi children with acute diarrhoea and persistant diarrhoea syndrome." *J Pediatr Gastroenterol Nutr*. 1992 Oct;15(3):289-96.

112. Shankar AH, Prasad AS. "Zinc and immune function: the biological basis of altered resistance to infection." *American Journal of Clinical Nutrition*. 1998, Vol 68 (suppl); pp.447S-448S.

113a. Singh KP, Zaidi SI, Raisuddin S, Saxena AK, Murthy RC, Ray PK. "Effect of zinc on immune functions and host resistance against infection and tumor challenge." *Immunopharmacol Immunotoxicol*. 1992;14:813-40.

113b. Salvin SB, Horecker BL, Pan LX, Rabin BS. "The effect of dietary zinc and prothymosin on cellular immune responses of RF/J mice." *Clin Immunol Immunopathol*. 1987 Jun;43:281-8.

114. Duke JA, Ph.D. *The Green Pharmacy*. Rodale Press, Emmaus, PA 1997 p.87.

115. Samonina G, Lyapina L, Kopylova G, Pastorova VV, Bakaeva Z, Jeliaznik N, Zuykova S, Ashmarin I I. "Protection of gastric mucosal integrity by gelatin and simple proline-containing peptides." *Pathophysiology*. 2000 Apr;7(1):69-73.

116. Howell E. Dr. *Enzyme Nutrition*. Avery Publishing, 1985. pp.9, 52-53.

117. Thompson EH, Wolf ID, Allen CE. "Ginger rhizome: A new source of proteolytic enzyme." *Journal of Food Science* 38, no. 4 (1973): pp.652-55.

118. Cichoke AJ. *The Complete Book of Enzyme Therapy*. Avery Publishing, New York, NY 1999. pp.30-31.

119. Howell E. *Enzyme Nutrition*. Avery Publishing, 1985. p.120

120. Howell E. *Enzyme Nutrition*. Avery Publishing, 1985. pp.12,27-29, 147-148.

121a. Katz D, Hollander D, Said HM, Dadufalza V. "Aging-associated increase in intestinal permeability to polyethylene glycol 900." *Dig Dis Sci*. 1987;32(3):285-88.

121b. Hollander D, Tarnawski H. "Aging-associated increase in intestinal absorption of macromolecules." *Gerontology*. 1985;31(3):133-37.

122. Galland L. "Intestinal Parasites, Bacterial Dysbiosis and Leaky Gut." Foundation for Integrated Medicine. Accessed 3/14/2008. <http://www.mdheal.org/parasites.htm>.

123. Duke JA, Ph.D. *The Green Pharmacy*. Rodale Press, Emmaus, PA 1997 pp.455-457.

124. Galland L. "A Healthy Home." Foundation for Integrated Medicine. Accessed 3/27/2008. <http://www.mdheal.org/protecti.htm>.

125a. Paganelli R, Fagiolo U, Cancian M, Scala E. "Intestinal permeability in patients with chronic uticaria-angioedema with and without arthralgia." *Ann Allergy.* 1991 Feb;66(2): 181-4.

125b. Tatsuno K. "[Intestinal permeability in children with food allergy]." *Arerugi.* 1989 Dec;38(12):1311-8.

125c. Schreiber RA, Walker WA. "Food allergy: facts and fiction." *Mayo Clinic Proc.* 1989 Nov;64(11):1381-91.

125d. Andre C, Andre F, Colin L, Cavagna S. "Measurement of intestinal permeability to mannitol and lactulose as a means of diagnosing food allergy and evaluating therapeutic effectiveness of disodium cromoglycate." *Ann Allergy.* 1987 Nov;59(5 Pt 2):127-30.

125e. Butkus SN, Mahan LK. "Food allergies: immunological reactions to food." *J Am Dietetic Assoc.* 1986 May;(5): 601-08.

126. Benard A, Desreumeaux P, Huglo D, Hoorelbeke A, Tonnel AB, Wallaert B. "Increased intestinal permeability in bronchial asthma." *J Allergy Clin Immunol.* 1996 Jun;97(6):1173-8.

127a. Caffarelli C, Cavagni G Menzies IS, Bertolini P, Atherton DJ. "Elimination diet and intestinal permeability in atopic eczema: a preliminary study." *Clin Exp Allergy.* 1993 Jan;23(1):28-31.

127b. Dupont C, Barau E, Molkhou P, Raynaud F, Barbet JP, Dehennin L. "Food-induced alterations of intestinal permeability in children with cow's milk-sensitive enteropathy and atopic dermatitis. *J Pediatr Gastroenterol Nutr.* 1989 May;8(4):459-65.

127c. Pike MG, Heddle RJ, Boulton P, Turner MW, Atherton DJ. "Increased intestinal permeability in atopic eczema." *J Invest Dermatol.* 1986 Feb;86(2):101-4.

128. Pearson AD, Eastham EJ, Laker MF, Craft AW, Nelson R. "Intestinal permeability in children with Crohn's disease and coeliac disease." *Br Med J (Clin Res Ed).* 1982 Jul 3;285(6334): 20-1.

129a. Olaison G, Sjodahl R, Tagesson C. "Abnormal intestinal permeability in Crohn's disease. A possible pathogenic factor." *Scand J Gastroenterol.* 1990 Apr;25(4):321-8.

129b. Pearson AD, Eastham EJ, Laker MF, Craft AW, Nelson R. "Intestinal permeability in children with Crohn's disease and coeliac disease." *Br Med J (Clin Res Ed).* 1982 Jul 3;285(6334): 20-1.

129c. Sanderson IR, Boulton P, Menzies I, Walker-Smith JA. "Improvement of abnormal lactulose/rhamnose permeability in active Crohn's disease of the small bowel by an elemental diet." *Gut* 1987 Sep;28(9): 1073-6.

130a. Brogan PA, Malik M, Shah N, Kilday JP, Ramsay A, Shah V, Murch SH, Thomson MA, Walker-Smith JA, Lindley KJ, Milla PJ, Dillon MJ. "Systemic vasculitis: a cause of indeterminate intestinal inflammation." *J Pediatr Gastroenterol Nutr.* 2006 Apr;42(4):405-15.

130b. Pagnoux C, Mahr A, Cohen P, Guillevin L. "Presentation and outcome of gastrointestinal involvement in systemic necrotizing vasculitides: analysis of 62 patients with polyarteritis nodosa, microscopic polyangiitis, Wegener granulomatosis, Churg-Strauss syndrome, or rheumatoid arthritis-associated vasculitis." *Medicine* (Baltimore). 2005 Mar;84(2):115-28.

130c. Koc B, Aymelek S, Sonmez A, Yilmaz MI, Kocar H. "Increased sucrose permeability in Behcet's disease." *Rheumatology International.* Volume 24, Number 6, 2004. pp.347-350.

130d. Humbert P, Monnier G, Billerey C, Birgen C, Dupond JL. "Polyneuropathy: an unusual extraintestinal manifestation of Crohn's disease." *Acta Neuro Scand.* 1989 Oct;80(4):301-6.

131a. Mielants H, De Vos M, Goemaere S, Schelstraete K, Cuvelier C, Goethals K, Maertens M, Ackerman C, Veys EM. "Intestinal mucosal permeability in inflammatory rheumatic diseases. II. Role of disease." *J Rheumatol.* 1991 Mar;18(3): 394-400.

131b. Mielants H. "Reflections on the link between intestinal permeability and inflammatory joint disease." *Clin Exp Rheumatol.* 1990 Sep-Oct;8(5): 523-4.

131c. Rooney PJ, Jenkins RT, Buchanan WW. "A short review of the relationship between intestinal permeability and inflammatory joint disease." *Clin Exp Rheumatol.* 1990 Jan-Feb;8(1):75-83.

131d. Katz KD, Hollander D. "Intestinal mucosal permeability and rheumatological diseases." *Baillieres Clin Rheumatol.* 1989 Aug;3(2): 271-84.

131e. Smith MD, Gibson RA, Brooks PM. "Abnormal bowel permeability in ankylosing spondylitis and rheumatoid arthritis." *J Rheumatol.* 1985 Apr;12(2): 299-305.

132. Howell E. *Enzyme Nutrition.* Avery Publishing, 1985. pp.29, 134-5.

133a. Vaile JH, Meddings JB, Yacyshyn BR, Russell AS, Maksymowych WP. "Bowel permeability and CD45RO expression on circulating CD20+ B cells in patients with ankylosing spondylitis and their relatives." *J Rheumatol.* 1999 Jan;26(1):128-35.

133b. Smith MD, Gibson RA, Brooks PM. "Abnormal bowel permeability in ankylosing spondylitis and rheumatoid arthritis." *J Rheumatol.* 1985 Apr;12(2): 299-305.

134. "Fibromyalgia and the Leaky Gut Syndrome." Accessed 1/6/2005. <http://www.ukfibromyalgia.com/nutrition/leakygut.html>.

CHAPTER 13

Fish and Flax Oils and the Oil Shortage

THERE is a widespread oil shortage that could be a crisis for many people. I'm not talking about the oil that is pumped from the ground and used to fill our gas tanks. I'm talking about a special type of oil that is neglected in our modern diet yet is very necessary for optimum health and maximum mental performance. Specifically, there is a major shortage of a very special group of oils called omega-3 essential fatty acids, abbreviated omega-3 EFAs. They are essential because our body cannot produce them, and, therefore, they must be obtained from our diet. Fish, fish oil, and flaxseed oil are nature's richest sources of omega-3 EFAs.

EFAs are the building blocks of our cells' membranes. The membrane is the outer skin of each cell and is involved in just about every function of the cell, such as transmitting signals, providing energy, and fighting off diseases.[1] Omega-3 EFAs make the membranes flexible so our cells can function properly.

Let's look at EFAs another way. Our brain and nerves make up the "electrical wiring" in our body. EFAs are critical components of nerve cells and brain cells (also called neurons).[2] Some neurons are 3 feet long and the electrical signals travel over 200 miles per hour! Omega-3 EFAs in our diet can help us have good electrical wiring in our body.

We don't want faulty electrical wiring in our house, our car, or the jet plane we are flying in, yet we can allow bad wiring in our body by neglecting to eat foods that contain proper amounts of omega-3 essential fatty acids.

One source estimates that only 20% of Americans get emough EFAs.[3]

Let's look at the importance of oils, fats, and fatty acids in our bodies:

1. Since fatty acids form the building blocks of our cells' membranes, omega-3 EFAs are especially important for proper function of brain cells, nerve cells, and our overall mental performance.[4]

2. Since the brain is 50% to 60% fats and fatty acids by weight,[5] it makes perfect sense that the types of fats and oils we eat affect the function of our brain. Multiple studies indicate that the following conditions may have links to omega-3 EFA deficiency: *degraded memory and cognition, increased anger and anxiety,*[6] *attention deficit disorder,*[7] *depression,*[8] *postpartum depression,*[9] *bipolar disorder,*[10] *increased psychological stress,*[11] degraded vision in preterm infants,[12] increased violence,[13] Alzheimer's disease,[15] and multiple sclerosis.[16]

3. EFAs play a huge role in cell-to-cell signaling, which allows cells to communicate with each other. The types of fatty acids in our nerve and brain cells determine how well these cells talk to each other.[17] EFAs are highly concentrated in the synapse membranes of each nerve cell,[18] where chemical neurotransmitters must jump a tiny gap, called the synapse or synaptic cleft, to pass on signals to neighboring nerve cells. A typical nerve cell can have 15,000 synapses![19]

4. Many inflammatory illnesses have been linked to omega-3 deficiency, including arthritis, Crohn's disease, ulcerative colitis, lupus, cancer,[20] asthma, inflammatory bowel disease, psoriasis,[21] atherosclerosis (hardening of the arteries), heart disease, and stroke.[22] More and more studies are showing that omega-3

supplements can be helpful for some of these inflammatory conditions. For instance, one study showed that enteric-coated fish oil tablets significantly reduced relapse of Crohn's disease.[23] (Crohn's disease is inflammation of the intestine. An enteric coating assures the fish oil is released in the intestine, not the stomach.)

5. Unhealthy inflammation is linked to many chronic illnesses. Note how many of the aforementioned illnesses involve inflammatory processes. This is no surprise since inflammation in our body depends on the various types of fats in the cell membranes and their ratios with each other. Omega-3 EFAs in sufficient amounts can help reduce unhealthy and unnecessary inflammation in our bodies.[24] Inflammation is not needed if our body is not injured or not being attacked. A lot of research has been directed to omega-3 EFAs and how they can help fight against unnecessary inflammation.

6. Omega-3 EFAs enable cell membranes to function properly so needed nutrients can get into each cell for proper function and growth. Cell membranes must also function as barriers to keep unwanted substances out. Omega-3 EFAs also help control energy production within each cell.[25]

7. Omega-3 EFAs promote better circulation by making the blood "less sticky."[26] Fish oil taken along with garlic has been shown to help lower LDL cholesterol, the bad type of fat that can clog our arteries.[27] Fish oil can help protect against heart attack.[28]

8. Omega-3 EFAs can also help with weight management by making our bodies burn more calories and take in more oxygen.[29] Remember from chapter 4 that ginger also makes our bodies burn more calories by increasing metabolism. This is called thermogenesis. This is helpful to know if you are trying to lose weight.

9. Adequate amounts of omega-3 EFAs in the diet may help prevent bone loss in later years.[30]

10. Certain countries and regions where seafood consumption is high have far fewer incidences of aggression, homicide, and suicide.[31] Fish and other seafood have generous amounts of omega-3 EFAs called EPA and DHA (EPA is short for eicosa-pentaenoic acid and DHA is short for docosahexaenoic acid. These are final forms of omega-3 EFAs that our body uses). Flaxseed oil is very rich in ALA (alpha-linolenic acid), which our bodies can transform into lesser amounts of EPA and DHA. A large portion of ALA is burned as energy by our bodies.

WHY THE OIL SHORTAGE?

Omega-3 EFAs come from green leafy plants and certain seeds and beans. They also come from algae and other vegetation that grows in rivers, lakes, and the sea, which are eaten by fish and other aquatic life. Before the industrial revolution, our ancestors ate more fruits and vegetables. Our ancestors also hunted wild game animals and ate more wild-caught fish, all of which feed upon green, leafy vegetation or algae. Fish and animals in the wild receive plenty of omega-3 EFAs from feeding on vegetation; these EFAs, in turn, are passed to the humans who hunt and eat the animals and plants.

Today, much of the food we eat contains the all-too-common omega-6 EFAs which are abundant in common grains such as corn and animal livestock and poultry that have also been fed corn and other grains that are high in omega-6 EFA's. Omega-6 EFAs are very impor-tant; however, most of us get too many because of their abundance in so many of the foods we eat.

The oil shortage is with omega-3 EFAs. A severe shortage of omega-3 EFAs in our diet is unhealthy and can result in unnecessary inflammation in our bodies. The problem is made worse when we also eat too many saturated fats (which are abundant in red meat and dairy products) and manufactured trans fats.

TRANS FATS ARE BAD

Trans fats have been used for many years in many snack foods, prepared foods, fast foods, and margarines because they resist spoiling, have a very long shelf life, and are an alternative to animal fats. Trans fats are manufactured from vegetable oils by forcing hydrogen atoms into the carbon links, which destroys the flexible bonds and produces new fatty molecules that are saturated (filled up) with hydrogen atoms. This process makes trans fats stiff, stable, and resistant to spoiling. Trans fats also have a similar "mouth feel" to animal fats and are solid at room temperature.

Trans fats are very durable. In fact, they are so durable that our bodies cannot break them down. Many experts label them as toxic. Note that natural soybean oil has some omega-3s; however, for the last 50 years, soybean oil has been largely turned into hydrogenated trans fats. Thankfully, trans fats are gradually being removed from margarines, snack foods, prepared foods, and fast foods.

SIGNS OF OMEGA-3 EFA DEFICIENCY

Signs of omega-3 deficiency may include the following symptoms:

- Skin problems[32]
- Dry, itchy skin
- Dry, cracked feet or weight gain[33]
- Bumpy skin resembling that of chicken skin, most commonly on the thighs and back of the arms (called follicular keratosis)[34]
- Brittle hair and nails
- Joint pain
- *Inability to concentrate*, fatigue, and *depression*[35]

Other symptoms of omega-3 deficiency may include the following:

- Dandruff, hair loss

- Cradle cap in babies
- Mixed oily and dry skin (combination skin)
- Dry eyes, excessive thirst, frequent urination
- *Impaired memory*
- Craving for fatty foods[36]

One study involving children with ADHD (attention deficit hyper-activity disorder) showed about 40% of these children had low blood levels of omega-3 EFAs. The following symptoms were observed:

- Dry skin, dry hair
- Excessive thirst
- Frequent need to urinate[37]

Studies in the early 1960s involving infants who were fed a skim milk formula (that contained *no* EFAs) showed the following illnesses:

- Skin lesions, decreased skin pigmentation
- Loss of muscle tone
- Malfunction of the kidneys, lungs, and liver
- Increased susceptibility to infection[38]

You may review some case studies of EFA deficiency at Dr. Leo Galland's Web site for Integraded Medicine: mdheal.org/fatty.htm.

FIX THE SHORTAGE THIS WAY: THREE GRAMS OF OMEGA-3S EVERY DAY!

Three grams of omega-3 EFAs every day are strongly recommended by several nutrition experts for the average adult. (Currently, the United States has no recommended daily amounts. Canada recommends 1.2–1.6 grams per day.)[39] This can easily be accomplished by taking 2 or 3 capsules of fish oil per day plus taking some flaxseed every 2 or 3 days.

Fish oil and flaxseed oil contain different types of omega-3 EFAs, and the reason for taking both types will be discussed later.

Three grams of omega-3s are believed to be an optimal amount when we also eat other foods that contain 6 to 7 grams of omega-6 EFAs each day. These amounts will give an omega-6 to omega-3 ratio of about 2.3 to 1 based on an intake of 2,000 calories per day (8,360 kilo-Joules). This ratio has been shown to provide maximum conversion of EFAs to the final forms EPA and DHA, which are especially needed by nerve cells and brain cells.[40] The average American diet is way out of balance, ranging from 10 to 1 to 20 to 1 when comparing the amount of omega-6 EFAs to omega-3 EFAs. These high ratios lead to unhealthy and unnecessary inflammation in our bodies,[41] which can set the stage for chronic disease.[42]

Omega-6 EFAs are abundant in common grains (especially corn, corn oil, cottonseed oil, peanut oil, safflower oil, and sunflower oil). Omega-6s are also abundant in dairy products, poultry, and meat from animals that were fed grains. Most of us need to reduce the amount of omega-6s in our diets. For now, let's just work on getting 3 grams of omega-3s. For me, the easiest way to get omega-3s into my diet is to take fish oil supplements (1 or 2 with breakfast or supper) and to make delicious fruit flax smoothies. We can also get small amounts of omega-3 EFAs from green, leafy vegetables; walnuts; soybean oil; and canola oil.

FRUIT FLAX SMOOTHIES— A DELICIOUS WAY TO GET OMEGA-3S!

My favorite way to use flaxseeds is to make fruit flax smoothies for my family of five. These cold drinks make a wonderful dessert because they taste almost like a milk shake. Here is what I do:

1. Put 1/2 cup of flaxseeds in an electric blender and grind up (1/2 cup = 90 grams flaxseed = 125 mL). Note: Golden flaxseeds work best for smoothies.

2. Add 3 to 4 cups of ice water that still has ice in it (750 to 1000 mL).

3. Add 1/2 cup of low-fat cottage cheese (or 3 times as much yogurt or a combination of both).

4. Add fresh or frozen fruit (such as strawberries), a banana, or even an orange.

5. I like to add 1/4 teaspoon of stevia, a natural herbal sweetener; or you can add honey or ice cream as other options (1/4 teaspoon = 1 mL). Add a teaspoon of vanilla flavoring too.

6. With a blender on high speed, blend everything together. The water-soluble fiber from the flaxseeds will cause the drink to thicken, almost like a milk shake. This is your super omega-3 drink! If you are a chocolate fan, substitute 1/8 cup of cocoa and 1/8 cup of chocolate malt (or even chocolate protein powder) in place of the fruit (1/8 cup = 30 mL). Enjoy!

Note: 1/2 cup of flaxseeds (125 mL or 90 grams) contains about 20 grams of omega-3 EFAs in the form of ALA (alpha-linolenic acid).[43] I divide this up for my family of five, which works out to about 4 grams of ALA in each serving. I have to confess that my serving is about two to three times larger than the serving I give my kids. I make flax smoothies just about two or three times a week. I also take 2 or 3 capsules of fish oil just about every day.

Note: I don't have a lot of time to calculate precise amounts and ratios of omega-3 EFAs. I am thrilled to have found such an easy and delicious way to get more omega-3s with the least amount of disruption to my busy schedule and my family. Consult a nutritionist for more exact amounts for your diet.

Note: Combining flaxseeds with cottage cheese (when mixed together thoroughly) incorporates Dr. Budwig's discovery that omega-3 EFAs become water soluble and can be readily absorbed by our bodies.[44] Yogurt, skim milk, or nuts can be used in place of cottage cheese (you must use 3 times the amount of yogurt as cottage cheese because yogurt has a lower protein density.) If desired, you may use 3 table-spoons (45 mL) of flaxseed oil instead of 1/2 cup of whole flaxseeds.[45]

The late Dr. Johanna Budwig (pronounced "bood vig") was one of the world's leading authorities on fats and devoted her life to studying the relationship between harmful fats, cancer, and other diseases. She also was a world-renowned researcher, biologist, pharmacologist, medical doctor, and seven-time nominee for the Nobel Prize. It is amazing that her complex research led to such a simple way to get omega-3 EFAs into our body! She also warned of the dangers of trans fats back in the 1950s. More about her amazing research later.

3-D IS THE KEY!

Think of fats as long chains of carbon atoms linked together. Saturated fats have hydrogen atoms attached alongside each of the carbon atoms, which makes the carbon chain stiff. On the other hand, EFAs are missing some hydrogen atoms and in their place have multiple flexible double bonds. The absence of some hydrogen atoms and the presence of these double bonds allows the chain to be very flexible. Because omega-3 EFAs have multiple flexible double bonds, they can take on a wide array of 3-dimensional shapes that enhance the flexibility and function of cell membranes.[46] Fish oil and natural seed and vegetable oils are liquids at room temperature because of their flexible double bonds. On the other hand, saturated fats and trans fats have a stiff, 2-dimensional shape and are solid at room temperature.

Cell membranes, like the tires on an automobile, must be flexible and resilient for proper function and maximum performance.

Too much saturated fats and trans fats in our bodies is like watching an old black-and-white television with rabbit ears. Do you remember the lousy picture and interference? Now, think of omega-3 EFAs as a new, high-definition television and all the extra things it can do. This is the difference our bodies see between bad fats and good fats.

FISH OIL AND FLAX OIL—WHAT'S THE DIFFERENCE?

Fish oil contains the two final forms of omega-3 EFAs called EPA and DHA, which are especially important for our brain, nerves, and circulatory system. (EPA has 5 flexible double bonds, while DHA has 6 flexible double bonds.)

What makes DHA so extremely important is this: *DHA is concentrated at the ends of our nerve and brain cells, where chemicals (called neurotransmitters) must jump a gap (called a synapse) in order to communicate with neighboring cells.*[47] Remember that a typical nerve cell can have 15,000 synapses.[48] EPA is used by cells but it is also acted on by special enzymes in our bodies, which add one more flexible double bond and more carbon links to produce … guess what—more DHA!

Flax oil and most other plant sources do not contain EPA or DHA; however, they do contain a special omega-3 EFA called ALA (alpha-linolenic acid), which has 3 flexible double bonds.[49] The unique chemical structure of ALA allows special enzymes in our bodies to add more carbon links and flexible double bonds, resulting in the production of some EPA and DHA—in a similar way that fish produce EPA and DHA except that fish are much more efficient. It is estimated that humans can convert 6% to 21% of ALA to EPA and 3.8% to 9% of ALA to DHA. Interestingly, the conversion rates are highest for young women of childbearing age.[50] When too many omega-6 EFAs are present, the conversion rate is reduced by as much as one-half.[51] This is why we need to reduce omega-6 EFAs, which are much too common in our Western diet.

As previously mentioned, the ideal ratio of omega-6 to omega-3 EFAs in our diet appears to be 2.3 to 1.[52] Our bodies also convert ALA into energy, burning off calories in the process.[53]

DETAILS! DETAILS! DETAILS!

Nutritional experts who recommend 3 grams of omega-3 EFAs per day further state that they should consist of about 2.2 grams of ALA (from flax oil, canola oil, and other sources) and 0.65 grams of combined EPA and DHA from fish oil.[54]

One gram of fish oil capsule typically contains about 300 milligrams (0.3 grams) of combined EPA and DHA. You may want to take 1 or 2 grams of fish oil every day (1 or 2 capsules) and make a fruit flax smoothie two or three times a week. Follow instructions on the bottle of fish oil. The amounts are for a 150-pound adult. Reduce amounts for children. For example, a 75-pound child would take half as much as a 150 pound adult.

OMEGA-3 EFAs FROM FISH— THE GOOD AND THE BAD

Wild fish feed on smaller fish, which in turn feed on plants and algae. Plants and algae are the original sources of omega-3 EFAs and are passed up the food chain to larger fish and then to humans. Oily, cold water fish have the largest amounts of omega-3 EFAs. These fish include herring, halibut, mackerel, wild-caught salmon, oysters, crab, shrimp, mussels, and white tuna.[55]

Dr. Floyd Chilton, PhD, a leading expert on inflammation and author of *Win the War Within*, warns that some farm-raised salmon may not have sufficient amounts of omega-3 EFAs and could possibly have dangerous levels of arachidonic acid, a final form of omega-6 EFA that our bodies readily transform into inflammatory chemicals. If farm-raised fish have been fed omega-6 grains, the fish meat will contain large amounts of arachidonic acid. Therefore, he recommends eating wild-caught salmon in his dietary program. Other foods with large amounts of arachidonic acid include egg yolks, pork fat, and turkey fat. His testing showed farm-raised trout and oysters appear to have sufficient omega-3

EFAs similar to those in the wild.[56] Refer to his book for specific dietary instructions for reducing inflammation on a therapeutic basis.

Note: I have reviewed other studies that show some farm-raised salmon do have sufficient amounts of omega-3 EFAs. It depends on the type of feed the fish received.

Be aware that most fish probably contains mercury. Smaller fish, like sardines, generally have less mercury than larger fish. Remember from chapter 7 that chlorella and cilantro can help remove mercury from our body. It may be a good idea to take a few chlorella tablets when eating fish. Generally, fish oil supplements may be safer than eating fish meat because mercury accumulates in the muscle, not in the fat from which fish oil is obtained, although certain toxins could be present in some fish oil supplements. Because most fish probably contains some mercury and other contaminants, consumption of fish should be limited to once or twice a month for women of childbearing age and adolescent girls[57] or even avoided altogether when planning for pregnancy, during pregnancy, or when breast-feeding and avoided for young children, according to some experts.[58] Consult your medical practitioner for further guidance. Avoid large fish, which tend to have higher levels of mercury, such as shark, swordfish, king mackerel, and tilefish.[59]

Another concern with fish and fish oil supplements is possible contamination with PCBs (polychlorinated biphenyls) and other environmental toxins. These toxins build up in the fish's fat deposits just underneath the skin. As with mercury, the larger and older the fish, the more likely it is to have a higher concentration of some toxins.[60] Refer to the following Web sites for more information:

- www.epa.gov/waterscience/fish United States Environmental Protection Agency, National Listing of Fish Advisories
- lpi.oregonstate.edu/infocenter/othernuts/omega3fa/ Linus Pauling Institute at Oregon State University, Micronutrient Information Center
- www.psr.org Physicians for Social Responsibility Web site

OTHER PRACTICAL WAYS TO GET OMEGA-3 EFAS

Here are some other suggestions to help get your three grams of omega-3 EFAs each day:

1. Take omega-3 EFA supplements, which usually contain fish oil and/or flax oil. Supplements are available that contain a blend of fish, flax, and borage oils. Dr. Mercola, expert nutritionist and medical doctor, recommends krill oil as the best source of omega-3 EFAs. Krill are tiny shrimp-like sea animals that feed on plankton and algae. See his Web site, www.mercola.com, for more details. Note that krill oil is more costly than fish oil. Several references say to take 400 milligrams of vitamin E along with fish oil to prevent lipid peroxidation (deterioration) of the omega-3 EFAs.

2. Grind up flaxseeds but be sure to mix thoroughly with cottage cheese or yogurt right after grinding in accordance with Dr. Johanna Budwig's requirements so the flax oil becomes water soluble.[61] Use equal amounts of cottage cheese and flaxseeds. If you are substituting, remember to use 3 times the amount of yogurt as cottage cheese because of its lower protein density.

3. Flaxseed oil can also be used. Mix 1 tablespoon of flaxseed oil with 3 tablespoons of cottage cheese.[62] Several sources suggest letting the mixture rest for 15 minutes, which will help decrease the oily taste.

4. Other sources of omega-3s include canola oil, walnuts, walnut oil, and soybean oil.[63] Wheat germ and oat germ also have some omega-3 EFAs.[64] For comparison, flaxseeds contain 23 times the amount of omega-3 EFAs as walnuts. Flaxseed oil contains about 6 times more omega-3 EFAs than canola oil and walnut oil and 8 times more than soybean oil. Perilla oil has a bit more omega-3 EFAs than flax oil[65] but is more costly.

Perilla is in the mint family and has been extensively studied in China.

5. Eat purslane, a green, leafy plant that has the highest omega-3 content among all green leafy plants. Purslane has 4 milligrams of omega-3 EFAs per gram of fresh leaves. In the United States, purslane is considered a weed but is making its way into some resturaunts as a trendy green and is a food source in many other countries. Purslane is fairly easy to grow and is a good source of vitamins C, E, and other antioxidants.[66] Purslane can be added to salads or eaten alone. The plant has thick, red stems and oval-shaped green leaves. Once purslane is established and has seeded itself, plenty should grow the following season. I planted some purslane seeds but was disappointed with the small harvest. A second year should yield a better crop.

6. Eat kale, spinach, and other green, leafy vegetables that contain some omega-3 EFAs. Kale has about 1/2 the amount of omega-3 EFAs as purslane, but kale produces many times the harvest of most other green, leafy vegetables. Kale grows in spring, summer, throughout fall, and into winter. Kale plants often survive the winter and produce leaves in early spring for a second season until blossoms appear, after which they produce only tiny leaves. Spinach has about 1/3 as much omega-3 EFAs as purslane.[67] It is generally believed that green, leafy plants cannot provide therapeutic amounts of EFAs; however, every bit helps. Remember that many plants also provide abundant amounts of important phytochemicals.

7. Other sources of omega-3 EFAs are tofu, soybeans, shrimp, scallops, and winter squash.[68]

8. The effectiveness of omega-3 EFAs are maximized when certain vitamins and minerals are present, including vitamins B, C, and E; folic acid; selenium; zinc; and coenzyme Q10.[69]

OUR WESTERN DIET IS FAR TOO SKIMPY ON OMEGA-3S

The typical Western diet provides about 0.1 to 0.2 grams (100 to 200 milligrams) of EPA and DHA per day.[70] This is a pitiful amount. We should be getting 3 to 6 times more. *The decreasing consumption of omega-3s throughout the twentieth century may be related to increased rates of depression.*[71] Now we are seeing dramatic increases of depression in children![72]

OMEGA-3 EFAS HELP WITH DEPRESSION AND ALZHEIMER'S

One study reported that just 1 gram of EPA per day was the most effective dose for improving symptoms of depression over a twelve-week study.[73] Zinc supplements were also helpful for treating depression at a dose of 25 milligrams per day.[74] Other helpful supplements for depression are folic acid[75] and selenium.[76]

A study involving 815 elderly people in Chicago showed that those who ate fish once a week had 60% less risk of Alzheimer's disease.[77]

OMEGA-3 EFAS ARE GOOD FOR OUR JOINTS

At least 3 grams of combined EPA and DHA are required in order to reduce morning stiffness and decrease tenderness of the joints associated with rheumatoid arthritis.[78]

OMEGA-3 EFAS ARE GOOD FOR OUR HEART

The American Heart Association recommends taking 1 gram of combined EPA and DHA per day for patients with coronary heart disease and 2 to 4 grams per day for patients who need to lower triglycerides, under the care of a physician.[79] (Triglycerides are fats in the blood that get stored in fat cells unless they are burned for energy.) High levels of triglycerides in the blood have been linked to coronary artery disease in some people or may be a consequence of another disease.[80]

It is known that omega-3 EFAs can help thin the blood; however, one leading researcher states, "There is little evidence to suggest that an intake less than 3 grams per day of omega-3 fatty acids would cause clinically significant bleeding."[81]

Just 1 gram of combined EPA and DHA per day may be helpful in reducing risk of major heart attack.[82]

The native Eskimos of Greenland were first studied in the 1970s because of their extremely low rates of heart disease resulting from a diet of meats and fats from fish and seal, which are high in omega-3 EPA and DHA.[84]

PREGNANCY, INFANTS, AND OMEGA-3 EFAS

It is known that a developing baby needs large amounts of EFAs from its mother, especially during the last trimester, as the brain rapidly increases in size and the retinas in the eyes develop.[85] (The retina is a highly sensitive membrane in the back of the eye that allows for sharp focus of objects.) It is also known that omega-3 EFAs in the mother's blood decrease during the later stage of pregnancy. Low levels of omega-3 EFAs in the mother's blood following birth have been linked to postpartum depression.[86] Omega-3 supplements may help to guard the mother against postpartum depression and promote a positive mood,[87] although more studies are needed.[88]

EFAs are passed from mother to child through the umbilical cord and by breast-feeding. Human breast milk contains DHA and an omega-6 EFA called arachidonic acid, a final form of omega-6 EFA that is abundant in the Western diet but is also important to the developing baby. One study concludes, "The DHA content of human milk varies over tenfold, being lowest in women with no intake of DHA and highest in women with high intakes of DHA, which is found predominately in fatty fish."[89] It is probably a good idea for every mother-to-be to include omega-3 supplements in her diet, especially during the third trimester of pregnancy and during breast-feeding.

Studies generally show increased mental development and better visual alertness in infants who were either breast-fed or given a formula fortified with omega-3 DHA.[90] As expected, infants who were fed formula with *no* DHA had poorer visual function, lower cognitive scores, and slower learning than those infants who received adequate amounts of DHA.[91] However, other sources of information indicate little or no advantage to infants who received formula fortified with EFAs and suggest waiting until further evidence is accumulated.[92] Formulas fortified with EFAs are available in the United States and over sixty countries. At the time of this writing, the FDA does not require that baby formulas contain EFAs.[93] Consult your health care practitioner and pediatrician for guidance.

USE OTHER OILS WISELY

Olive oil is great in salads and dressings. One source says not to use olive oil for cooking because of its abundant supply of oleic acid, which could have some harmful effects after being heated.[94] Olive oil consists mostly of monounsaturated fatty acids. (Monounsaturated means it has only one flexible double bond.) James A. Duke, PhD author of *The Green Pharmacy*, highly recommends using olive oil for salad dressings in place of corn or other vegetable oils. Dr. Duke admits that although the explanation is complex, all we need to know is that olive oil is much better for us than most other common vegetable oils.[95]

Virgin olive oil is a major component of the Mediterranean diet, which shows a decreased risk of cardiovascular disease and lower risk factors for cancer and other illnesses. Virgin olive oil also has some antioxidant and anti-inflammatory properties.[96] In fact, olive oil and its importance in the Mediterranean diet is believed to have many benefits as affirmed in 2005 by the International Conference on the Healthy Effect of Virgin Olive Oil."[97] Virgin olive oil is obtained from the first squeezing of olives.

In addition to olive oil, the Mediterranean diet includes an abundance of fresh fruit, vegetables, whole grains and whole grain breads, fish, lamb, and wine along with lesser amounts of eggs, cheese, and other meats.[98] Many foods in the Mediterranean diet were considered peasant food because the grains were simple and unrefined.

Coconut oil appears to be best for cooking because of its abundance of saturated fat, which makes it very stable and more resistant to breakdown during cooking.[99] Coconut oil has many healthful benefits such as antibacterial, antiviral, and anti-inflammatory actions. Coconut oil can help our heart and blood vessels by increasing levels of good HDL cholesterol in our blood.[100]

Dr. Budwig was one of the early researchers who affirmed the many benefits of coconut oil and used it in many of her recipes in *The Oil Protein Diet Cookbook*. She found coconut oil especially helpful for her patients who were very sick and weak, but it is also good for healthy persons and even athletes when served on bread, rice, grains, and lightly cooked or steamed vegetables.[101] Coconut oil contains approximately 86% saturated fat. (Saturated fats have no flexible double bonds and are very stable.)

Butter also is a good choice for cooking for many people, according to Sally Fallan and Mary Enig, PhD, in their book *Nourishing Traditions: The Cookbook That Challenges Politically Correct Nutrition and the Diet Dictocrats*. These experts emphasize the many benefits of natural butter and the importance of cholesterol in our bodies to help give our cell walls sufficient stiffness, help with absorption of vitamin D for healthy bones, help with proper function of the immune system, and many other important benefits.[102] Butter contains over 66% saturated fat and 30% monounsaturated fat. (Remember that monounsaturated fats have only one flexible double bond and, therefore, are more stable than polyunsaturated fats, which have two or more flexible double bonds.)

Coconut oil and butter appear to be the better choices for cooking because they are more stable because of their large amounts of saturated fats.

Whichever fat you use, try to keep your cooking temperature well below the smoking point. Here is a list of smoking point temperatures of various oils: butter 350°F (177°C), canola oil (refined) 400°F (204°C), coconut oil 350°F (177°C), and extra virgin olive oil 406°F (208°C).[103]

Do not use flax oil for cooking or baking because the omega-3 EFAs are very reactive and deteriorate quickly when heated. Oils such as flax oil, canola oil, corn oil, safflower oil, and soy oil have significant amounts of polyunsaturated fatty acids that break down at high temperatures and form harmful compounds called lipid peroxides.[104] Lipid peroxides are produced when the double bonds in unsaturated fats are damaged by free radicals, heat, light and oxygen.

REDUCE OMEGA-6 EFAS

Omega-6 EFAs are also important; however, they are abundant in many common foods and vegetable oils, including most meats and organ foods from land animals, egg yolks, and some farm-raised fish.[105]

Most vegetable and seed oils have omega-6 EFAs, including corn oil, peanut oil, safflower oil, sunflower oil, soybean oil, sesame seed oil, and cottonseed oil. (Note that soybean oil also contains significant amounts of omega-3 EFAs.[106]) Omega-6 EFAs are abundant in the meat of animals that have been fed grains. Experts agree the typical Western diet has too much omega-6s but not enough omega-3s. Too many omega-6 EFAs in our diet, along with too many animal fats, increases inflammation in our bodies, which can lead various inflammatory illnesses[107] and promote the development of various types of cancer.[108] Inflammation and omega-6 EFAs are also discussed in chapter 16.

ELIMINATE TRANS FATS

Trans fats are saturated fats that are manufactured from vegetable oils by destroying the flexible double bonds and replacing them with extra hydrogen atoms along the carbon links. The process is called hydrogenation and uses heat and pressure in the presence of hydrogen and a metal catalyst. The result is a very stable, straight and rigid fat molecule that is solid at room temperature and very resistant to spoiling and turning rancid.

Because trans fats have a very long shelf life, they were widely used during the 1980s (and are still used as of this writing) in the manufacture of many snacks and prepared foods, including cookies, chips, cereals, cake mixes, donuts, French fries, desserts, frozen foods, and many fast foods. Originally, they were thought to be a better substitute for animal fats. This proved wrong. In fact, because trans fats are so rigid and durable, our bodies cannot break them down. As a result, trans fats end up in the arteries and around the heart muscle, a ticking time bomb for heart disease.

A survey in 2005 revealed about 40 percent of supermarket foods contained trans fats. The survey also stated that the fast food industry was one of the biggest users of trans fats. The survey reported that a large order of French fries could contain as much as seven grams of trans fat.[109] As of this writing, manufacturers are finally reducing or eliminating trans fats from prepared foods. Many menus now list the amount of trans fats in a food item.

Dr. Budwig warned of the dangers of these unnatural fats back in the 1950s even though she was criticized by special interest groups in her native Germany,[110] where trans fats were first developed and commercialized. Many experts in nutrition label trans fats as toxic and claim trans fats are responsible for tens of thousands of premature deaths in the United States.[111] Be aware that small amounts of trans fats do occur naturally in some beef and dairy products and some other animal sources; however, these natural trans fats occur in small amounts and may actually reduce certain risk factors associated with heart disease, diabetes, and obesity.[112]

After years of research, debate, and economic analysis, many food manufacturers and fast food restaurants are finally doing the right thing by reducing or abolishing the use of trans fats. As of 2006, food labels must show the amount of trans fats in food; however, if one serving of the food contains less than 0.5 grams of trans fat, the FDA allows the food label to read "0 grams trans fat."[113] Other names of trans fats are hydrogenated oil, partially hydrogenated oil, shortening, margarine, and modified fats.

- *Trans fats are bad for the brain.* Animal studies show that trans fats make their way into nerve cells, brain cells, and microvessels in the brain.[114] Rats that were fed a diet high in trans fats and saturated fats had impaired memory and more memory errors.[115]

- Human and animal studies show that trans fats that are eaten by mothers are passed on to their babies during pregnancy and breast-feeding.[116]

- Trans fats inhibit our body's utilization of EFAs. Trans fats are not water soluble and have no electrons—Dr. Budwig described them as "a battery that is empty." Dr. Budwig also reported that humans and animals ate 6 times as much food when fed trans fats.[117]

- Trans fats become incorporated into our cell membranes, making the membranes denser and, in turn, reducing the receptor activation[118]—in other words, degrading the cell's function.

- *Trans fats are especially bad for the heart and blood vessels.* Trans fats have been shown to increase LDL—bad cholesterol—and also to decrease HDL—good cholesterol. High levels of LDL plus low levels of HDL have been linked to diseases of the heart and circulatory system.[119] (LDL cholesterol is bad because high levels in the blood can lead to the buildup of fatty plaque deposits in the arteries. HDL cholesterol is good because it picks up LDL in our blood and transports it back to the liver for removal from the body.) Coronary heart disease is the leading cause of death in the United States. It is caused by narrowing of the blood vessels that supply blood and oxygen to the heart, which occurs from the buildup of fatty deposits.

NATURAL SATURATED FATS SERVE A PURPOSE

Natural saturated fats come from animal meats and dairy products and are important for our bodies; however, these foods are easily obtained in the typical Western diet, except for some vegetarian diets. Some saturated fats are needed to give some rigidity to our cell walls.[1206]

Remember that fats are made up of many links of carbon atoms that form a chain. The links of saturated fats are completely filled up with hydrogen atoms, which makes them stiff and solid at room temperature. Saturated fats have no flexible double bonds. On the other hand, most natural seed oils and vegetable oils have one or more flexible double bonds, which makes them remain liquid at room temperatures.

Sources of saturated fats are the following: animal fats and meats (even fish), milk, butter, other dairy products, and tropical oils including coconut oil, palm oil, and cottonseed oil. Our bodies know how to use these naturally occurring saturated fats. In fact, the liver even manufactures saturated fats from carbohydrates we eat! Saturated fats are very important to our bodies because they provide energy and, like EFAs, are the building blocks of cell walls. Cell membranes contain about 50% saturated fats.

Mary Enig PhD, international expert in fats chemistry, explains that natural saturated fats have been given a bad rap because they have been shoved into the same category as trans fats. Natural saturated fats, like other fats, are bad when oxidized by frying at high temperatures. It appears that slower cooking at lower temperatures is best.[121]

Extended diets that avoid fats may be dangerous, especially for children and expecting mothers,[122] and are not recommended unless under the strict care of a medical expert. On the other hand, eating too many saturated fats can also feed the inflammation cycle and lead to other problems.

Natural saturated fats also do other important jobs such as protecting the liver and strengthening the immune system.[123]

DR. JOHANNA BUDWIG AND HER DISCOVERIES

The late Dr. Johanna Budwig was one of the world's leading authorities on fats and devoted her life to studying the relationship between harmful fats, cancer, and other diseases. She also was a world-renowned researcher, biologist, pharmacologist, medical doctor, and seven-time nominee for the Nobel Prize. During the 1950s, her research on cancer cells revealed that a major difference between cancer cells and healthy cells was the presence of isolated fats within cancer cells.[124] Dr. Budwig's groundbreaking research throughout the 1950s and 1960s pointed out that the lack of omega-3 EFAs could be at the core of the cancer problem. Her treatment program includes a special diet of simple foods like fresh fruits and vegetables and flax oil mixed with cottage cheese along with exercise, some sunlight, and eliminating various foods.[125] Her treatment program became known as the "Budwig Protocol" and is "far and away the most successful anti-cancer diet in the world," as re-examined in 1990 by Dr. Dan Roehm, MD (oncologist and former cardiologist).[126]

The centerpiece of Dr. Budwig's research is very simple—when flax oil is combined with a sulfur-containing protein such as cottage cheese, the proteins in the cottage cheese combine with the flax oil and make it water soluble, so our bodies can readily absorb the vitally important omega-3 EFAs. EFAs are required to convert the saturated fats we eat into energy and also to transport oxygen to our bodies' cells.[127]

Her book, *Flax Oil as a True Aid Against Arthritis, Heart Infarction, Cancer, and Other Diseases* (Apple Publishing Company), includes several of Dr. Budwig's lectures explaining some of the chemistry and science (including quantum physics) behind her protocol in treating cancer, dissolving tumors, and treating other conditions such as psoriasis and joint problems. She has published several other books including *The Oil Protein Diet Cookbook* and *Cancer—The Problem and Solution*. Be sure to consult your health care provider before starting a special diet.

Budwig provided many reasons why we need to add omega-3 EFAs to our diet:

- **Improved nerve and brain function:** Dr. Budwig witnessed children with below-average school performance who had improved their report cards by two marks after following a simple diet and supplements of flax oil mixed with cottage cheese.[128] Since EFAs are the building blocks of the central nervous system and cell signaling systems, it follows that a deficiency of EFAs has been linked to various psychological and neurological conditions as discussed at the beginning of this chapter.

- **Increased uptake of oxygen into cells:** Dr. Budwig explained that when the flax oil/cottage cheese mixture is eaten, a negative electric charge (due to an abundance of electrons in the flax oil) is passed to the blood and to the cells of the body. This negative charge strongly attracts oxygen, improving the respiration of each cell.[129]

Omega-3 EFAs bring more oxygen into our body's cells, kind of like a turbocharger that sends more oxygen into an engine, boosting its horsepower and performance.

- **Anti-inflammatory properties:**[130] Reducing inflammation is extremely important to healing LGS, fighting off diseases, and keeping a clear head. There appears to be a strong connection between inflammation and cancer[131] and many other diseases. Inflammation is further discussed in chapter 16.

- **Can help remove toxins from our body:**[132] Electron-rich foods such as flaxseed are extremely important for proper secretion of mucus and lymph fluid—both of which are vital for a strong immune system and ridding the body of toxins. Dr. Budwig showed that rats that were fed flaxseed did not become ill after being exposed to large amounts of cigarette smoke.[133]

- **Better circulation:** Omega-3 EFAs make red blood cells more flexible so they can pass through even the smallest capillaries. On the other hand, trans fats are rigid and cause blood to thicken and may lead to circulation problems.[134] Even though omega-3 EFAs may increase bleeding time, there is no evidence of excessive bleeding by investigators in any studies.[135]

- **May help fight disease:** Animal studies suggest that including flaxseeds in the diet may help reduce the incidence of certain cancers. The lignans from the shells of flaxseeds appear to have some anticancer actions against breast cancer,[136] colon cancer,[137] prostate cancer,[138] and skin cancer.[139] The hulls of flaxseeds are nature's richest sources of lignans, which are believed to enhance the anticancer actions of the oil. Lignans are also found in fruits, vegetables, whole grains, and beans; however, flaxseed contains over 75 times more than any other plant source.[140] Lignans are transformed in the digestive tract into estrogen-like chemicals that are shown to have anticancer properties in animal studies;[141] however, more research is needed to determine actual benefits to humans. Producers of high-quality flax oil add lignans to their bottled oil.

GUIDELINES FOR USING FLAX OIL AND FLAXSEEDS

1. A general recommendation is to eat 1 tablespoon (15 mL) of flax oil per day per 100 pounds (45 kg) of body weight mixed with *4 times* that amount of low-fat cottage cheese or about 1/4 cup of cottage cheese for each tablespoon of flax oil.[142] Add milk or water to facilitate mixing with a hand mixer or electric blender. It must be mixed until no traces of oil remain in order for the flax oil to be water soluble.

2. You must use *3 times* the amount of ground flaxseeds to get the same amount of omega-3 ALA as in flax oil.[143]

3. Various sources suggest that yogurt can be substituted for cottage cheese, but use *3 times* as much yogurt because of its lower protein density. Other sources say skim milk and tofu may also be combined with flax oil to make it water soluble. Another option is a supplement called "Companion Nutrients," which is especially helpful if you cannot eat dairy products. These supplements can be purchased from Bionatures at 800-624-7114 or via the Web site bionatures.com.

4. The seeds must be broken or ground up to release their EFAs. Whole seeds merely pass through the body with little benefit.[144]

5. Dr. Budwig instructed to mix cottage cheese or yogurt with the ground-up seeds immediately after grinding because EFAs deteriorate within 10 to 15 minutes of exposure to oxygen, light, and heat. Seeds that have been ground up and left for a long time (without proper sealing) may contain some altered compounds that could do more harm than good, according to Dr. Budwig.[145]

6. Recent studies show that ground flaxseeds can be stored at

room temperature in a plastic bag that is sealed tightly and enclosed by a paper bag to block out light.[146]

7. In her book *The Oil Protein Diet Cookbook*, Dr. Budwig treated patients who were seriously ill with up to 8 tablespoons of flaxseed oil daily, divided among meals. She also advised her seriously ill patients to eat abundant amounts of fruits and steamed vegetables. For the first four weeks, she forbids eating animal fats, pastries, margarine, salad oils, and butter.[147]

8. Because the flax oil/cottage cheese mixture may be distasteful to many people (including myself), here are some suggestions to make it easier to eat: Wait 15 minutes after mixing and the oily taste should go away. Add pineapple or applesauce to help cover up the taste. Dr. Budwig recommends adding fruit, nuts, and coconut. My suggestion is to make fruit flax smoothies.

9. As previously stated, do not use flax oil for cooking. Polyunsaturated oils such as flax oil are too reactive for cooking and may produce harmful compounds upon heating.[148] Some studies indicate that ground flaxseed can be used in baked products with little degradation.[149] I prefer to adhere to Dr. Budwig's instructions to mix the ground flaxseeds with cottage cheese or yogurt rather than cooking or baking flaxseed.

10. Flax oil and flaxseeds should have a natural nutty flavor. Do not use if there is a bitter taste, which indicates the presence of lipid peroxides.[150] After a new bottle of flax oil is opened, it must be refrigerated.

11. Keep whole flaxseeds in a tightly sealed bag or container until you are ready to grind and use them. Flaxseeds and flax oil can be frozen for two years and still retain the omega-3 EFAs.[151]

12. Other terms used when referring to flaxseed oil are highly unsaturated, polyunsaturated, and alpha-linolenic acid, from which the name linseed oil is derived. Commercial linseed oil is used to preserve wood and is unsuitable for human consumption whereas flaxseed oil produced for human consumption must be processed by cold pressing in the

absence of oxygen because the EFAs are quickly destroyed by heat, light, and oxygen.

13. The University of Maryland has an excellent Web site that gives recommended amounts of flaxseed and flaxseed oil along with some cautions. Flaxseeds or flaxseed oil could possibly interact with blood-thinning medications, diabetic medications, oral contraceptives, hormonal replacement therapy, and other medications.[152] You may visit their Web site at www. umm.edu/altmed/articles/flaxseed.

14. Note that most oils are a combination of saturated, monounsaturated, and polyunsaturated fatty acids. Many oils are also a combination of omega-3 and omega-6 EFAs. It is the amount of each type of EFA that gives certain oils special benefits.

15. EFAs are labeled omega-3, -6, or -9 depending on whether the first double bond occurs at the third, sixth, or ninth carbon atom from the end (omega means *the end*).

ADDITIONAL INFORMATION FROM DR. BUDWIG'S RESEARCH

Dr. Budwig died in 2003 at the age of ninety-five. She devoted her life to her research and helping people. She actively educated many people and gave many lectures, even into her later years. I place a great amount of trust in her writing, her amazing research, her methods, and her explanations. I believe she carried out her work with the highest standards of integrity and truthfulness.

1. Dr. Budwig lectured on the importance of electrical charges in the body and how flax oil helps the body to function properly like a well-charged battery. Our body is an electrical system. Every muscle and every heartbeat is controlled by electrical charges. Heartbeat is measured by an electrocardiogram (EKG). Brain activity is also measured by electrical activity via an electroencephalograph. Dr. Budwig explained that flax oil

carries a strong negative charge (from an abundance of electrons captured with the help of sunlight), which can be quickly conducted into the body, causing a "recharging of the living substance, especially the brain and nerves."[153]

2. For the proper growth of new cells, electrical charges are very important. Budwig explained that the membrane (outer skin) of growing cells has a high concentration of EFAs, which gives it a negative charge, while the nucleus (center) has an opposing positive charge. When a cell divides, the daughter cell must contain enough electron-rich EFAs to divide off completely from the mother cell. If this process is interrupted, the body begins to die. Dr. Budwig points out that "this can be reversed by eating simple foods, cottage cheese and flaxseed oil, which revises the stagnated growth process. This naturally causes the tumor to dissolve and the whole range of symptoms which indicates a dead battery are cured."[154]

3. Omega-3 oils have flexible double bonds that are missing hydrogen atoms. The first double bond is located at the third carbon link, hence the name omega-3. Omega-3 oils have at least two flexible double bonds, each missing hydrogen atoms and are also called unsaturated and polyunsaturated. When these flexible double bonds are close together (as in flaxseed oil), it creates an electron cloud that gets released in the body. These electron clouds are vital for attracting oxygen into our bodies' cells, according to Dr. Budwig.[155]

4. Dr. Budwig offered her patients a "three-day challenge" to try her program of diet and supplementation with flax oil and cottage cheese, after which people would say they "suddenly feel so light … no longer so heavy" and would not want to return to their previous eating habits.[156]

5. Dr. Budwig also believed that diabetes was a basic problem of "fats metabolism" and that the assimilation of sugar is secondary.[157] It is interesting that several recent studies (about forty years after Dr. Budwig's original research) show that

sensitivity to insulin is increased when dietary omega-3 EFAs are increased.[158] Another study showed that sensitivity to insulin could also be increased by increasing monounsaturated fats (as in olive oil) and decreasing saturated fats.[159] (Increased sensitivity to insulin is desirable because most diabetics are resistant to insulin.)

6. One may wonder why such a breakthrough in knowledge came up against resistance by various establishments. One can only speculate by looking back into her lectures and correspondence with her colleagues, which may provide some clues:

- Was it because her powerful explanation, which combined complex physics, pharmacology, biology, and chemistry, translated into a protocol consisting of simple therapies, including a simple diet, simple foods, exercise, and sunlight?

- Or was it that her methods could not be patented nor provide significant profit incentives for corporations since her methods consisted only of natural elements? (Profits are necessary and good for the free enterprise system and innovation. Huge profits are not good when greed overruns moral judgement and character.)

- Or was it because she was one of the few scientists who recognized that humans are very different from animals because of the "extra metabolism involved in constant thinking," which did not fit the "evolutionary develop-ment from animals model" popular with the scientific and medical institutions of that time? (It is reported that we humans expend about three times more energy to sustain our brain than monkeys and gorillas.[160])

- Or was it because she was a brilliant scientist and a woman with multiple doctorate degrees who was far ahead of the current thinking of the establishments of that time?

- Oh, yeah, guess how your doctor measures cholesterol levels in your blood. You guessed it—by measuring the *proteins* attached to the fats; LDL (low-density lipo*proteins*) and HDL (high-density lipo*proteins*)—just as Dr. Budwig explained back in the 1950's by combining cottage cheese with flax oil. More about blood and circulation in chapter 19.

OTHER SOURCES OF INFORMATION

Web sites:

- www.barleans.com Barleans Organic Oils
- www.cancure.org The Cancer Cure Foundation
- www.healingcancernaturally.com Healing Cancer Naturally!!! (locate Dr. Johanna Budwig's Protocol)
- www.efaeducation.nih.gov U.S. Department of Health & Human Services, National Institutes of Health

REFERENCES FOR CHAPTER 13

1a.   Hulbert AJ, Turner N, Storlien LH, Else PL. "Dietary fats and membrane function: implications for metabolism and disease." *Biol Rev Camb Philos Soc.* 2005 Feb;80(1):155-69.

1b.   Budwig, Johanna. *Flax Oil as a True Aid Against Arthritis, Heart Infarction, Cancer and Other Diseases.* Apple Publishing Co. Ltd. 1994

2.   Haag, Marianne MSc, DSc. "Essential Fatty Acids and the Brain." *Canadian Journal Psychiatry.* Vol. 48, No. 3. April 2003.

3.   Web site: Bionatures Flaxseed Oil Products. Article: Frequently Asked Questions. <http://www.budwigflax.com/FAQs/questions.htm>. Accessed 6/7/06.

4a.   Fontani G, Corradeschi F, Felici A, Alfatti F, Migliorini S, Lodi L. "Cognitive and physiological effects of Omega-3 polyunsaturated fatty acid supplementation in healthy subjects." *Eur J Clin Invest.* 2005 Nov;35(11):691-9.

4b.   Haag, Marianne MSc, DSc. "Essential Fatty Acids and the Brain." *Canadian Journal Psychiatry.* Vol. 48, No. 3. April 2003. p.1.

4c.   Andrew L. Stoll, M.D. *The Omega-3 Connection.* Simon & Schuster, 2001. pp 44-47.

4d.   Budwig, Johanna. *Flax Oil as a True Aid Against Arthritis, Heart Infarction, Cancer and Other Diseases.* Apple Publishing Co. Ltd. 1994 pp.8-9, 12, 40-41.

5.   Haag, Marianne MSc, DSc. "Essential Fatty Acids and the Brain." *Canadian Journal Psychiatry.* Vol. 48, No. 3. April 2003. p.1.

6a.   Fontani G, Corradeschi F, Felici A, Alfatti F, Migliorini S, Lodi L. "Cognitive and physiological effects of Omega-3 polyunsaturated fatty acid supplementation in healthy subjects." *Eur J Clin Invest.* 2005 Nov;35(11):691-9.

6b.   Stoll Andrew L. M.D. *The Omega-3 Connection.* Schuster & Schuster. New York, NY 10020. pp.172-178.

7a.   Young GS, Conquer JA, Thomas R. "Effect of randomized supplementation with high dose olive, flax or fish oil on serum phospholipid fatty acid levels in adults with attention deficit hyperactivity disorder." *Reprod Nutr Dev.* 2005 Sep-Oct;45(5):549-58.

7b.   Burgess JR, Stevens L, Zhang W, Peck L. "Long chain polyunsaturated fatty acids in children with attention deficit hyperactivity disorder." *Am J Clin Nutr.* 2000;71:327S-330S.

8a.   Alan C Logan. "Omega-3 fatty acids and major depression: A primer for the mental health professional." Lipids Health Dis. 2004; 3: 25. Published online 2004 November 9.

8b.   Kobayakawa M, Yamawaki S, Hamazaki K, Akechi T, Inagaki M, Uchitomi Y. "Levels of omega-3 fatty acid in serum phospholipids and depression in patients with lung cancer." *Br J Cancer.* 2005 Dec 12;93(12):1329-33.

8c.   Frasure-Smith N, Lesperance F, Julien P. "Major depression is associated with lower omega-3 fatty acid levels in patients with recent acute coronary syndromes." *Biol Psychiatry.* 2004 May 1;55(9):891-6.

8d.   Suzuki S, Akechi T, Kobayashi M, Taniguchi K, Goto K, Sasaki S, Tsugane S, Nishiwaki Y, Miyaoka H, Uchitomi Y. "Daily omega-3 fatty acid intake and depression in Japanese patients with newly diagnosed lung cancer." *Br J Cancer.* 2004 Feb 23;90(4):787-93.

8e.   Colin A, Reggers J, Castronovo V, Ansseau M. "[Lipids, depression and suicide]." *Encephale.* 2003 Jan-Feb;29(1):49-58. Article in French.

8f.   Edwards R, Peet M, Shay J, Horrobin D. "Omega-3 polyunsaturated fatty acids levels in the diet and in red blood cell membranes of depressed patients." *J Affect Disord.* 1998;48:149-55.

9.   Andrew L. Stoll, M.D. *The Omega-3 Connection.* Simon & Schuster. 2001, pp.100-103.

10a.   Stoll AL. Severus WE, Freeman MP, Rueter S, Zboyan HA, Diamond A, and others. "Omega-3 Fatty acids in bipolar disorder." *Arch Gen Psychiatry.* 1999;56:401-12.

10b.   Patrick Perry. "Omega-3 for bipolar disorder - Restoring the balance". Web site: www.fabresearch.org. 01 September 2001 USA. Handout - courtesy of Food And Behaviour Research.

11.   Maes M, Christophe A, Bosmans E, Lin A, Neels H. "In humans, serum

polyunsaturated fatty acid levels predict the response of pro-inflammatory cytokines to psychological stress." *Biol Psychiatry* 2000;47:910-20.

12. SE Carlson, SH Werkman and EA Tolley. "Effect of long-chain n-3 fatty acid supplementation on visual acuity and growth of preterm infants with and without bronchopulmonary dysplasia." *American Journal of Clinical Nutrition.* 1996 Vol 63, 687-697.

13. "Aggression, Homicide and Suicide." Web site: National Institutes of Health. Accessed 7/8/2008. <http://efaeducation.nih.gov/sig/aggretion.html>.

14. Not used.

15a. Ma QL, Teter B, Ubeda OJ, Morihara T, Dhoot D, Nyby MD, Tuck ML, Frautschy SA, Cole GM. "Omega-3 fatty acid docosahexaenoic acid increases SorLA/LR11, a sorting protein with reduced expression in sporadic Alzheimer's disease (AD): relevance to AD prevention." *J Neurosci.* 2007 Dec 26;27(52):14299-307.

15b. Morris MC, Evans DA, Biejias JL, Tangney CC, Bennett DA, Wilson RS, Aggarwal N, Schneider J. "Consumption of fish and n-3 fatty acids and risk of incident Alzheimer disease." *Arch Neurol.* 2003 Jul;60(7):940-6.

16. Holman R, Johnson S, Kokmen E. "Deficiencies of polyunsaturated fatty acids and replacement by non-essential fatty acids in plasma lipids in multiple sclerosis." *Proc Natl Acad USA.* 1989;86:4720-4.

17a. Jose A Matta, Rosa L Miyares, and Gerard P Ahem. "TRPV1 is a novel target for omega-3 polyunsaturated fatty acids". *J Physiol.* 2007 January 15; 578 (Pt 2): 397-411. Published online 2006. October 12.

17b. Haag, Marianne MSc, DSc. "Essential Fatty Acids and the Brain." *Canadian Journal Psychiatry.* Vol. 48, No. 3. April 2003. pp.199-201.

17c. Litman BJ, Niu SL, Polozova A. Mitchell DC. "The role of docosahexaenoic acid containing phospholipids in modulating G protein-coupled signaling pathways: visual transduction". *J Mol Neurosci.* 2001 Apr-Jun;16(2-3):237-42.

18a. McNamara RK, Sullivan J, Richtand NM, Jandacek R, Rider T, Tso P, Campbell M, Lipton J. "Omega-3 fatty acid deficiency augments amphetamine-induced behavioral sensitization in adult DBA/2J mice: Relationship with ventral striatum dopamine concentrations." *Synapse.* 2008 Jul 23;62(10):725-735. [Epub ahead of print].

18b. Haag, Marianne MSc, DSc. "Essential Fatty Acids and the Brain." *Canadian Journal Psychiatry.* Vol. 48, No. 3. April 2003. p.1.

19. "Alzheimer's Disease: Unraveling the Mystery". Web site: U.S. National Institutes of Health, National Institute on Aging. "Neurons and Their Jobs". Accessed 6/24/2008. <http://www.nia.nih.gov/Alzheimers/Publications/UnravelingTheMystery/Part1NeuronsAndTheirJobs>.

20. Simopoulos AP. "Omega-3 fatty acids in inflammation and autoimmune diseases." *J Am Coll Nutr.* 2002 Dec;21(6):495-505.

21.   Grimble RF, Tappia PS. "Modulation of pro-inflammatory cytokine biology by unsaturated fatty acids." *Z Ernahrungswiss.* 1998;37 Suppl 1:57-65.

22.   Mori TA, Beilin LJ. "Omega-3 fatty acids and inflammation." *Curr Atheroscler Rep.* 2004 Nov;6(6):461-7.

23.   Belluzzi A, Brignola C, Campieri M, Pera A, Boschi S, Migliolo M. "Effect of an enteric-coated fish-oil preparation on relapses in Crohn's disease." *N Engl J Med.* 1996 Jun 13;334(24):1557-60.

24a.   Simopoulos AP. "The omega-6/omega-3 fatty acid ratio, genetic variation, and cardiovascular disease." *Asia Pac J Clin Nutr.* 2008; 17 Suppl 1:131-4.

24b.   Haag, Marianne MSc, DSc. "Essential Fatty Acids and the Brain." *Canadian Journal Psychiatry.* Vol. 48, No. 3. April 2003.

24c.   Chilton FH, Tucker L. *Win the War Within.* Rodale Inc. 2006.

24d.   Zhao G, Etherton TD, Martin KR, Gilliew PJ, West SG, Kris-Etherton PM. "Dietary alpha-linolenic acid inhibits proinflammatory cytokine production by peripheral blood mononuclear cells in hypercholesterolemic subjects." *Am J Clin Nutr.* 2007 Feb;85(2):385-91.

24e.   Mori TA, Beilin LJ. "Omega-3 fatty acids and inflammation." *Curr Atheroscler Rep.* 2004 Nov;6(6):461-7.

25.   Andrew L. Stoll, M.D. *The Omega-3 Connection.* Simon & Schuster. 2001, p.37.

26a.   von Schacky C. "A review of omega-3 ethyl esters for cardiovascular prevention and treatment of increased blood triglyceride levels." *Vasc Health Risk Manag.* 2006;2(3):251-62.

26b.   Mori TA, Woodman RJ, Burke V, Puddey IB, Croft KD, Beilin LJ. "Effect of eicosapentaenoic acid and docosahexaenoic acid on oxidative stress and inflammatory markers in treated-hypertensive type 2 diabetic subjects." *Free Radic Biol Med.* 2003 Oct 1;35(7):772-81.

26c.   Mori TA, Beilin LJ, Burke V, Morris J, Ritchie J. "Interactions between dietary fat, fish, and fish oils and their effects on platelet function in men at risk of cardiovascular disease." Arterioscler Thromb Vasc Biol. 1997 Feb;17(2):279-86.

26d.   Agren JJ, Vaisanen S, Hanninen O, Muller AD, Hornstra G. "Hemostatic factors and platelet aggregation after a fish-enriched diet or fish oil or docosahexaenoic acid supplementation." *Prostaglandins Leukot Essent Fatty Acids.* 1997 Oct;57(4-5):419-21.

27.   Mao, Joseph L. "Dietary Influences on Cardiovascular Disease and Female Cancer Risk." *Clinical Nutrition Insights.* 1997 by Advanced Nutrition Publications, Inc. Rev. 4/99.

28a.   Rupp H, Wagner D, Rupp T, Schulte LM, Maisch B. "Risk stratification by the "EPA+DHA level" and the "EPA/AA ratio" focus on anti-inflammatory and antiarrythmogenic effects of long-chain omega-3 fatty acids."

28b.   Das UN. "Beneficial effect(s) of n-3 fatty acids in cardiovascular diseases:

but, why and how?" Prostaglandins Leukot Essent Fatty Acids. 2000 Dec;63(6):351-62.

29a. Jade Beutler RRT, RCP. "Flax and Figures." Web site: Barleans. Accessed 5/28/06. <http://www.barleans.com/literature/flax/17-flax-and-figures.html>.

29b. Andrew L. Stoll, M.D. *The Omega-3 Connection.* Simon & Schuster. 2001, pp.80-81.

30. Griel AE, Kris-Etherton PM, Hilpert KF, Zhao G, West SG, Corwin RL. "An increase in dietary n-3 fatty acids decreases a marker of bone resorption in humans." *Nutr J.* 2007 Jan 16;6:2.

31. "Agression, Homicide and Suicide." Web site: National Institutes for Health. Accessed 4/19/2007. <http://efaeducation.nih.gov/sig/aggretion.html>.

32. Palle B Jeppesen, Carl-Erik Hoy, and Per B Mortensen. "Essential fatty acid deficiency in patients receiving home parenteral nutrition." *Am J Clin Nutr.* 1998;68:126-33.

33. "Omega-3 is Essential to the Human Body". Web site: Mercola.com Accessed 8/2/2008. <http://articles.mercola.com/sites/articles/archive/2001/09/08/omega-3-part-one.aspx>.

34. Bhat KS, Belavady B. "Biochemical studies in phyrnoderma (follicular hyperkeratosis). II. Polyunsaturated fatty acid levels in plasma and erythrocytes of patients suffering from phrynoderma." *Am J Clin Nutr.* 1967 May;20(5):386-92.

35. "omega-3 fatty acids". Web site: the world's healthiest foods. George Mateljan Foundation. Accessed 6/12/2008. <http://www.whfoods.com/genpage.php?pfriendly=1&tname=nutrient&dbid=84>.

36. Blake Graham. "Omega-3 Fatty Acids". Articles from web site: Nutritional Healing, A resource for nutritional medicine. Accessd 6/2/2008. <http://www.nutritional-healing.com .au/content/articles-content. php?heading=Omega-3%2...>

37. Andrew L. Stoll, M.D. *The Omega-3 Connection.* Simon & Schuster. 2001. pp.94-103, 158-160.

38. Andrew L. Stoll, M.D. *The Omega-3 Connection.* Simon & Schuster. 2001. p.94.

39. Kris-Etherton PM, Taylor DS, Yu-Poth S, Huth P, Moriarty K, Fischell V, Hargrove RL, Shao G, Etherton TD. "Polyunsaturated fatty acids in the food chain in the United States." *Am J Clin Nutr.* 2000 Jan;71(1 Suppl):179S-88S.

40a. PM Kris-Etherton, Denise Shaffer Taylor, Shaomei Yu-Poth, Peter Huth, Kristen Moriarty, Valerie Fishell, Rebecca L Hargrove, Guixiang Shao and Terry D Etherton. "Polyunsaturated fatty acids in the food chain in the United States." *American Journal of Clinical Nutrition*, Vol. 71, No. 1, 179S-188S, January 2000.

40b. Masters C. "Omega-3 fatty acids and the peroxisome." *Mol Cell Biochem.* 1996 Dec 20;165(2):83-93.

41a.   Simopoulos AP. :The omega-6/omega-3 fatty acid ratio, genetic variation, and cardiovascular disease." *Asia Pac J Clin Nutr.* 2008;17 Suppl 1:131-4.

41b.   Simopoulos AP. "Omega-3 fatty acids and athletics." *Curr Sports Med Rep.* 2007 Jul;6(4):230-6.

41c.   Simopoulos AP. "Omega-3 fatty acids in health and disease and in growth and development." *Am J Clin Nutr.* 1991 Sep;54(3):438-63.

42.   Simopoulos AP. "The omega-6/omega-3 fatty acid ratio, genetic variation, and cardiovascular disease." *Asia Pac J Clin Nutr.* 2008;17 Suppl 1:131-4.

43.   "FLAX - A Health and Nutrition Primer" Web site: Flax Council of Canada. p.11. Accessed 9/12/2008. <http://www.flaxcouncil.ca>.

44.   Budwig, Johanna. *Flax Oil as a True Aid Against Arthritis, Heart Infarction, Cancer and Other Diseases.* Apple Publishing Co. Ltd. 1994. pp.11, 30-31.

45.   Budwig, Johanna. *The Oil-Protein Diet.* Apple Publishing Co, Ltd. Vancouver BC. Canada. 1994 pp.vi, 15.

46.   Haag, Marianne MSc, DSc. "Essential Fatty Acids and the Brain." *Canadian Journal Psychiatry.* Vol. 48, No. 3. April 2003.

47a.   McNamara RK, Sullivan J, Richtand NM, Jandacek R, Rider T, Tso P, Campbell N, Lipton J. "Omega-3 fatty acid deficiency augments amphetamine-induced behavioral sensitization in adult DBA/2J mice: Relationship with ventral striatum dopamine concentrations." *Synapse.* 2008 Jul 23;62(10):725-735. [Epub ahead of print].

47b.   Edwards R, Peet M, Shay J, Horrobin D. "Omega-3 polyunsaturated fatty acid levels in the diet and in red blood cell membranes of depressed patients." *J Affect Disord.* 1998 Mar;48(2-3):149-55.

48.   "Alzheimer's Disease: Unraveling the Mystery". "Neurons and Their Jobs". Web site: U.S. National Institutes of Health, National Institute on Aging. Accessed 6/24/2008. <http://www.nia.nih.gov/Alzheimers/Publications/UnravelingTheMystery/Part1NeuronsAndTheirJobs>.

49.   Dr. Diane H. Morris. "New Flax Facts, Metabolism of Alpha-Linolenic Acid" by Dr. Diane H. Morris. Web site: Flax Council of Canada. Accessed 7/15/2008. <http://www.flaxcouncil.ca>.

50a.   Burdge GC, Wootton SA. "Conversion of alpha-linolenic acid to eicosapentaenoic, docosapentaenoic and docosahexaenoic acids in young women." *Br J Nutr.* 2002 Oct;88(4):411-20.

50b.   Gerster H. "Can adults adequately convert alpha-linolenic acid (18:3n-3) to eicosapentaenoic acid (20:5n-3) and docosahexaenoic acid (22:6n-3)?" *Int J Vitam Nutr Res.* 1998;68(3):159-73.

51.   Gerster H. "Can adults adequately convert alpha-linolenic acid (18:3n-3) to eicosapentaenoic acid (20:5n3) and docosahexaenoic acid (22:6n3)?" *Int J Vitam Nutr Res.* 1998;68(3):159-73.

52.   Kris-Etherton PM, Taylor DS, Yu-Poth S, Huth P, Moriarty K, Fischell V,

Hargrove RL, Shao G, Etherton TD. "Polyunsaturated fatty acids in the food chain in the United States." *Am J Clin Nutr.* 2000 Jan;71(1 Suppl):179S-88S.

53.   Gerster H. "Can adults adequately convert alpha-linolenic acid (18:3n-3) to eicosapentaenoic acid (20:5n-3) and docosahexaenoic acid (22:6n-3)?" *Int J Vitam Nutr Res.* 1998;68(3):159-73.

54.   Kris-Etherton PM, Taylor DS, Yu-Poth S, Huth P, Moriarty K, Fischell V, Hargrove RL, Shao G, Etherton TD. "Polyunsaturated fatty acids in the food chain in the United States." *Am J Clin Nutr.* 2000 Jan;71(1 Suppl):179S-88S.

55.   "Omega-3 Fatty Acids and Fish Consumption" Web site: Physicians for Social Responsibility. Accessed 6/10/2008. <http://www.psr.org>.

56.   Floyd H. Chilton, Ph.D., with Laura Tucker. *Win the War Within.* Rodale Inc. 2006. pp.92-95, 202-203.

57.   "Fish Consumption to Promote Good Health and Minimize Contaminants. A Quick Reference Guide for Clinicians." Web site: Physicians for Social Responsibility. Accessed 6/10/2008. <http://www.psr.org>.

58.   Penny M. Kris-Etherton, William S. Harris, Lawrence J. Appel. "Fish Consumption, Fish Oil, Omega-3 Fatty Acids, and Cardiovascular Disease". *Circulation.* 2002;106;2747-2757. Accessed 7/8/08. <http://circ.ahajournals. org/cgi/content/full/106/21/2747>.

59.   "Fish Consumption to Promote Good Health and Minimize Contaminants. A Quick Reference Guide for Clinicians." Web site: Physicians for Social Responsibility. Accessed 6/10/2008. <http://www.psr.org>.

60.   "Fish Consumption to Promote Good Health and Minimize Contaminants. A Quick Reference Guide for Clinicians." Web site: Physicians for Social Responsibility. Accessed 6/10/2008. <http://www.psr.org>.

61.   Budwig, Johanna. *Flax Oil as a True Aid Against Arthritis, Heart Infarction, Cancer and Other Diseases.* Apple Publishing Co. Ltd. 1994 pp.10-11, 30-35.

62.   Budwig, Johanna. *The Oil-Protein Diet.* Apple Publishing Co, Ltd. Vancouver BC. Canada. 1994 p.15.

63.   "Essential Fats in Food Oils". Web site: National Institutes of Health. Accessed 5/14/2007. <http://efaeducation.nih.gov/sig/esstable.html>.

64.   Karen Schroeder, MS, RD. "Good Food Sources of Omega-3 Fatty Acids." Accessed 8/30/06. <http://healthlibrary.epnet.com>.

65a. "Flax Nutrition Profile" Web site: Flax Council of Canada. Accessed 7/15/2008. <http://www.flaxcouncil.ca/english/print.php?p=g3>.

65b. "Essential Fats in Food Oils". Web site: National Institutes of Health. Accessed 5/14/2007. <.http://efaeducation.nih.gov/sig/esstable.html>.

65c. "Walnuts Rank High on New Nutrition Scales." Press Release: [Folsom, CA] February 19, 2008. Accessed 6/12/2008. <http://www.walnuts.org>.

66a. Simopoulos AP, Norman HA, Gillaspy JE, Duke JA. "Common purslane: a source of omega-3 fatty acids and antioxidants." J Am Coll Nutr. 1992 Aug;11(4):374-82.

66b.   "Purslane". Web site: Drugs.com. Accessed 6/2/2008. <http://www.drugs. com/npp/purslane.html?printable=1>.

67a.   "Kale, raw." Web site: NutritionData.com. Accessed 7/12/2008. <http://www. nutritiondata.com/facts/vegetables-and-vegetable-products/2461/2>.

67b.   "Spinach, raw." Web site: NutritionData.com. Accessed 7/12/2008. <http:// www.nutritiondata.com/facts/vegetables-and-vegetable-products/2626/2>.

67c.   Simopoulos AP, Norman HA, Gillaspy JE, Duke JA. "Common purslane: a source of omega-3 fatty acids and antioxidants." *J Am Coll Nutr.* 1992 Aug;11(4):374-82.

68.   "omega-3 fatty acids". Web site: www.whfoods.org. George Mateljan Foundation. Accessed 5/2/2009. <http://whfoods.com/genpage.php?pfriendly =1&tname=nutrient&dbid=84>.

69.   Andrew L. Stoll, M.D. *The Omega-3 Connection.* Simon & Schuster. 2001. pp.223-224.

70.   Kris-Etherton PM, Taylor DS, Yu-Poth S, Huth P, Moriarty K, Fischell V, Hargrove RL, Shao G, Etherton TD. "Polyunsaturated fatty acids in the food chain in the United States." *Am J Clin Nutr.* 2000 Jan;71(1 Suppl):179S-88S.

71.   Colin A, Reggers J, Castronovo V, Ansseau M. "[Lipids, depression and suicide]" *Encephale.* 2003 Jan-Feb;29(1):49-58.

72.   "Depression". Web site: Children's Hospital Boston. Accessed 12/12/2009. <http://www.childrenshospital.org/patientsfamilies/Site1393/mainpag- eS1393P201sublevel154Flevel162.html>

73.   Peet M, Horrobin DF. "A dose-ranging study of the effects of ethyl-eicosap- entaenoate in patients with ongoing depression despite apparently adequate treatment with standard drugs." 2000;59:913-919.

74.   Nowak G, Siwek M, Dudek D, Zieba A, Pilc A. "Effect of zinc supple- mentation on antidepressant therapy in unipolar depression: a preliminary placebo-controlled study." *Pol J Pharmacol.* 2003 Nov-Dec;55(6):1143-7.

75.   Paul RT, McDonnell AP, Kelly CB. "Folic acid: neurochemistry, metabo- lism and relationship to depression." *Hum Psychopharmacol.* 2004 Oct;19(7):477-88.

76.   Benton D. "Selenium intake, mood and other aspects of psychological func- tioning." *Nutr Neurosci.* 2002 Dec;5(6):363-74.

77.   Morris MC, Evans DA, Biejias JL, Tangney CC, Bennett DA, Wilson RS, Aggarwal N, Schneider J. "Consumption of fish and n-3 fatty acids and risk of incident Alzheimer disease." *Arch Neurol.* 2003 Jul;60(7):940-6.

78.   Covington MB. "Omega-3 fatty acids." *Am Fam Physician.* 2004 Jul 1:70(1):133-40. *Am Fam Physician.* 2005 Jul 15;72(2):226.

79.   "Fish and Omega-3 Fatty Acids". Web site: American Heart Association. Accessed 9/21/2008. <http://www.americanheart.org/presenter. jhtml?identifier=4632>.

80.   "Triglycerides". Web site: American Heart Association. Accessed 9/23/2008.
        <http://www.americanheart.org/presenter.jhtml?identifier=4778>.

81.   Penny M. Kris-Etherton, William S. Harris, Lawrence J. Appel and for the
        Nutrition Committee. "Fish Consumption, Fish Oil, Omega-3 Fatty Acids,
        and Cardiovascular Disease." *Circulation.* 2002;106;2747-2757.

82a.   von Shacky C. "A review of omega-3 ethyl esters for cardiovascular prevention
        and treatment of increased blood triglyceride levels." *Vasc Health Risk Manag.*
        2006;2(3):251-62.

82b.   Covington MB. "Omega-3 fatty acids." *Am Fam Physician.* 2004 Jul
        1:70(1):133-40. *Am Fam Physician.* 2005 Jul 15;72(2):226.

83.   Not used.

84.   Dyerberg J, Bang HO, Hjorne N. "Fatty acid composition of the plasma lipids
        in Greenland Eskimos." *Am J Clin Nutr.* 1975 Sep;28(9):958-66.

85.   Innis SM. "Polyunsaturated fatty acids in human milk: an essential role in
        infant development." *Adv Exp Med Biol.* 2004;554:27-43.

86a.   Andrew L. Stoll, M.D. *The Omega-3 Connection.* Simon & Schuster. 2001.
        pp.100-102, 111-112.

86b.   Hibbein JR. "Seafood consumption, the DHA content of mother's milk and
        prevalence rates of postpartum depression: a cross-national, ecological anal-
        ysis." *J Affect Disord.* 2002 May;69(1-3):15-29.

86c.   "Aggression, Homicide and Suicide". Web site: National Institutes of Health.
        Accessed 7/08/2008. <http://efaeducation.nih.gov/sig/aggretion.html>.

87a.   Fontani G, Corradeschi F, Felici A, Alfatti F, Migliorini S, Lodi L. "Cognitive
        and physiological effects of Omega-3 polyunsaturated fatty acid supplementa-
        tion in healthy subjects." Eur J Clin Invest. 2005 Nov;35(11):691-9.

87b.   Andrew L. Stoll, M.D. *The Omega-3 Connection.* Simon & Schuster. 2001.
        pp.100-102.

88.   Miyake Y, Sasaki S, Yokoyama T, Tanaka K, Ohya Y, Fukushima W, Saito
        K, Ohfuji S, Kiyohara; Osaka Maternal and Child Health Study Group.
        "Risk of postpartum depression in relation to dietary fish and fat intake in
        Japan: the Osaka Maternal and Child Health Study." Psychol Med. 2006
        Dec;36(12):1727-35. Epub 2006 Aug 29.

89.   Innis SM, "Polyunsaturated fatty acids in human milk: an essential role in
        infant developmnent." *Adv Exp Med Biol.* 2004;554:27-43.

90a.   Fleith M, Clandinin MT. "Dietary PUFA for preterm and term infants: review
        of clinical studies." *Crit Rev Food Sci Nutr.* 2005;45(3):205-29.

90b.   Birch EE, Garfield S, Hoffman DR, Uauy R, Birch DG. "A randomized
        controlled trial of early dietary supply of long-chain polyunsaturated fatty
        acids and mental development in term infants." *Dev Med Child Neural.* 2000
        Mar;42(3):174-81.

90c.   Carlson SE, Werkman SH. "A randomized trial of visual attention of preterm infants fed docosahexaenoic acid until two months." *Lipids.* 1996 Jan;31(1):85-90.

91.   Moriguchi, Toru; Salem, Norman Jr. "Recovery of brain docosahexaenoate leads to recovery of spatial task performance." *Journal of Neurochemistry.* 87(2):297-309, October 2003.

92.   Gal Dubnov-Raz, MD MSc, Yaron Finkelstein, MD, and Gideon Koren, MD FRCPC. "w-3 fatty acid supplementation during pregnancy For mother, baby, or neither?" Can Fam Physician. 2007 May;53(5): 817-818.

93.   Andrew L. Stoll, M.D. *The Omega-3 Connection.* Simon & Schuster, 2001. pp 99-100.

94.   Dr. Joseph Mercola with Rachael Droege. "What Oil Should You be Cooking With, and Which Should You Avoid?" Web site: Mercola.com. Accessed 9-21-2008. <http://articles.mercola.com/sites/articles/archive/2003/10/15/cooking-oil.aspx>.

95.   James A. Duke, Ph.D. *The Green Pharmacy. Rodale Press.* Emmaus, Pennsylvania. 1997. p.25.

96a.   Fito M, Cladellas M, de la Torre R, et al. "Anti-inflammatory effect of virgin olive oil in stable coronary disease patients: a randomized, crossover, controlled trial." *Eur J Clin Nutr.* 2008 Apr;62(4):570-4. Epub 2007 Mar 21.

96b.   Perez-Jimenez F, Alvarez de Cienfuegos G, et al. "International conference on the healthy effect of virgin olive oil." *Eur Clin Invest.* 2005 Jul;35(7):421-4.

96c.   Beauchamp GK, Keast RS, Morel D, Lin J, Pika J, Han Q, Lee CH, Smith AB, Breslin PA. "Phytochemistry: ibuprofen-like activity in extra-virgin olive oil." *Nature.* 2005 Sep 1;437(7055):45-6.

97.   Perez-Jimenez F, Alvarez de Cienfuegos G, et al. "International conference on the healthy effect of virgin olive oil." *Eur Clin Invest.* 2005 Jul;35(7):421-4.

98a.   Sarah Yang. "The Mediterranean Diet". Web site: WebMD.com Accessed 7/17/2008. <http://www.webmd.com/content/pages/10/1671_50594.htm>.

98b.   "Mediterranean Diet". Web site: American Heart Association. Accessed 9/8/2008. <http://www.americanheart.org/print_presenter.jhtml;jsessionid=5 HPJGR4DKI44OCQFCXP...>.

99.   Dr. Joseph Mercola with Rachael Droege. "What Oil Should You be Cooking With, and Which Should You Avoid?" Web site: Mercola.com. Accessed 9/21/2008. <http://articles.mercola.com/sites/articles/archive/2003/10/15cooking-oil.aspx>.

100.   Mary Enig, PhD. F.A.C.N. "Coconut: On Support of Good Health in the 21st Century" Nutritional Sciences Division, Enig Associates, Inc. 1201 Prosperity Drive, Suite 340, Silver Spring, MD 20904-1689.

101.   Budwig, Johanna . *The Oil-Protein Diet Cookbook.* Apple Publishing Co Ltd. 199 p.7.

102.   Mary Enig, PhD and Sally Fallon. "The Skinny on Fats" *Nourishing Traditions: The Cookbook that Challenges Politically Correct Nutrition and the Diet*

Dictocrats. Second Edition. 1999 New Trends Publishing, Inc. Article accessed from web site on 9/16/2008. <http://www.westonaprice.org/knowyourfats/skinny.html>.

103.   "Cooking Oil Smoke Points". Accessed 5/2/2009. <http/www.goodeatsfanpage.com/CollectedInfo/OilSmokePoints.htm>.

104.   "Research Report - Flaxseed." "Health Perspectives". Web site: Barlean's. Accessed 7/11/2008. <http://www.barleans.com/literature/flax/29-flaxseedbest-source.html>.

105.   Floyd H. Chilton, Ph.D., with Laura Tucker. Win the War Within. Rodale Inc. 2006. pp.92-97, 101-104.

106.   "Essential Fats In Food Oils". Web site: National Institutes of Health. Accessed 6/16/2008. <http://efaeducation.nih.gov/sig/esstable1.html>.

107.   Floyd H. Chilton, Ph.D., with Laura Tucker. Win the War Within. Rodale Inc. 2006. pp. forward, 3-4, 64, 114-124.

108.   Schacter E, Weitzman SA. "Chronic Inflammation and Cancer." Oncology. Vol 16, No 2 (February 2002). pp. 104, 114-116, 124-128.

109.   Mary Enig, PhD. "The Deadliest Fats" BottomLine health. September 2005. pp.3-4.

110.   Budwig, Johanna. Flax Oil as a True Aid Against Arthritis, Heart Infarction, Cancer and Other Diseases. Apple Publishing Co. Ltd. 1994 p.8-9.

111.   Ascherio A. "Trans fatty acids and blood lipids." Atheroscler Suppl. 2006 May;7(2):25-7. Epub 2006 May 19.

112.   Flora Wang. "Natural Trans Fats Have Health Benefits, New Study Finds". University of Alberta. Web site: ScienceDaily (Apr. 5, 2008). Accessed 9/22/2008. <http://www.sciencedaily.com/releases/2008/04/080402152140.htm>.

113.   Eller FJ, List GR, Teel JA, Steidley KR, Adlof RO. "Preparation of spread oils meeting U.S. Food and Drug Administration Labeling requirements for trans fatty acids via pressure-controlled hydrogen." J Agric Fod Chem. 2005 Jul 27;53(15):5982-4.

114.   Grandgirard A, Bourre JM, Julliard F, Homayoun P, Dumont O, Piciotti M, Sebedio JL. "Incorporation of trans long-chain n-3 polyunsaturated fatty acids in rat brain structures and retina." Lipids. 1994 Apr;29(4):251-8.

115.   Ann-Charlotte Granholm, Heather A Bimonte-Nelson, Alfred B Morre, Matthew E. Nelson Linnea R. Freeman, Kumar Sambamurti. "Effects of a Saturated Fat and High Cholesterol Diet on Memory and Hippocampal Morphology in the Middle-Aged Rat." Journal of Alzheimer's Disease. 1387-2877 (Print) 1875-8908 (Online), Volume 14, Number 2 / 2008 133-145.

116a. Pisani LP, Oyama LM, Bueno AA, Biz C, Albuquerque KT, Ribeiro EB, Oller do Nascimento CM. "Hydrogenated fat intake during pregnancy and lactation modifies serum lipid profile and adipokine mRNA in 21-day-old rats." Nutrition. 2008 Mar;24(3):255-61. Epub 2008 Jan 4.

116b. Tinoco SM, Sichieri R, Setta CL, Moura AS, do Carmo MG. "Trans fatty acids from milk of Brazilian mothers of premature infants." *J Paediatr Child Health*. 2008 Jan;44(1-2):50-6. Epub 2007 Jul 19.

116c. Marhol P, Dlouhy P, Rambousková J, Pokorny R, Wiererova O, Hrncírová D, Procházka B, Andel M. "Higher content of C18:1 trans fatty acids in early human milk fat of Roma breast-feeding women." *Ann Nutr Metab*. 2007;51(5):461-7. Epub 2007 Noiv 20.

116d. Albuquerque KT, Sardinha FL, Telles MM, Watanabe RL, Nascimento CM, Tavares do Carmo MG, Ribeiro EB. "Intake of trans fatty acid-rich hydrogenated fat during pregnancy and lactation inhibits the hypophagic effect of central insulin in the adult offspring." *Nutrition*. 2006 Jul-Aug;22(7-8):820-9.

116e. Mojska H, Socha P, Socha J, Soplinska E, Jaroszewska-Balicka W, Szponar L. "Trans fatty acids in human milk in Poland and their association with breast-feeding mothers' diets." *Acta Paediatr*. 2003 Dec;92(12):1381-7.

117. Budwig, Johanna . *Flax Oil as a True Aid Against Arthritis, Heart Infarction, Cancer and Other Diseases*. Apple Publishing Co. Ltd. 1994 pp.8-9, 18.

118. Shui-Lin Niu, Drake C. Mitchell, and Burton J. Litman. "Trans Fatty Acid Derived Phospholipids Show Increased Membrane Cholesterol and Reduced Receptor Activation as Compared to Their Cis Analogs." *Biochemistry*. 2005 March 22; 44(11): 4458-4465.

119a. Siguel EN, Lerman RH. "Trans-fatty acid patterns in patients with angiographically documented coronary artery disease." *Am J Cardiol*. 1993 Apr 15;71(11):916-20.

119b. Mozaffarian D, Abdollahi M, Campos H, Houshiarrad A, Willett WC. "Consumption of trans fats and estimated effects on coronary heart disease in Iran." *Eur J Clin Nutr*. 2007 Aug;61(8):1004-10. Epub 2007 Jan 31.

119c. Hodgson JM, Wahlqvist ML, Boxall JA, Balazs ND. "Platelet trans fatty acids in relation to angiographically assessed coronary artery disease." *Atherosclerosis*. 1996 Feb;120(1-2):147-54.

120. "Molecular Biology of the Cell". "IV. Internal Organization of the Cell". "10. Membrane Structure". Web site: National Institutes of Health. Accessed 9/21/2008. <http://www.ncbi.nlm.gov/books/bv.fcgi?rid=mboc4. section.1864>.

121. Mary Enig, PhD and Sally Fallon. "The Skinny on Fats" *Nourishing Traditions: The Cookbook that Challenges Politically Correct Nutrition and the Diet Dictocrats*. Second Edition. 1999 New Trends Publishing, Inc. Article accessed on web site 9/16/2008. <http://www.westonaprice.org/knowyourfats/skinny. html>.

122. Chet Day. "Strict Vegan Diets May Be Dangerous, Especially for Expectant Mothers and Children." July 14, 2000. Updated October 22, 2002. Web site: Chet Day's Health & Beyond. Accessed 9/18/2008. <http://chetday.com/ vegandietdangers.htm>.

123. Mary Enig, PhD and Sally Fallon. "The Skinny on Fats" *Nourishing Traditions: The Cookbook that Challenges Politically Correct Nutrition and the Diet Dictocrats*. Second Edition. 1999 New Trends Publishing, Inc. Article accessed on web site 9/16/2008. <http://www.westonaprice.org/knowyourfats/skinny.html>.

124. Budwig, Johanna . *Flax Oil as a True Aid Against Arthritis, Heart Infarction, Cancer and Other Diseases*. Apple Publishing Co. Ltd. 1994 p.4.

125. Budwig, Johanna . *Flax Oil as a True Aid Against Arthritis, Heart Infarction, Cancer and Other Diseases*. Apple Publishing Co. Ltd. 1994 pp.11, 18-20,34, 43-44.

126. Chris Turner. "Budwig Flax Oil Diet." Web site: Positive Health. Accessed 7/3/2006. <http://www.positivehealth.com/PERMIT/ARTICLES/Nutrition/turner60.htm>.

127. Budwig, Johanna. *Flax Oil as a True Aid Against Arthritis, Heart Infarction, Cancer and Other Diseases*. Apple Publishing Co. Ltd. 1994 pp.7, 11.

128. Budwig, Johanna. *Flax Oil as a True Aid Against Arthritis, Heart Infarction, Cancer and Other Diseases*. Apple Publishing Co. Ltd. 1994 pp.12-13.

129. Budwig, Johanna. *Flax Oil as a True Aid Against Arthritis, Heart Infarction, Cancer and Other Diseases*. Apple Publishing Co. Ltd. 1994 pp.32-33, 35.

130a. Guixiang Zhao, Terry D Etherton, Keith R Martin, Peter J Gillies, Sheila G West and Penny M Kris-Etherton. "Dietary alpha-linolenic acid inhibits proinflammatory cytokine production by peripheral blood mononuclear cells in hypercholesterolemic subjects". *American Journal of Clinical Nutrition*. Vol. 85, no. 2, 385-391, February 2007.

130b. GE Caughey, E Mantzioris, RA Gibson, LG Cleland and MJ James. "The effect of human tumor necrosis factor alpha and interleukin 1 beta production of diets enriched in n-3 fatty acids from vegetable oil or fish oil." *American Journal of Clinical Nutrition*, Vol 63, 116-122.

131a. Brower V. "Feeding the Flame: New Research Adds to Role of Inflammation in Cancer Development." *Journal of the National Cancer Institute*. Vol 97, No 4, February 16, 2005.

131b. Schacter E, Weitzman SA. "Chronic Inflammation and Cancer." *Oncology*. Vol 16, No 2 (February 2002).

132. Budwig, Johanna. *Flax Oil as a True Aid Against Arthritis, Heart Infarction, Cancer and Other Diseases*. Apple Publishing Co. Ltd. 1994 p.35.

133. Budwig, Johanna. *Flax Oil as a True Aid Against Arthritis, Heart Infarction, Cancer and Other Diseases*. Apple Publishing Co. Ltd. 1994 p.35.

134. Budwig, Johanna. *Flax Oil as a True Aid Against Arthritis, Heart Infarction, Cancer and Other Diseases*. Apple Publishing Co. Ltd. 1994 pp.9,14.

135. Simopoulos AP. "Summary of the NATO advanced research workshop on dietary omega 3 and omega 6 fatty acids: biological effects and nutritional essentiality." *J Nutr*. 1989 Apr;119(4):521-8.

136a. Chen J, Tan KP, Ward WE, Thompson LU. "Exposure to flaxseed or its purified lignan during suckling inhibits chemically induced rat mammary tumorigenesis." *Exp. Biol Med* (Maywood). 2003;228:951-958.

136b. Chen J, Thompson LU. "Lignans and tamoxifen, alone or in combination, reduce human breast cancer cell adhesion, invasion and migration in vitro." *Breast Cancer Res Treat.* 2003 Jul;80(2):163-70.

136c. Dabrosin C, Chen J, Wang L, Thompson LU. "Flaxseed inhibits metastasis and decreases extracellular vascular endothelial growth factor in human breast cancer xenografts." *Cancer Lett.* 2002 Nov 8;185(1):31-7.

136d. Chen J, Stavro PM, Thompson LU. "Dietary flaxseed inhibits human breast cancer growth and metastasis and downregulates expression of insulin-like growth factor and epidermal growth factor receptor." *Nutr Cancer.* 2002;43:187-192.

136e. Thompson LU, Rickard SE, Orcheson LJ, Seidl MM. "Flaxseed and its lignan and oil components reduce mammary tumor growth at a late stage of carcinogenesis." *Carcinogenesis.* 1996 Jun;17(6):1373-6.

136f. Thompson LU, Seidl MM, Richard SE, Orcheson LJ, Fong HH. "Antitumorigenic effect of a mammalian lignan precursor from flaxseeds." Nutr. Cancer. 1996;26(2):159-65.

136g. Serraiano M, Thompson LU. "The effect of flaxseed supplementation on early risk markers for mammary carcinogenesis." *Cancer Lett.* 1991 Nov;60(2):135-42.

136h. Trentin GA, Moody J, Torous DK, Thompson LU, Heddle JA. "The influence of dietary flaxseed and other grains, fruits and vegetables on the frequency of spontaneous chromosomal damage in mice." *Mutat Res.* 2004 Jul 13;551(1-2):213-22.

137. Serraino M, Thompson LU. "Flaxseed supplementation and early markers of colon carcinogenesis." *Cancer Lett.* 1992 Apr 15;63(2):159-65.

138a. Demark-Wahnefried W, Robertson CN, Walther PJ, Polascik TJ, Paulson DF, Vollner RT. "Pilot study to explore effects of low-fat, flaxseeds-supplemented diet on proliferation of benign prostatic epithelium and prostate-specific antigen." *Urology.* 2004 May;63(5):900-4.

138b. Lin X, Gingrich Jr, Bao W, Li J, Haroon ZA, Demark-Wahnefried W. "Effect of flaxseed supplementation on prostatic carcinoma in transgenic mice." *Urology.* 2002;60:919-924.

138c. Demark-Wahnefried W, Price DT, Polascik TJ, Robertson CN, Anderson EE, Paulson DF, Walther PJ, Gannon M, Vollmer RT. "Pilot study of dietary fat restriction and flaxseed supplementation in men with prostate cancer before surgery: exploring the effects on hormonal levels, prostate-specific antigen, and histopathologic features." *Urology.* 2001 Jul;58(1):47-52.

139. Yan L, Yee JA, Li D, McGuire MH, Thompson LU. "Dietary flaxseed supple-

mentation and experimental metastasis of melanoma cells in mice." *Cancer Lett.* 1998;124:181-186.

140.   "Questions and Answers". Web site: Flax Lignan Information Bureau. Accessed 9/19/2008. <http://www.flaxlignaninfo.com/rsg_flax/didifolder.nsf/ htmlViewDocuments/40517D975C...>.

141a. Thompson LU, Richard SE, Orcheson LJ, Seidl MM. "Flaxseed and its lignan and oil components reduce mammary tumor growth at a late stage of carcinogenesis." *Carcinogenesis.* 1996,17:1373-1376.

141b. Thompson LU, Seidl MM, Rickard SE, Orcheson LJ, Fong HH. "Antitumorigenic effect of a mammalian lignan precurser from flaxseed." *Nutr Cancer.* 1996, 26:159-165.

142.   "Tips on Using Flax oil". Beckwith Family web site. Accessed 9/21/2008. <http://www.beckwithfamily.com/usage.html>.

143.   "FLAX - A Health and Nutrition Primer". "TABLE 1". "Proximate composition of flax based on common measures". Web site: Flax Council of Canada. Accessed 9/12/2008. <http://www.flaxcouncil.ca>.

144.   Budwig, Johanna. *Flax Oil as a True Aid Against Arthritis, Heart Infarction, Cancer and Other Diseases.* Apple Publishing Co. Ltd. 1994 pp.22-23.

145.   Budwig, Johanna. *Flax Oil as a True Aid Against Arthritis, Heart Infarction, Cancer and Other Diseases.* Apple Publishing Co. Ltd. 1994 p.22.

146a. Duan JK. "Additional Data on the Storage Stability of Milled Flaxseed." *Journal of American Oil Chemists Society.* 78 no. 1(2001): 105-106.

146b. Malcolmson LJ, Przybylski R, Duan JK. "Storage Stability of Milled Flaxseed." *Journal of American Oil Chemists Society.* 77 no. 3 (2000): 235-238.

147.   Budwig, Johanna. *Flax Oil as a True Aid Against Arthritis, Heart Infarction, Cancer and Other Diseases.* Apple Publishing Co. Ltd. 1994 pp.6-9.

148.   "Research Report - Flaxseed". Web site: Barleans.com. Accessed 9/26/2008. <http://barleans.com/literature/flax/29-flaxseed-best-source.html>.

149a. Nesbitt PD, Lamy, Thompson LU. "Human metabolism of mammalian lignan precursors in raw and processed flaxseed." *American Journal of Clinical Nutrition.* 36 (1999)L 549-555.

149b. Cunnane SC, Hamadeh MJ, Liede AC, Thompson LU, Wolever TM, Jenkins DJ. "Nutritional attributes of traditional flaxseed in healthy young adults." *American Journal of Clinical Nutrition.* 61 (1995): 62-68.

149c. Cunnane SC, Ganuli S, Menard C, Liede C, Hamadeh MJ, Chen Z-Y, Wolever TM, Jenkins DJ. "High alpha-linolenic acid flaxseed: some nutritional properties in humans." *British Journal of Nutrition.* 69 (1993): 443-453.

149d. Chen Z-y, Ratnayake WMN Cunnane SC. "Stability of flaxseed during baking." *Journal of American Oil Chemists Society.* 71 (1992): 629-632.

150.   "Research Report - Flaxseed". Web site: Barleans.com. Accessed 9/26/2008. <http://barleans.com/literature/flax/29-flaxseed-best-source.html>.

151.   "Frequently Asked Questions". "Can the flax oil be frozen?" Web site accessed
       9/21/2008. <http://www.budwigflax.com/Articles/FAQs.html>.
152.   "Flaxseed". Web site: University of Maryland. Accessed 10/18/2007. <http://
       www.umm.edu/altmed/articles/flaxseed>.
153.   Budwig, Johanna. *Flax Oil as a True Aid Against Arthritis, Heart Infarction,
       Cancer and Other Diseases.* Apple Publishing Co. Ltd. 1994 p.8.
154.   Budwig, Johanna. *Flax Oil as a True Aid Against Arthritis, Heart Infarction,
       Cancer and Other Diseases.* Apple Publishing Co. Ltd. 1994 pp.16-20.
155.   Budwig, Johanna. *Flax Oil as a True Aid Against Arthritis, Heart Infarction,
       Cancer and Other Diseases.* Apple Publishing Co. Ltd. 1994 pp.46-50.
156.   Budwig, Johanna. *Flax Oil as a True Aid Against Arthritis, Heart Infarction,
       Cancer and Other Diseases.* Apple Publishing Co. Ltd. 1994 pp.20-21, 33.
157.   Budwig, Johanna. *Flax Oil as a True Aid Against Arthritis, Heart Infarction,
       Cancer and Other Diseases.* Apple Publishing Co. Ltd. 1994 p.12.
158a. Dubnov G, Berry EM. "Polyunsaturated Fatty acids, insulin resistance, and
       atherosclerosis: is inflammation the connecting link?" *Metab Syndr Relat
       Disord.* 2004 Jun;2(2):124-8.
158b. Simopoulos AP. "is insulin resistance influenced by dietary linoleic acid and
       trans fatty acids?" *Free Radic Biol Med.* 1994 Oct;17(4):367-72.
159.   Bessby B, Unsitupa M, Mermansen K, et al. "Substituting dietary saturated for
       monounsaturated fat impairs insulin sensitivity in healthy men and women:
       The KANWU Study." *Diabetologia.* 2001 Mar;44(3):312-9.
160.   William R. Leonard, Marcia L. Robertson, J.Josh Snodgrass, Christopher
       W. Kuzawa. "Metabolic correlates of homonid brain evolution" *Comparative
       Biochemistry and Physiology* Part A 136 (2003) 5-15.

CHAPTER 14

Candida Overgrowth— The Silent Thief of This Modern Age

If our car has a leaky exhaust pipe, it allows the waste products to pollute the air inside the car—it will make us sick.

LIKE a leaky exhaust pipe, a similar condition can happen in our bodies when *Candida* overgrowth spews out its toxic waste products and pollutes our bodies. *Candida* overgrowth can poke holes in the digestive tract, allowing undigested food particles and waste products to enter our bloodstream. Inflammation in our body and a multitude of various symptoms and syndromes may result. You must listen to what your body is telling you and pay attention to the warning lights. The good news is that your body has the ability to heal itself if you take the proper action. The bad news is that for some of us, we have gone for many, many years sputtering along, our mind and body operating at far less than our full potential. The cost to ourselves and those around us is huge; it can make the price of a new automobile seem small. The cost really adds up when we consider such things as underperformance at work, lost career opportunities, accidents that could have been prevented, related health problems, and damaged relationships in our family and personal lives. This condition demands serious attention. It is amazing that *Candida* overgrowth has been overlooked by many medical professionals however, it is increasingly being recognized as an illness. Practitioners who recognize and treat this condition indicate it is more widespread than originally thought.

John Parks Trowbridge, MD, author of *The Yeast Syndrome*, writes, "Almost everyone in the world exhibits some minor complication from the disease, but large numbers of people show signs and symptoms that have them functioning at very low levels of wellness, if not outright sickness. Approximately 30% of all persons around the world above the age of twelve—mostly females—are suffering with yeast-related illness caused by the fungus within us known as *Candida albicans*." Trowbridge is referring to the industrialized, or modernized, countries of the world.[1]

Everybody has a form of this yeast, but it is normally kept in check by our immune system. However, a weakened immune system and other factors can allow *Candida* yeast to overgrow and change into an aggressive fungus infection called candidiasis, or *Candida* overgrowth. *Candida* overgrowth is a nasty, hard-to-detect infection and a common cause of LGS (Leaky Gut Syndrome). The fungus can become anchored inside the intestine wall where it can grow thread-like tentacles that poke holes through the intestine wall, allowing undigested food particles, toxins, and waste products to pass directly into the bloodstream.

FOUR WAYS CANDIDA OVERGROWTH DEGRADES OUR HEALTH

1. *Candida* overgrowth degrades our health by causing improper digestion. This stresses the body and challenges the immune system. Because nutrients are not properly absorbed, our bodies may be deprived of certain nutrients no matter how healthy we eat.

2. *Candida* overgrowth degrades our health by dumping its toxins and bacteria into the bloodstream. Candida affects other organs and tissues, impairing their function. *Candida* poisons

the body by releasing its own toxins and allowing other toxins and harmful bacteria to enter the bloodstream. Over 100 waste products given off by *Candida albicans* have been recognized,[2] some of which are highly toxic and can damage tissues.[3] The liver works extra hard trying to clean up the overload of toxins in the blood but cannot keep up. The whole body becomes sick.

Once in the bloodstream, these toxins and bacteria affect other organs and tissues, including the brain, and may result in many psychological symptoms. Dr. C. Orian Truss, author of *The Missing Diagnosis*, describes many symptoms, including *anxiety, loss of self confidence, depression, memory loss, difficulty concentrating and reasoning, impaired intellectual function, and various emotional abnormalities such as uncontrollable crying (in women).*[4] *Candida* overgrowth can also alter hormone balance (especially in women).[5] Dr. Truss recently published his second book, *The Missing Diagnosis II*, in 2009 which he provides a recommended diet, more studies and charts based on his 56 years of medical experience and research with *Candida*. He states that *Candida's* toxins stiffens cell membranes, likely reducing the transport of nutrients into our cells. He further states how stiffened membranes makes cells resistant to insulin. Insulin is secreted by the pancreas, released into the blood stream and allows the glucose (blood sugar) to enter cells in order to produce energy. He believes insulin resistance is a key cause of fatigue and problems with short-term memory and concentration. (This condition also provides some insight into type II diabetes mellitus which is cell's resistance to insulin).[6] His patients show significant improvement in these conditions following anti-*Candida* therapy.

3. *Candida* overgrowth degrades our health by suppressing the immune system.[7] This opens the door for other illnesses and

diseases to develop. *Candida* overgrowth can also mimic other illnesses or be a factor in their cause.[8]

4. *Candida* overgrowth degrades our health and well-being by causing people to be *irritable, less mentally alert, less coordinated, and, in turn, more likely to underperform at work, more likely to cause an accident, or simply more likely to say and do stupid things.*

SYMPTOMS OF CANDIDA OVERGROWTH

The three most common symptoms as reported by the late Dr. William Crook are *fatigue, headache, and depression.*[9] Dr. Crook is credited with educating the general public about this illness in his popular 1983 book, *The Yeast Connection Handbook.* Crook devoted his career and the rest of his life to helping children and adults overcome *Candida*, even when it meant going against popular medical opinion. He wrote 14 books and published numerous medical articles.

Dr. C. Orian Truss explains that testing for *Candida* is unreliable and therefore, relies on multiple symptoms and signs for his clinical picture.[10] He lists additional symptoms of *Candida* overgrowth, most of which improved or went away following anti-*Candida* treatment:

- *Explosive irritability, fatigue, lethargy, "inability to cope," dizziness, clumsiness, "spacey or foggy feelings,"* insomnia or excessive sleepiness, hypothyroidism (the thyroid gland not producing enough hormones resulting in feeling tired and weak)
- Migraine and sinus headaches; postnasal drainage; low blood sugar (hypoglycemia); digestion problems such as heartburn, indigestion, "sour stomach," abdominal bloating, rectal itch, diarrhea, constipation, or both
- Acne, asthma, hives, hay fever, sensitivities to food
- Chemical intolerances to odors such as colognes, exhaust fumes, hair sprays, cigarette smoke, and chemical odors

- Feeling worse on damp or muggy days or in moldy places[11]

Other sources list the following symptoms:

- sugar cravings, *"fogged in"* or *"isolated"* feeling, *dizziness, recurring depression,* gas, urinary tract infections, prostatitis, hay fever, postnasal drip, habitual coughing, frequent colds, sore throat, athlete's foot, skin rash, psoriasis, cold extremities, arthritis-like symptoms,[12] sensitivity to perfume and fabric odors, *"ringing in the ears",* and *"fuzzy thinking."*[13]

One informative Web site describes more symptoms:

- "Incapacitating fatigue and *problems with concentration* and *short-term memory,"* "flu-like symptoms such as pain in the joints and muscle, extreme tightness in shoulders and neck," acid reflux, brown mucus in the back of the throat, blisters in the mouth/tongue/throat, white-coated tongue, *"an aversion to being touched or jumping,"* crawling skin, and chronic dental problems
- "Chronic sinus problems and headaches including migraines"
- "Visual disturbances may include blurring, sensitivity to light, and eye pain"
- *"Panic attacks, personality changes,* and *mood swings"* (irrational rage or crying for no reason)
- *"Fear of talking to people or any kind of confrontation"*[14]

Refer to the books and Web sites listed later in this chapter for additional symptoms and information on *Candida.*

In women, the condition is more common due to monthly hormonal fluctuations, use of the birth control pill, and past antibiotic treatment. *Candida* has been blamed for severe premenstrual tension and recurring vaginal and bladder infections. *Candida* can also cause abnormal hormone function. Its effects on the brain include *bouts of depression, "uncontrollable crying," and "explosive irritability."*[15] A woman may be told time and time again she has a psychological problem and needs to undergo psychiatric therapy. It can be devastating to her role as wife and mother and to her career. A marriage may become seriously strained if a woman's husband (or ex-husband) views her as "not the person I married," and he may feel he married the wrong person. The tragedy is that a proper diagnosis and simple antifungal treatment may have prevented the ruin of some of the best years of some people's lives. Endometriosis also appears in a large number of women with *Candida* overgrowth.[16] Endometriosis occurs when uterus-like tissue grows in locations outside the uterus. It can also be a cause of infertility.

Because men do not experience wide hormonal fluctuations and are less likely to seek medical attention, *Candida* symptoms move in slowly and may go undetected unless specifically looked for. Most men do not display the emotional swings seen in women. *Candida's* effect on a man's brain may cause him to have *"chronic ill-temper"* or *"bad disposition," "low-grade depression,"* and *chronic fatigue.*[17] The people who know him may say, "That's just the way he is and he won't change." In addition, it may impair his memory and concentration and may reduce his ability to communicate. At times he may be out of touch with himself and reality. He may have a lot of repressed anger but cannot explain why he feels angry. He may simply blame those around him for his unhappiness and failures. His marriage and family suffers, and his career may suffer. Life is much more difficult for him than it should be. Past failures and the fear of more failures multiply the pain. Likewise, his wife (or ex-wife) expresses, "He's not the man I married."

In teenage boys, *Candida* is just as devastating. He may appear *depressed or ill tempered* or may be lethargic and lack motivation. Because his memory and concentration are impaired, his schoolwork suffers. School dropouts, both boys and girls, show these symptoms. On the other hand, even if the teen boy is motivated, he will underperform in his achievements despite his maximal efforts. If his acne is severe, he may have been put on tetracycline, a very strong antibiotic that stimulates the growth of *Candida*.[18] Physical weakness and impaired physical coordination will degrade his performance in gym class and athletics.

Teenage girls are particularly susceptible to *Candida* because of fluctuating hormones at puberty. Symptoms of improper hormone balance include excessive cramping and frequent vaginal yeast infections, which provide additional clues to solving the *Candida* puzzle. Psychological effects may include *"abrupt personality change"* accompanied by *depression, "uncontrollable crying" (for no reason), and "explosive irritability"* as each menstrual period draws near.[19]

Dr. Truss tells of a girl who had been healthy for the first 12 years of her life until she was treated for mild acne with the antibiotic tetracycline for 2 1/2 months. "She promptly developed acute yeast vaginitis, constipation, and headache, none of which had been problems prior to this time." Her physical and mental health had become so poor she had to drop out of school. Tetracycline was stopped for 4 1/2 months. Upon restarting tetracycline, her brain function suffered in the form of *depression, anxiety,* and *crying* that same day. Within 4 days of restarting tetracycline, she broke out in hives and developed severe bronchial asthma and had 2 periods a month. She also had great *difficulty with memory and concentration and talked of suicide.* After taking the antifungal medication Nystatin, the asthma and hives cleared up quickly. There was a gradual improvement in her mental confusion and abnormal emotions. She later was able to return to school. This case illustrates *Candida's* combined effect on the brain, emotions, and body.[20]

In children, various symptoms of *Candida* overgrowth may follow after the first use of antibiotics. These symptoms may include *hyperactivity, irritability, short attention span, learning difficulties,* and behavior problems. Fungus also has been linked to problems with the nervous system in some autistic children.[21] Other manifestations of *Candida* include restlessness, discontentment, recurrent ear infections, diaper rash, diarrhea, constipation, poor appetite, erratic sleep patterns, runny nose (with clear discharge), and oral thrush (white fungal infection on the tongue).[22]

We owe much gratitude to C. Orian Truss for his pioneering work in discovering *Candida albicans* as the missing diagnosis for many people's suffering. He successfully treated many patients using anti-*Candida* therapy. His treatment of choice is the prescription antifungal medication Nystatin, and, in some cases, a *Candida* vaccine.

Nystatin was discovered by two women researchers as a naturally occurring fungus in the soil that would knock out all other fungus on contact. It was named after the New York State Health Department, after its discovery in 1950; it has proven over the years to be highly effective against *Candida* with little or no side effects.[23] The two discoverers, Elizabeth Lee Hazen and Rachel Fuller Brown, were inducted into the National Inventors Hall of Fame in 1994.[24] More of Dr. Truss's cases' studies are described at the end of the chapter.

Drunkenness—Without Drinking?

In the 1970s, Japanese researcher Dr. Kazuo Iwata at the University of Tokyo discovered something quite strange—that *Candida* overgrowth can cause the body to become an "automatic brewery," creating its own alcohol (ethanol) by fermentation of sugars within the digestive tract.[25] This condition became known as "drunk syndrome" because these people "feel drunk" and can have blood alcohol levels several times beyond the legal limit for driving even though they consumed no alcohol.[26]

Toxic Effects of Candida Infection

One of the most toxic chemicals given off by *Candida* is acetaldehyde. Acetaldehyde is the chemical most responsible for hangover symptoms when excessive alcohol is consumed, including headache, nausea, and increased heart rate. Acetaldehyde *impairs brain function, impairs memory and concentration,*[27] and is believed to be about 6 times more toxic than alcohol.[28] Acetaldehyde is highly reactive and contributes to liver damage in alcoholics.[29] New research indicates acetaldehyde may also increase the risk of certain cancers if the body is not detoxified.[30] Acetaldehyde is produced when the body metabolizes (breaks down) alcohol. Acetaldehyde is also found in cigarette smoke, car exhausts, and is very similar to the embalming fluid formaldehyde (hence the drinking term "getting embalmed").[31]

It is also believed that *Candida* toxins played a part in the tragic deaths of women during the 1970s from toxic shock syndrome. It was discovered that *Candida* can increase the toxicity of staphylococcal infections by as much as 100,000 times, which gives some insight into this tragedy.[32]

Another toxic chemical given off by *Candida* is tartaric acid, which inhibits the production of glucose (blood sugar), the main fuel for the brain. This can result in hypoglycemia (low blood sugar), which can lead to *brain fog* because there is not enough fuel for the brain.[33] Tartaric acid causes muscle weakness, can damage the muscles and kidneys, and may play an important role in autism and fibromyalgia. (Fibromyalgia is a disease with symptoms of "foggy thinking," depression, and pain in the muscles and joints.)[34] You can read more about it at www.greatplainslaboratory.com/yeast.html.

It is no wonder *Candida* sufferers feel "sick all over" and often have several mental and physical issues going on at the same time. More on this later.

CAUSES OF CANDIDA INFECTION

The causes of Candida overgrowth may be many; however, physicians who recognize this condition and have treated many patients point to the use of broad-spectrum antibiotics as the chief cause.[35] Antibiotics strip the digestive tract of both good and bad bacteria. With much of the beneficial bacteria destroyed, *Candida* grows rapidly unless the immune system is strong enough to stop it.

Some experts suggest that antibiotics used during infancy or a mother's yeast infection during pregnancy may result in the child's immune system tolerating *Candida* rather than fighting it.[36] This would explain why some people's immune systems do *not* fight *Candida*, giving it an opportunity to take over and run its ugly course.

Other contributors to *Candida* overgrowth include the following:

- Having had thrush, a "yeasty diaper rash," or cradle cap as a baby[37]
- Low stomach acid[38]
- Hormonal changes in women[39]
- Use of the birth control pill[40]
- Too much sugar in the diet[41] along with too many empty carbohydrates (foods made of refined white flour, lots of sugar, but very little vitamins and fiber)
- Drinking fermented beverages—especially wine and beer[42]
- Steroid medications[43]
- A weakened immune system caused by chemotherapy, radiation, a major injury, surgery, radiation, or other medications[44]
- Exposure to herbicides,[45] environmental toxins, chemicals, molds, cigarette smoke, and heavy metals, particularly lead from old lead water pipes and automobile exhaust from leaded gasoline (lead is no longer added to gasoline); some studies suggest mercury (from amalgam tooth fillings) can also weaken the immune system[46]

RECOGNIZING AND DIAGNOSING CANDIDA OVERGROWTH

Entire books, publications, web sites, and treatment programs are devoted to this complex subject, some of which I have listed in this chapter. You should discuss a treatment program with your medical practitioner. Be aware that many medical practitioners have not been trained to recognize and treat *Candida* overgrowth, so you may have to be assertive in presenting your case. The U.S. Centers for Disease Control and Prevention (CDC) recognizes candidiasis as an illness[47] while the American Association of Allergy, Asthma, and Immunology (AAAI) in 1986 issued the following statement: "The concept is speculative and unproven … There is no published proof that *Candida albicans* is responsible for the syndrome."[48]

The important issue is for you to get well. In addition to the symptoms previously described, the most common test is a questionnaire available on several Web sites: www.yeastconnection.com and www.candidasupport.org. You and your health practitioner can discuss what testing is right for you. See www.genovadiagnostics.com and www.greatplainslaboratory.com for additional tests.

OVERCOMING CANDIDA

Overcoming *Candida* involves attacking it several ways:

1. Reduce its food supply—sugar, empty carbohydrates (foods made from refined white flour), and alcohol. This alone will help starve and kill off some *Candida*.
2. Take probiotic supplements to replenish the beneficial bacteria in the digestive tract. Beneficial bacteria crowds out *Candida* and bad bacteria.
3. After 1 week of cutting out sugar, take antifungal supplements or medications to kill off more *Candida* and keep it under control.
4. Take enzymes and other supplements to help with digestion and boost the immune system.

Getting *Candida* under control is a gradual process and will take at least 3 to 4 months.[49]

Here are the steps in more detail:

1. **No sugar! No alcohol!** Since *Candida* thrives on sugar and alcohol, you must do your best to cut off its food supply. Special diets such as the Feingold diet attempt to eliminate all forms of sugar.
   A 1993 study at St. Jude Children's Hospital in Memphis, Tennessee, showed that mice that were fed dextrose (a liquid

form of sugar) had *200 times greater growth* of *Candida albicans* as compared to mice that were fed only water.[50]

There is disagreement among health practitioners about how extreme a diet is required. Some practitioners say to cut out all forms of sugar, including all fruits, for a period of time. Other practitioners say to eliminate foods with added sugars (including many processed foods). Small amounts of these foods may be added as healing progresses. You and your practitioner must decide on a treatment program that will work for you.

Other forms of sugar to avoid are anything that ends with *-ose*, such as dextrose, fructose, and sucrose. Remember that milk contains the sugar lactose, and, therefore, you may have to reduce your milk consumption for a period of time. Commercially produced fruit juices often contain a lot of sugar.

I prefer to sweeten foods with stevia, a natural herbal sweetener. Just 1/2 teaspoon of stevia powder has the equivalent sweetness of 1 cup of sugar. Note: Stevia has recently been approved by the FDA as a food additive.

2. *Do* **follow the steps for healing Leaky Gut Syndrome.**
Reduce dried fruits, canned fruit juice, and refined white flour products (bread, pasta, and pastries). Try to eat whole grain foods unless you suspect gluten may be a problem. Gluten is present in wheat and other grains as discussed in chapter 12. There is dispute among health professionals whether yeast-containing foods should be avoided or not. Many yeasts are good for you and are rich in vitamins and enzymes.

3. **Take probiotic supplements such as *acidophilus*, *Bifidobacteria*, and *Lactobacillus bulgaricus*.** Dr. Atkins calls these "The Three Musketeers" of friendly flora probiotics,[51]

and they can help re-establish the beneficial bacteria in the digestive tract.

You can also eat yogurt, but make sure it contains active bacteria cultures. Many sources advise eating plain yogurt on a regular basis to help restore the beneficial bacteria but to avoid flavored yogurt because of the added sugar. Dr. William Crook always recommended probiotic supplements to all his patients, especially those with yeast-related health problems.[52]

Some fruits and vegetables contain a special type of sugar called fructooligosaccharides (FOS) that can help nurture the growth of beneficial bacteria. Bananas have the highest amounts of FOS. Garlic, onions, and some other vegetables also have this special sugar.[53] (Remember that you may have to reduce some fruits for a time in order to reduce sugar.)

4. **After 1 week of cutting out sugar, begin taking antifungal supplements or medications.** The 1-week wait is recommended for this reason: *Candida* fungi will begin to die off as the food supply (sugar) is cut off. Taking supplements and/or medications increases the die-off. If too much die-off occurs, then large amounts of debris and toxins are released and may make your symptoms worse. This is called "die-off" or "Hexheimer reaction."[54] Reactions to die-off can be minimized by taking antifungal supplements or medications in small doses first, then gradually increasing the dose as time goes on. Dr. Truss's medication of choice is oral Nystatin.[55] Other prescription anti-fungal medications include Diflucan, Lamisil, Sporanox, and Nizoral.

Because testing for *Candida* can be inconclusive, Dr. Truss recommends taking Nystatin for 5 to 6 weeks along with a strict diet that avoids sugar, yeasts and reduces carbohydrates. If a patient's condition improved, then *Candida* was a probable cause. He recommends taking 1/8 teaspoon of oral Nystatin powder after each meal and at bed time and for women, using vaginal Nystatin two times a day. He doubles the dose of oral Nystatin each week until symptoms improve up to a limit of 2 teaspoons four times a day.[56] Note that some liquid forms of Nystatin medications may contain large amounts of sucrose (sugar) which is bad for the teeth and works against the treatment.

Herbal antifungal supplements and programs can be obtained from these Web sites: www.yeastconnection.com, www.candidafree.net, www.candidapage.com, www.arthritistrust.org, and www.greatplainslaboratory.com.

Foods and supplements that have antifungal actions include the following: ginger,[57] garlic,[58] caprylic acid,[59] virgin olive oil,[60] goldenseal,[61] citrus seed extract (some experts believe citrus seed extract to be as effective as Nystatin and caprylic acid),[62] aloe vera,[63] cranberry, Echinacea, goldenrod, licorice, lemongrass, taheebo tea (pau-d'arco), purslane, sage, turmeric,[64] cinnamon, oregano, thyme,[65] alfalfa,[66] barberry, fennel, ginseng, rosemary,[67] and anise.[68] You can use stevia, anise, and licorice for sweeteners instead of sugar.

Caprylic acid is a naturally occurring fatty acid that is derived from coconut oil and was discovered in the 1960s by Dr. Irene Neuhauser at the University of Illinois. It has strong antifungal properties and, since it is a food product, does not require a prescription and can be easily obtained from mail-order vitamin stores. Some professionals claim caprylic acid is just as effective as the prescription drug Nystatin. Dr. Neuhauser also recommends taking psyllium powder supplements with caprylic acid. This helps the caprylic acid remain in the digestive tract for a longer time, increasing its effectiveness.[69] Also, psyllium will help to scrape away *Candida* and other toxins from the digestive tract. Some people have had success taking coconut oil to fight off *Candida*.

Goldenseal was used by Native Americans for fighting infections and is effective against *Candida albicans*.[70] Many references say that goldenseal should only be used for a short time and avoided if pregnant.

Extracts of fresh ginger have been shown to have strong anti-fungal actions in at least 5 studies and therefore, it would be wise to include some fresh ginger in your wellness program. I also recommend drinking plenty of fresh ginger tea. (It is the gingerols in fresh ginger that kill *Candida*.)[71] In addition, ginger's potent antioxidant actions also help fight against *Candida*'s toxins and its oxidative effect on the liver and kidneys. We will explore ginger's amazing antioxidant actions in chapter 17.

I got my life back by eating 5 to 10 slices of fresh ginger per day, taking 1 or 2 grams of dried ginger powder per day, and reducing sugary foods, junk foods, and milk products. Although I had undergone allergy testing (no major allergies were reported), the allergist did report I had no resistance to *Candida* but gave no indication of *Candida*'s relationship to *brain fog* and many other health problems. I wish my health care practitioners would have told me to read *The Missing Diagnosis* by C. Orian Truss and *The Yeast Connection* by William Crook.

5. **Take enzyme supplements.** Digestive enzyme supplements help with digestion, and enteric-coated enzymes fight inflammation and boost the immune system. Refer to chapter 15 for more information on enzymes.

6. **Take other supplements to boost the immune system.** These include vitamins B, C, and E. Vitamin B and zinc are extremely important for restoring proper function of the brain. *Candida* overgrowth and alcohol use produce acetaldehyde, which can cause a major deficiency of vitamin B1. Dr. Crook strongly advised taking CoQ10 (coenzyme Q10) for boosting the immune system and he gives references of CoQ10's other

actions such as strengthening the heart and fighting breast cancer.[72] CoQ10 works with our bodies' enzymes to produce cell energy and is also a strong antioxidant. Zinc is very crucial to the immune system and will help fight *Candida* over-growth.[73] Additionally, folic acid, selenium, and molybdenum will help prevent ethanol in the body from being converted to acetaldehyde. These supplements will help convert the ethanol into acetic acid, which is then excreted out of the body.[74]

7. **Remember that *Candida* and other fungal infections can spread to other areas of the body.** *Candida* can spread under the arms, in the mouth (thrush),[75] to fingernails and toenails (thick yellowish nails, called onycholysis), in the reproductive organs of females (vulvovaganitis, moniliasis, or genital candidiasis), and in the groin for men (jock itch). Caprylic acid is helpful for fungal skin infections and can be taken as a supplement and used externally on the skin. Another good skin treatment can be made by adding 5 drops of clove oil and 5 drops of oregano oil to 1 tablespoon of coconut oil. Several websites state that yellowish nails can be helped by soaking fingernails or toenails in vinegar everyday and applying Vicks VapoRub to the nail. New nail growth should be clear.

8. **Some of us may have to use several forms of anti-*Candida* prevention for the rest of our lives.** It is probably a good idea to take several herbal supplements on a regular basis, limit sugary foods and junk foods and try to eat more fruits, vegetables and other wholesome foods as practical. Also, don't be afraid to have a special treat from time to time for being good! Recent studies show that *Candida* can hide within the folds of the intestine and even become a part of our bodies' cells by attaching itself to the DNA within each cell and therefore will always have a tendency to take over. Dr. Truss writes of a 60-year-old man who remained well for 12 years while on

Nystatin, but when the man stopped using Nystatin he had a reoccurrence of lethargy and constipation. Truss also writes that many other patients were able to discontinue Nystatin and remain well.[76]

Truss theorizes why some of us have little or no resistance to *Candida*. He describes the 1970s as "the antibiotics generation" and gives the following explanation: "A hypothetical young person 16 years of age in 1977 ... Typically, his mother would have used birth control pills for a year or more prior to conception. Already weakened in her response to yeast, she enters the yeast-associated condition of pregnancy. Any of the 79 yeast antigens that cross the placental barrier will result in intra-uterine exposure with its tolerance-reducing influence on the unborn child. It is almost a certainty that antibiotics would have been prescribed intermittently during these years of pregnancy and 'the pill.' Should she have had asthma, arthritis, or any one of a number of other conditions, cortisone or other immunosuppressant drugs might have added their influence. Soon after birth, yeast enters the newborn child, establishes itself permanently, and perpetuates the state of partial tolerance established in utero. If his immune response (IR) genes dictate a reasonably strong resistance, he may overcome this situation as his immune system matures. If on the other hand he has inherited genes that allow him a limited defense at best against *Candida*, he has little chance of overcoming the state of responsiveness. Antibiotics soon after birth and intermittently thereafter continue to stimulate the yeast. Allergic membranes with frequent infections are common, increasing the need for antibiotics."[77]

9. **Consider the need for heavy metal detoxification.** Certain metals such as mercury can promote the growth of *Candida*. Refer back to chapter 7.

10. Read other publications, Web sites, and books on digestive healing that suggest other supplements and medications.

Obtain a copy of Dr. Truss's *the Missing Diagnosis II* or the late Dr. Crook's *The Yeast Connection* or his latest book, *Tired, So Tired* and his book coauthored with Marjorie Hurt Jones, *The Yeast Connection Cookbook.*

Pertinent Web sites include the following: www.arthritistrust. org, www.candidafree.net, www.candida-yeast.com, www. greatplainslaboratory.com, www.genovadiagnostics.com, and www.yeastconnection.com (this last site was set up by Dr. Crook's daughter).

CANDIDA AND OTHER ILLNESSES

Candidiasis has been linked to the activity and flare-ups of other illnesses, including asthma,[78] psoriasis,[79] mitral valve prolapse,[80] and multiple sclerosis.[81]

Dr. Truss reports that *Candida* appears to be linked to a variety of illnesses because of its "involvement of a variety of tissues in the body." Some of these illnesses include Crohn's disease, erythematosus, myasthenia gravis, multiple sclerosis, systematic lupus, and other auto-immune diseases.[82]

Dr. Crook, in his book *The Yeast Connection,* states that *chronic fatigue syndrome* (CFS) and candidiasis appear to be related conditions. Out of 1,100 patients diagnosed with CFS, 84% had recovered to the point where they were working 30 to 40 hours per week when put on a sugar-free diet and antifungal medication.[83]

Dr. William Shaw, founder of the Great Plains Laboratory in Kansas, has for years reported that yeasts and fungus play a role in the following diseases:[84] Alzheimer's disease, attention deficit disorder (ADD), autism, child psychosis, chronic fatigue syndrome, colitis, Crohn's disease, depression, fibromyalgia, inflammatory bowel disease, migraine headache, obsessive-compulsive disorder (OCD), Rett syndrome, schizophrenia, seizures, Tourette's syndrome, and ulcerative colitis.

CANDIDA AND CANCER

Candida overgrowth often appears in patients with acute leukemia after receiving anti-cancer therapy. (Acute leukemia occurs when too many immature blood cells are produced by the bone marrow). One remarkable study in 1999 showed that all 3 patient's leukemia went into remission following aggressive antifungal therapy. (The anti-cancer therapy had to be reduced for these patients because of complications from *Candida* overgrowth).[85] Coincidence? Maybe, maybe not. It is known that exposure to large amounts of the chemical preservative formaldehyde has been linked to leukemia.[86] As previously stated, *Candida* gives off acetaldehyde which is similar in chemical composition to formaldehyde. It makes one wonder if *Candida* and its many toxins might be a possible link to leukemia.

CASE STUDIES OF *CANDIDA* INFECTION BY C. ORIAN TRUSS

Here is a sample of the range of illnesses treated by Dr. Truss and the fascinating success of his theory and treatments as detailed in his book *The Missing Diagnosis*:

A 28-year-old man who had been a champion marathon runner in excellent health suddenly become weak, debilitated, had anxiety attacks and bouts of depression, and was labeled a "psychoneurotic" with a nerve disorder. He developed severe chemical intolerances to food, drugs, and odors in homes and motels. This became the dominant problem, as it often does with *Candida* infection. He was diagnosed as "totally allergic to foods—chemicals due to immune deficiency." He found some relief by avoiding carbohydrates and eating only meat (removing carbohydrates removes some of *Candida*'s food source). He was unable to run for 4 years. Following 6 months of treatment for *Candida* and allergies, his health was completely restored and he was able to run almost as fast as he did in his prime days. Also, he reported that 95% of all his chemical intolerances disappeared, and he was able to attend a basket-ball game "in a smokey coliseum."[87]

A highly motivated 21-year-old pre-med student had to drop out of college because of nasal allergies, poor memory, and an inability to concentrate. His grades suffered, especially during the fall and winter terms. He usually did well in courses that required reasoning but performed poorly in courses that required a lot of memorization. After receiving 6 months of allergy treatment (*Candida albicans* yeast extract), he returned to college, improved his grades, and was later accepted into medical school. (He was required to attend 2 extra semesters to prove his high mental performance could be sustained.) This case illustrates the subtle effect of chronic allergy on the brain and how it degrades intel-lectual ability despite a person's maximum effort to succeed. As a child, he had received antibiotics for allergies and nasal obstruction.[88]

A 44-year-old woman with Crohn's disease who suffered from intes-tinal bleeding, severe diarrhea, and abdominal pain had undergone 3 operations to remove an 8-foot section of her small intestine. She aver-aged 12 to 15 bowel movements per day accompanied by extreme weakness and frequent infections. Her condition quickly improved within 1 week of treatment with Nystatin and a low-carbohydrate diet. This woman's case illustrates an autoimmune attack on the digestive tract and how *Candida* can make an existing illness even worse. Prior to being diagnosed with Crohn's disease, she had experienced heartburn for several years and constipation since childhood.[89]

Two women had been repeatedly diagnosed with schizophrenia (split personality). Both women improved quickly with anti-*Candida* treatment with no relapse. Recovery was complete.[90]

A young woman had been diagnosed with multiple sclerosis for 7 years. She suffered from numbness in her hands, feet, and over her entire trunk for 3 years prior to treatment by Truss. One month before treatment, she had a delay in initiating bladder emptying (about 10 minutes, which is typical of multiple sclerosis patients). Three days after starting Nystatin, her bladder functioned normally. Following 7 months of Nystatin, she was completely free of symptoms. Truss writes that the cases of the aforementioned three women suggest, in theory, that *Candida* appears to "mimic" other illnesses, particularly in the case of psychosis and autoimmune diseases, even to the degree of being misdiagnosed by competent professionals; *Candida* may possibly be a factor in the cause of some illnesses.[91]

Many sufferers become very frustrated because they feel they can't cope with life, underperform at their jobs, and are faced with multiple health issues all at the same time. Some give up all hope of getting well. Truss writes of a 36-year-old registered nurse who had attempted suicide with a gun but had narrowly survived. Prior to this she had suffered multiple health problems, severe hormonal dysfunction, and increasing depression. Her once excellent memory became poor. As she is quoted in *The Missing Diagnosis*: "I despise my husband and child when I'm like this; as soon as they come in the door I scream at them over just anything; I don't appreciate anything." Her health problems included urinary bleeding; kidney stones; wide weight fluctuations; abnormal menstrual cycles since age 14 with clots, cramps, and premenstrual tension; and stuffy nose in the fall and winter along with multiple allergies. Although her treatment by Truss did involve some setbacks, she eventually became well enough to work regularly at a nursing home and was later promoted to administrator. Eleven years later, she still receives *Candida* vaccine weekly with no recurrence of her old symptoms. This case illustrates how *Candida* can cause major disruption of the central nervous system and much mental anguish and physical suffering. This woman had colitis (inflammation of the large intestine) as an infant, had received antibiotic treatment at age 9 for oral thrush, and received antibiotics again for vaginitis after pregnancy.[92]

A 3-year-old boy with low red blood cell count (autoimmune

hemolytic anemia) required blood transfusions and cortisone drugs to prevent death. (His problems started at age 11 months after receiving a 3-week round of ampicillin, an antibiotic). Truss put the 3-year-old on Nystatin, which quickly corrected his extreme hyperactivity, temper tantrums, and chronic diarrhea. After 5 months of Nystatin, his red blood cell count was back to normal. This case illustrates how *Candida* might be turning off protective actions by the immune system.[93]

A 16-month-old baby boy with chronic diarrhea, runny nose, irritability, difficulty sleeping, pus in his ears, and frequent infections was treated by Truss. (His problems began at age 3 months and he received many rounds of different antibiotics between the age of 3 and 11 months.) His health recovered after 4 months of treatment with Nystatin.[94]

We owe much gratitude to Dr. Truss for his dedication and brilliance in putting together the complex pieces of a confusing puzzle. He accurately concluded that it was the *toxins* given off by *Candida albicans* (not the *Candida* infection itself) that impaired other organs and tissues and led to a multitude of syndromes and illnesses.[95] Note in these case studies how *Candida* affects different people in different ways.

WHAT WE CAN LEARN FROM PICKLES...

Recall that acetaldehyde is a nasty toxin given off by *Candida* and is also a by-product from the break-down of alcohol in our body. Acetaldehyde is also produced in small amounts in canned pickles as oxygen slowly seeps into the plastic jar, resulting in an undesirable off-flavor. Turmeric, added for yellow coloring, also reduces the formation of acetaldehyde inside the jar of pickles by its potent anti-oxidant actions.[96]

In our bodies, acetaldehyde can have the effect of "pickling" or stiffening cell membranes and tissues in our bodies, similar to the effect of formaldehyde,[97] a preservative used for embalming. Formaldehyde is also given off by tobacco smoke; unvented, fuel-burning appliances, like gas stoves or kerosene space heaters; and is used in the manufacture of permanent-press clothing and fabrics and pressed wood construction products and furniture.[98] You may see the name formalin which is another name for a mixture of formaldehyde and water.

Dr. Truss points out that *Candida* also stiffens cell membranes another way—by causing a deficiency of long-chain EFAs,[99] possibly by decreasing the absorption of omega-3 EFAs that we studied in chapter 13. It is no wonder that *Candida* produces such a wide variation of symptoms and behaviours in many people.

WHAT WE CAN LEARN FROM ALCOHOLISM...

It is known that acetaldehyde from the break-down of alcohol forms morphine-like compounds.[100] This may be a major factor in alcohol addiction. *Candida* also makes one crave for more alcohol and sugar, feeding the vicious cycle that produces even more acetaldehyde and toxins. Interestingly, Chinese and Japanese people have a gene mutation that makes it very difficult for their bodies to get rid of acetaldehyde. As a result, acetaldehyde builds up quickly, resulting in headaches, nausea and many other undesirable effects. This mutant gene discourages these Asian people from heavy drinking and alcoholism.[101]

After learning of the effects of alcetaldehyde on the brain, it is no longer a mystery that my alcoholic friend, after 20 years of addiction, became well after eating chunks of fresh ginger (like it was candy) and was able to conquer his alcohol addiction. I believe the fresh ginger played a big part in killing off *Candida* overgrowth, helped to detoxify his liver of acetaldehyde and other toxins, reduced inflammation in his digestive tract and helped him to have a clear enough head to want to stop his addiction and improve his life. Let's look at some more amazing actions of ginger and other simple foods in the next chapter.

208   Lynn Smith

REFERENCES FOR CHAPTER 14

1. Towbridge, John Parks, MD, Walker, Moton, DPM. *The Yeast Syndrome.*
    Bantam Books, New York, NY. 1986. p.9.
2. Rochlitz S. *Allergies and Candida, with the 21st Century Solution.* Human
    Ecology Balancing Sciences Inc., New York, 1988.
3a. Hasumura Y, Teschke R, Lieber CS. "Characteristics of acetaldehyde oxidation
    in rat liver mitochondria." *J Biol Chem.* 1976 Aug 25;251(16):4908-13.
3b. Dr. William Shaw. "Yeast Overgrowth - The Yeast Problem & Bacteria
    Byproducts: Info" The Great Plains Laboratory, Inc. Accessed 9/27/2005.
    <http://www.greatplainslaboratory.com/yeast.html>.
4. Truss, C. Orian, MD. *the Missing Diagnosis.* The Missing Diagnosis, Inc., PO
    Box 26508, Birmingham, AL 35226. 1985. p.15.
5. Truss, C. Orian, MD. *the Missing Diagnosis.* The Missing Diagnosis, Inc., PO
    Box 26508, Birmingham, AL 35226. 1985. p.15.
6. Truss, C. Orian, MD. *the Missing Diagnosis II.* The Missing Diagnosis, Inc.,
    2614 Highland Avenue, Birmingham, AL 35205. 2009. pp.103-112.
7. Iwata K, Uchida K. "Cellular Immunity in Experimental Fungal Infections in
    Mice" 1978. *Mykosen.* Suppl. 1, 72-81.
8. Truss, C. Orian, MD. *the Missing Diagnosis.* The Missing Diagnosis, Inc., PO
    Box 26508, Birmingham, AL 35226. 1985. pp.84-85.
9. Iwata K, Uchida K. "Cellular Immunity in Experimental Fungal Infections in
    Mice." 1978, *Mykosen, Suppl.* 1, 72-81.
10. Truss, C. Orian, MD. *the Missing Diagnosis II.* The Missing Diagnosis, Inc.,
    2614 Highland Avenue, Birmingham, AL 35205. 2009. pp.72-73.
11. Truss, C. Orian, MD. *the Missing Diagnosis.* The Missing Diagnosis, Inc., PO
    Box 26508, Birmingham, AL 35226. 1985. front cover & pp.14, 15, 38, 39, 40,
    41, 57.
12. "Candidiasis Symptoms" Web site: Enzymedica The Enzyme Experts. Accessed
    12/24/2004. <http://www.enzymedica.com/candidase.php>.
13. Lipski E. *Leaky Gut Syndrome.* Keats Publishing, Inc., New Canaan, CT, 1998.
    p.21.
14. Mark Cobb. "Eliminate The Underlying Cause" Web site: Candida Free.
    Accessed 1/6/2005. <http://www.candidafree.net/pages/1/index.htm>.
15. Truss, C. Orian, MD. *the Missing Diagnosis.* The Missing Diagnosis, Inc., PO
    Box 26508, Birmingham, AL 35226, 1985. pp.19-21, 28-30, 47, 48.
16. Truss, C. Orian, MD. *the Missing Diagnosis.* The Missing Diagnosis, Inc., PO
    Box 26508, Birmingham, AL 35226, 1985. p.39.
17. Truss, C. Orian, MD. *the Missing Diagnosis,* The Missing Diagnosis, Inc., PO
    Box 26508, Birmingham, AL 35226. 1985. pp.17, 55, 56.
18. Truss, C. Orian, MD. *the Missing Diagnosis,* The Missing Diagnosis, Inc., PO
    Box 26508, Birmingham, AL 35226. 1985. pp.55-56.

19. Truss, C. Orian, MD. *the Missing Diagnosis*, The Missing Diagnosis, Inc., PO Box 26508, Birmingham, AL 35226. 1985. pp.49, 50.

20. Truss, C. Orian, MD. *the Missing Diagnosis*. The Missing Diagnosis, Inc., PO Box 26508, Birmingham, AL 35226. 1985. pp.50-51.

21. Anthony di Fabio, *Psychiatric Pollution!*, The Rheumatoid Disease Foundation, Op.Cit. 1989.

22. Truss, C. Orian, MD. *the Missing Diagnosis*. The Missing Diagnosis, Inc., PO Box 26508, Birmingham, AL 35226. 1985. p.77.

23. Web site: Drugs.com. "Nystatin (Oral)" Accessed 12/3/2008. <http://www.drugs.com/cons/nystatin.html>.

24. Web site: About.com. Nystatin. Rachel Fuller Brown and Elizabeth Lee Hazen invented the worlds first useful antifungal antibiotic – nystatin. Accessed 1/22/2010. http://inventors.about.com/library/inventors/blnystatin.htm?p=1.

25. Iwata K. "A Review of the Literature on Drunken Symptoms Due to Yeast in the Gastrointestinal Tract." *Yeasts and Yeast-Like Microorganisms in Medical Science.* University of Tokyo Press. pp.260-8, 1976.

26. Crook, William D., M.D., *The Yeast Connection Handbook*, Professional Books, Inc., Box 3246, Jackson, TN, Copyright 2000, pp.195-7.

27. "Acetaldehyde: Alcohol's Most Toxic Metabolite". Web site: Rebound. Accessed 4/23/2005. <http://www.reboundhangover.com/acetaldehyde.htm>.

28. Gus J. Prosch, Jr., M.D. et al. "Candidiasis: Scourge of Arthritics" 1994. Article from Web site: The Arthritis Trust of America. Accessed 12/6/2008. <http://www.arthritistrust.org>. Birmingham, AL 35226, 1985, p.2.

29a. Dean J. Tuma, Ph.D., and Carol A. Casey, Ph.D. "Dangerous Byproducts of Alcohol Breakdown-Focus on Adducts." Web site: National Institute on Alcohol Abuse and Alcoholism. Accessed 8/28/05. <http://www.niaaa.nih.gov/publications/arh27-4/285-290.htm>.

29b. Hasumura Y, Teschke R, Lieber CS. "Characteristics of acetaldehyde oxidation in rat liver mitochondria." *J Biol Chem.* 1976 Aug 25;251(16):4908-13.

30. "Acetaldehyde: Alcohol's Most Toxic Metabolite". Web site: Rebound. Accessed 4/23/2005. <http://www.reboundhangover.com/acetaldehyde.htm>.

31. Shibutani S, (faculty member at the State University of New York at Stony Brook). Accessed 4/23/2005. <http://www.reboundhangover.com/acetaldehyde.htm>.

32. Raymond Keith Bown, M.D. *Aids, Cancer and the Medical Establishment.* Trizoid Press, New York, 1993. ISBN0-9639293-0-5.

33. Dr. William Shaw. "Yeast Overgrowth - The Yeast Problem & Bacteria Byproducts: Info". Web site: The Great Plains Laboratory, Inc. Accessed 5/8/05. <http://www.greatplainslaboratory.com/yeast.html>.

34. Dr. William Shaw. "Yeast Overgrowth - The Yeast Problem & Bacteria Byproducts: Info". Web site: The Great Plains Laboratory, Inc. Accessed 5/8/05. <http://www.greatplainslaboratory.com/yeast.html>.

35a.   Truss, C. Orian, MD. *the Missing Diagnosis*, The Missing Diagnosis, Inc., PO
        Box 26508, Birmingham, AL 35226. 1985. pp.64-65.

35b.   Towbridge JP, MD, Walker M, DPM. *The Yeast Syndrome*. Bantam Books, New
        York, NY. 1986. pp.42-53.

35c.   Crook, William D., M.D.. *The Yeast Connection Handbook*. Professional Books,
        Inc., Box 3246, Jackson, TN. 2000, p.61.

35d.   Ruiz-Sanchez D, Calderon-Romero L, Sanchez-Vega JT, Tay J. "Intestinal
        candidiasis. A clinical report and comments about this opportunistic pathology."
        Mycopathologia. 2003;156(1):9-11.

35e.   Witsell DL, Garrett CG, Yarbrough WG, Dorrestein SP, Drake AF, Weissler
        MC. "Effect of Lactobacillus acidophilus on antibiotic-associated gastro-
        intestinal morbidity: a prospective randomized trial." *J Otolaryngol*. 1995
        Aug;24(4):230-3.

35f.   Still JM Jr, Law EJ, Belcher KE, Spencer SA. "A comparison of susceptibility
        to five antifungal agents of yeast cultures from burn patients." *Burns*. 1995
        May;21(3):167-70.

35g.   MJ Kenedy and PA Volz. "Ecology of Candida albicans gut colonization:
        inhibition of Candida adhesion, colonization, and dissemination from the
        gastrointestinal tract by bacterial antagonism." *Infect Immun*. 1985 September;
        49(3): 654-663.

36.   Dr. William Shaw. "Yeast Overgrowth - The Yeast Problem & Bacteria
        Byproducts: Info". Web site: The Great Plains Laboratory, Inc. Accessed 5/8/05.
        <http://www.greatplainslaboratory.com/yeast.html>.

37.   "Children and Candida" Web site: Candida Support. Accessed 5/22/05. <http://
        www.candidasupport.org/childrenandcandi.html>.

38.   Lipski, E. Ph.D. *Digestive Wellness*. McGraw-Hill, New York, NY. 2004. p.192.

39.   Truss, C. Orian, MD. *the Missing Diagnosis*, The Missing Diagnosis, Inc., PO
        Box 26508, Birmingham, AL 35226. 1985. pp.29-31.

40.   Truss, C. Orian, MD. *the Missing Diagnosis*, The Missing Diagnosis, Inc., PO
        Box 26508, Birmingham, AL 35226. 1985. pp.65-66.

41.   Crook, William D., M.D., *The Yeast Connection Handbook*, Professional Books,
        Inc., Box 3246, Jackson, TN, Copyright 2000, p.62.

42a.   Truss, C. Orian, MD. *the Missing Diagnosis*, The Missing Diagnosis, Inc., PO
        Box 26508, Birmingham, AL 35226. 1985. p.64.

42b.   Crook, William D., M.D., *The Yeast Connection Handbook*, Professional Books,
        Inc., Box 3246, Jackson, TN, Copyright 2000, p.107.

43.   Towbridge, John Parks, MD, Walker, Moton, DPM. *The Yeast Syndrome*.
        Bantam Books, New York, NY. 1986. p.xvii.

44.   "Discovery of Genetic Pathways May Provide New Ways to Combat Candida
        Infections" Web site: Whitehead Institute for Biomedical Research. Accessed
        12/7/2008. <http://www.wi.mit.edy/news/archives/1997/gf_0905.html>.

45.   Crook, William D., M.D., *The Yeast Connection Handbook*, Professional Books, Inc., Box 3246, Jackson, TN, Copyright 2000, p.42.

46.   Crook, William D., M.D., *The Yeast Connection Handbook*, Professional Books, Inc., Box 3246, Jackson, TN, Copyright 2000, pp.189-190.

47.   "Candidiasis" Web site: U.S. Centers for Disease Control and Prevention, Department of Health and Human Services. Accessed 12/5/2008. <http://www.cdc.gov>.

48.   Towbridge, John Parks, MD, Walker, Moton, DPM. *The Yeast Syndrome*. Bantam Books, New York, NY. 1986. p.10.

49.   Gus J. Prosch, Jr., M.D. et al. "Candidiasis: Sourge of Arthritics" 1994. Article from Web site: The Arthritis Trust of America. Accessed 12/6/2008. <http://www.arthritistrust.org>.

50.   Vargas SL. Patrick CC, Ayers GD, and Hughes WT. "Modulating Effect of Dietary Carbohydrate Supplementation on *Candida albicans*, Colonization and Invasion in a Neutropenic Mouse Model" *Infection and Immunity*. February 1993; 61:619-626.

51.   Atkins Robert C., M.D. *Dr. Atkins' Vita-Nutrient Solution*. Simon & Schuster, New York, NY. 1998. pp.230-231.

52.   Crook, William D., M.D., *The Yeast Connection Handbook*, Professional Books, Inc., Box 3246, Jackson, TN, Copyright 2000, p.129.

53.   Lipski, E. Ph.D. *Digestive Wellness*. McGraw-Hill, New York, NY. 2004. pp.48-50.

54.   Towbridge, John Parks, MD, Walker, Moton, DPM. *The Yeast Syndrome*. Bantam Books, New York, NY. 1986. pp.367-368.

55.   Truss, C. Orian, MD. *the Missing Diagnosis*, The Missing Diagnosis, Inc., PO Box 26508, Birmingham, AL 35226. 1985. pp.68-69.

56.   Truss, C. Orian, MD. *the Missing Diagnosis II*. The Missing Diagnosis, Inc., 2614 Highland Avenue, Birmingham, AL 35205. 2009. pp.23, 24.

57a.   Nguefack J, Leth V, Amvan Zollo PH, Mathur SB, "Evaluation of five essential oils from aromatic plants of Cameroon for controlling food spoilage and myco-toxin producing fungi," *Int J Food Microbiol.*, 2004 Aug 1;94(3):329-34.

57b.   Jagetia GC, Baliga MS, Venkatesh P, Ulloor JN. "Influence of ginger rhizome (Zingiber officinale Rosc) on survival, glutathione and lipid peroxidation in mice after whole-body exposure to gamma radiation." *Radiat Res.* 2003 Nov;160(5):584-92.

57c.   Ficker C, Smith ML, Akpagana K, Gbeassor M, Zhang J, Durst T, Assabgui R, Arnason JT, "Bioassay-guided isolation and identification of antifungal compounds from ginger." *Phytother Res.* 2003 Sep;17(8):897-902.

57d.   Ficker CE, Arnason JT, Vindas PS, Alvarez LP, Akpagana K, Gbeassor M, De Souza C, Smith ML, "Inhibition of human pathogenic fungi by ethnobotani-cally selected plant extracts," *Mycoses*, 2003 Feb;46(1-2):29-37.

57e.   Martins AP, Salgueiro L, Goncalves MJ, da Cunha AP, Vila R, Canigueral S,

Mazzoni V, Tomi F, Casanova J. "Essential oil composition and antimicrobial activity of three Zingiberaceae from S. Tome e Principe." *Planta Med.* 2001 Aug;67(6):580-4.

58a. Crook, William D., M.D., *The Yeast Connection Handbook*, Professional Books, Inc., Box 3246, Jackson, TN, Copyright 2000, p.131.

58b. Yoshida S, Kasuga S, Hayashi N, Ushiroguchi T, Matsuura H, Nakagawa S. "Antifungal Activity of Ajoene Derived from Garlic." *Applied and Environmentsl Microbiology.* Mar 1987, p.615-617.

59. Crook, William D., M.D., *The Yeast Connection Handbook*, Professional Books, Inc., Box 3246, Jackson, TN, Copyright 2000. pp.129-130.

60. Gus J. Prosch, Jr., M.D. et al. "Candidiasis: Scourge of Arthritics" 1994. Article from Web site: The Arthritis Trust of America. Accessed 12/6/2008. <http://www.arthritistrust.org>.

61. Crook William D., M.D., *The Yeast Connection Handbook*, Professional Books, Inc., Box 3246, Jackson, TN, Copyright 2000. p.132.

62. Crook, William D., M.D., *The Yeast Connection Handbook*, Professional Books, Inc., Box 3246, Jackson, TN, Copyright 2000. p.130.

63. Crook, William D., M.D., *The Yeast Connection Handbook*, Professional Books, Inc., Box 3246, Jackson, TN, Copyright 2000. p.133.

64. Duke, James A., Ph.D. The Green Pharmacy. Rodale Press, Emmaus, PA 1997. pp.204, 462-464.

65. Pozzatti P, Scheil LA, Spader TB, Atayde ML, Santurio JM, Alves SH. "Invitro activity of essential oils extracted from plants used as spices against fluconazole-resistant and fluconazole-susceptible Candida spp. *Can J Microbiol.* 2008 Nov;54(11):950-6.

66. Itzhack Polacheck, Uri Zehavi, Michael Naim, Mordekhai Levy, and Ruth Evron. "Activity of Compound G2 Isolated from Alfalfa Roots against Medically Important Yeasts" *Antimicrobial Agents and Chemotherapy.* Aug. 1986. p.290-294.

67. "Candidiasis" Web site accessed 11/15/2004. <http://www.liferesearchuniversal.com/candidiasis3.html>.

68. Kosalec I, Pepeljnjak S, Kustrak D. "Antifungal activity of fluid extract and essential oil from anise fruits (Pimpinella anisum L., Apiaceae)." *Acta Pharm.* 2005 Dec;55(4):377-85.

69. Crook William D., M.D., *The Yeast Connection Handbook*, Professional Books, Inc., Box 3246, Jackson, TN, Copyright 2000, pp.129-130.

70. Duke, James A., Ph.D. The Green Pharmacy. Rodale Press, Emmaus, PA 1997. pp.203-204.

71a. Nguefack J, Leth V, Amvan Zollo PH, Mathur SB, "Evaluation of five essential oils from aromatic plants of Cameroon for controlling food spoilage and myco-toxin producing fungi," *Int J Food Microbiol.*, 2004 Aug 1;94(3):329-34.

71b. Jagetia GC, Baliga MS, Venkatesh P, Ulloor JN. "Influence of ginger rhizome

(Zingiber officinale Rosc) on survival, glutathione and lipid peroxidation in mice after whole-body exposure to gamma radiation." *Radiat Res.* 2003 Nov;160(5):584-92.

71c.   Ficker C, Smith ML, Akpagana K, Gbeassor M, Zhang J, Durst T, Assabgui R, Arnason JT, "Bioassay-guided isolation and identification of antifungal compounds from ginger," *Phytother Res.* 2003 Sep;17(8):897-902.

71d.   Ficker CE, Arnason JT, Vindas PS, Alvarez LP, Akpagana K, Gbeassor M, De Souza C, Smith ML, "Inhibition of human pathogenic fungi by ethnobotanically selected plant extracts," *Mycoses,* 2003 Feb;46(1-2):29-37.

71e.   Martins AP, Salgueiro L, Goncalves MJ, da Cunha AP, Vila R, Canigueral S, Mazzoni V, Tomi F, Casanova J. "Essential oil composition and antimicrobial activity of three Zingiberaceae from S. Tome e Principe." *Planta Med.* 2001 Aug;67(6):580-4.

72.   Crook, William D., M.D., *The Yeast Connection Handbook,* Professional Books, Inc., Box 3246, Jackson, TN, Copyright 2000. pp.164-166.

73a.   "Secrets of the Immune System" Web site: The Great Plains Laboratory, Inc. Accessed 12/6/2008. <http://www.greatplainslaboratory.com/immune-system. html>.

73b.   Singh KP, Zaidi SI, Raisuddin S, Saxena AK, Murthy RC, Ray PK. "Effect of zinc on immune functions and host resistance against infection and tumor challenge." *Immunopharmacol Immunotoxicol.* 1992;14(4):813-40.

73c.   Salvi SB, Horecker BL, Pan LX, Rabin BS. "The effect of dietary zinc and prothymosin alpha on cellular immune responses of RF/J mice." *Clin Immunol Immunopathol.* 1987 Jun;43(3):281-8.

74.   Dr. Stephen Cooter. "Molybdenum: Recycling Fatigue Into Energy," Townsend Letter for Doctors. 911 Tyler St., Port Townsend, WA 98368-6541, April 1994, p.332; excerpt from "Beating Chronic Illness: Fatigue, Pain Weakness, Insomnia, Foggy Thinking." Pro Motion Publishing, 10387 Friars Rd. San Diego, CA.

75.   Crook, William D., M.D., *The Yeast Connection Handbook,* Professional Books, Inc., Box 3246, Jackson, TN, Copyright 2000. pp.259-260.

76.   Truss, C. Orian, MD. *the Missing Diagnosis,* The Missing Diagnosis, Inc., PO Box 26508, Birmingham, AL 35226. 1985. p.136.

77.   Truss, C. Orian, MD. *the Missing Diagnosis,* The Missing Diagnosis, Inc., PO Box 26508, Birmingham, AL 35226. 1985. pp.144-145.

78.   Crook William D., M.D., *The Yeast Connection Handbook,* Professional Books, Inc., Box 3246, Jackson, TN, Copyright 2000, pp.44-45.

79.   Crook William D., M.D., *The Yeast Connection Handbook,* Professional Books, Inc., Box 3246, Jackson, TN, Copyright 2000, pp.45-46.

80.   Gus J. Prosch, Jr., M.D. et al. "Candidiasis: Scourge of Arthritics" 1994. Article from Web site: The Arthritis Trust of America. Accessed 12/6/2008. <http:// www.arthritistrust.org>.

81.   Crook William D., M.D., *The Yeast Connection Handbook*, Professional Books,
       Inc., Box 3246, Jackson, TN, Copyright 2000, pp.46-47.
82.   Truss, C. Orian, MD. *the Missing Diagnosis*, The Missing Diagnosis, Inc., PO
       Box 26508, Birmingham, AL 35226. 1985. pp.138-138.
83.   Crook William D., M.D., *The Yeast Connection Handbook*, Professional Books,
       Inc., Box 3246, Jackson, TN, Copyright 2000, pp.32-34.
84.   Dr. William Shaw. "Yeast Overgrowth - The Yeast Problem & Bacteria
       Byproducts: Info". The Great Plains Laboratory, Inc. Web site: Accessed
       12/06/2008. <http://www.greatplainslaboratory.com/home/eng/candida.asp>.
85.   Karthaus M. "Surprising Long-Term, Leukemia-Free Survival in Patients with
       Hepatosplenic Candidiasis Receiving Minimal Antileukemic Therapy." Abstr Intersci
       Conf Antimicrob Agents Chemother. 1999 Sep 26-29; 39: 575 (abstract no. 1645).
86.   Web site: National Cancer Institute. "Formaldehyde and Cancer Risk." Accessed
       1/15/2010. http://www.cancer.gov/cancertopics/factsheet/Risk/formaldehyde>
87.   Truss, C. Orian, MD. *the Missing Diagnosis*. The Missing Diagnosis, Inc., PO
       Box 26508, Birmingham, AL 35226. 1985. pp.57-61.
88.   Truss, C. Orian, MD. *the Missing Diagnosis*. The Missing Diagnosis, Inc., PO
       Box 26508, Birmingham, AL 35226. 1985. pp.101-107.
89.   Truss, C. Orian, MD. *the Missing Diagnosis*. The Missing Diagnosis, Inc., PO
       Box 26508, Birmingham, AL 35226. 1985. pp.88-89.
90.   Truss, C. Orian, MD *the Missing Diagnosis*. The Missing Diagnosis, Inc., PO
       Box 26508, Birmingham, AL 35226. 1985 pp.83-86, 94.
91.   Truss, C. Orian, MD. *the Missing Diagnosis*. The Missing Diagnosis, Inc., PO
       Box 26508, Birmingham, AL 35226. 1985. pp.83-86.
92.   Truss, C. Orian, MD. *the Missing Diagnosis*. The Missing Diagnosis, Inc., PO
       Box 26508, Birmingham, AL 35226. 1985. pp.134-135.
93.   Truss, C. Orian, MD. *the Missing Diagnosis*. The Missing Diagnosis, Inc., PO
       Box 26508, Birmingham, AL 35226. 1985. p.87.
94.   Truss, C. Orian, MD. *the Missing Diagnosis*. The Missing Diagnosis, Inc., PO
       Box 26508, Birmingham, AL 35226. 1985. pp.79-81.
95.   Truss, C. Orian, MD. *the Missing Diagnosis*. The Missing Diagnosis, Inc., PO
       Box 26508, Birmingham, AL 35226. 1985. p.63, 143.
96.   Cleary, KA, McFeeters, RF. 2006 "Effects of oxygen and turmeric on the forma-
       tion of oxidative aldehydes in fresh-pack dill pickles." Journal of Agricultural and
       Food Chemistry. 54:3421-3427.
97.   Towbridge, John Parks, MD, Walker, Moton, DPM. *The Yeast Syndrome*.
       Bantam Books, New York, NY. 1986. pp.274-275.
98.   Web site: U.S. Environmental Protection Agency. "An Introduction to Indoor
       Air Quality. Formaldehyde." Accessed 2/1/2010. <http://epa.gov/iaq/formalde.
       html>
99.   Truss, C. Orian, MD. *the Missing Diagnosis II*. The Missing Diagnosis, Inc.,
       2614 Highland Avenue, Birmingham, AL 35205. 2009. pp.76-77.

100.   Web site: Virtual Chembook, Elmhurst College. Charles E. Ophardt, 2003.
       "Alcohol Metabolism Effects." Accessed 1/22/2010. <http://www.elmhurst.
       edu/~chm/vchembook/642alcoholmet.html>
101.   Web site: Chemcases.com. "Alcohol, chemistry and You. Metabolism of Ethyl
       Alcohol in the Body." Dr. Bill Boggan. Accessed 1/22/2010. <http://www.chem-
       cases.com/alcohol/alc-06.htm>

CHAPTER 15

Enzymes and Phytochemicals—
Another Shortage!

MANY biological and chemical reactions are slow—much too slow to support life. Nature overcomes this problem by the amazing actions of enzymes. What are enzymes? Enzymes are specialized proteins that do very special jobs in all plants, animals, and humans: *Enzymes either start up or speed up the billions of biological and chemical processes in every system of the body.* Enzymes perform their work in the body, become worn out, and are dismantled by other enzymes. These worn-out enzymes must be replaced.[1]

Enzymes are produced by the pancreas, saliva glands, small intestine, and other organs. We have known for a long time that our bodies may not be able to produce adequate amounts of certain digestive enzymes—this is called pancreatic insufficiency.[2] Dr. Anthony J. Cichoke, in his book *The Complete Book of Enzyme Therapy*, writes that one of the first signs of enzyme deficiency is probably disturbed digestion, which includes indigestion, stomach upset, feeling bloated, and gas.[3] We may not be able to produce the specific enzymes for digesting certain foods—beans, for example, for which there are specific enzyme supplements such as Beano and Be Sure. Many people cannot digest lactose, a type of milk sugar, for which the enzyme supplement lactase can be taken.

Research shows that our bodies produce fewer enzymes as we age. Making matters worse, Dr. Edward Howell and Dr. Max Wolf, pioneers in enzyme research, showed that enzymes "can't do their jobs as well" as we grow older.[4] An interesting study showed that the enzyme activity of insects is limited and, when their supply runs out, the end result is death.[5]

Now, for some good news: our body tries to conserve and recycle enzymes as much as possible. You can help your body conserve its supply of enzymes by eating more fresh, uncooked fruits and vegetables so your body spends fewer enzymes for digestion of food. Fresh, uncooked fruits and vegetables come prepackaged with the enzymes needed to break down and digest that fruit or vegetable. Prolonged heating and cooking destroys these enzymes.[6] You can also get more enzymes into your body by taking oral enzyme supplements, which are available in capsules and tablets. Enzyme supplements are safe and are well tolerated by most people although some caution is necessary as with most other nutritional supplements and therapies.[7] Some cautions are given later in this chapter.

There are over 3,000 types of enzymes in our bodies with more being discovered as research progresses. We will consider 2 major jobs that enzymes perform:

1. Digestive enzymes break down the food we eat into tiny microscopic particles so nutrients can be absorbed into the bloodstream.
2. Metabolic enzymes run our bodies, repair tissues, fight illness and disease, get rid of toxins, and perform many other functions.

Much research is focused on a special group of enzymes that break down proteins. These enzymes are called proteolytic enzymes (also called proteases). Proteolytic enzymes have some amazing therapeutic actions that will be discussed shortly. Let's take a quick look at fresh ginger's potent supply of proteolytic enzymes.

Fresh Ginger's Enzymes

Fresh ginger happens to be one of nature's most concentrated, ready-to-eat sources of proteolytic (protein-digesting) enzymes. Zingibain, the proteolytic enzyme present in *fresh* ginger, is responsible for its enzyme action. The discovery of zingibain is fairly recent—it occurred in the early 1970s, in a food laboratory at the University of Minnesota, by Dr. Eugene Allen. Allen also showed that crushed fresh ginger is a very effective meat tenderizer when used in a marinade and put on meat before cooking.[8]

Fresh ginger aids digestion because it supplies an extremely large amount of proteolytic enzymes, which are an amazing *180 times more concentrated* than the enzyme papain in papaya. Papain is an enzyme derived from unripe papaya and is used in meat tenderizers.[9] Other foods that contain significant amounts of proteolytic enzymes are fresh, raw pineapple (contains the enzyme bromelain, also used in meat tenderizers);[10] figs (contains the enzyme ficin);[11] kiwi; and guava.[12]

When eaten with food, fresh ginger's potent enzymes break down food proteins for better digestion. It is mentioned in the writing of the great philosopher Confucius that he ate fresh ginger with every meal.[13] Proteolytic enzymes will not attack our bodies because our cells have built-in protective mechanisms to prevent self-digestion. However, if the body's natural defenses are broken down, irritation could result.[14] See the cautions later in this chapter.

You will want to keep in mind that when fresh ginger is heated above 140°F (60°C), its enzyme activity decreases. Higher temperatures will destroy the delicate enzymes.[15] Dried ginger powder and various ginger products may or may not have enzymes, depending on the various processing methods used and how much heating was involved and for how long.

An extract from fresh ginger was shown to destroy parasites and their eggs.[16] This is probably why the Japanese have a long tradition of serving pickled ginger slices with sushi, a favorite traditional food made from very fresh, uncooked fish. Actually, the study pointed out that the gingerols in the ginger extract were responsible for killing the parasites. Pickled ginger probably has no enzymes (do to boiling during the pickling process) however, fresh ginger's potent supply of enzymes also contribute to its antiparasite, antibacterial, and anti-inflammatory actions.

FRESH GINGER TEA

If you do not care to eat slices of fresh ginger, I suggest making a delicious tea by gently squeezing fresh ginger in a garlic press and allowing the juice to dribble into warm water. Remember to keep the water well below 140°F (60°C),[17] which preserves the delicate enzymes. Add honey for sweetness. (Do *not* make fresh ginger tea by steeping, which means bringing the water to a boil at 212°F (100°C). High temperatures destroy active enzymes.)

The beauty of fresh ginger tea is that we can serve it to those around us who may not realize (or are too stubborn to admit) they can be helped by this simple yet amazing food that provides a powerful supply of enzymes and phytochemicals.

A NEW WAY TO GET GINGER'S ENZYMES

A new supplement made from zingibain, ginger's potent enzyme, was developed by Dr. Cliff Hawkins at the University of Queensland, Australia. Hawkins discovered that zingibain snips apart specific proteins in food. These proteins are of the proline type that are present in most of the foods we eat including meat, cheese, dairy, vegetables, nuts, beans, soy, seeds, grains, wheat and gluten. (Gluten is the protein in wheat and other grains that can cause allergies in many people, especially those with celiac disease.) Hawkins has developed zingibain supplements that can aid digestion and reduce the potential for allergic reactions. Refer to his Web site, www.biohawk.com.au, for more information.

How Important are Food,
Enzymes and Diet?

The discovery of the actions of enzymes and their importance in sustaining life was such a huge breakthrough in the science of life that Eduard Buchner of Germany was awarded the Nobel Prize for Chemistry in 1907.[18] The U.S. National Research Council issued a report in 1998, _Diet, Nutrition, and Cancer_, that points out that diet is probably the single biggest factor in the incidence of cancer.[19] Experts who are knowledgeable about enzymes point to the lack of enzymes in our modern diet as a major contributor to the many types of degenerative diseases we face today.[20]

Much of the food in our modern diet is "dead"—there are no active enzymes to help digest the food we eat. Food enzymes occur naturally in fresh fruits and vegetables but are destroyed upon cooking, frying, microwaving, and canning (canned foods are cooked first). Frozen foods are usually blanched (heated enough to kill enzymes and bacteria) and, therefore, have few or no enzymes. Although freezing alone (without heating) slows down enzyme activity, many enzymes should become active upon thawing. However, this needs further research. Harvesting fruits and vegetables before ripening also destroys enzymes. If our food contains few or no enzymes, our bodies must produce the extra enzymes needed for digestion. An enzymeless diet requires that the pancreas produce extra enzymes by borrowing or stealing enzymes from other important processes (such as clearing out toxins and making needed repairs in the body).[21]

Many enzymes are produced by the pancreas, which is a small organ weighing only about 3 ounces—about the weight of 2 golf balls—yet it must produce approximately 1 1/2 liters of digestive juices per day for the average adult. In addition, the pancreas must also produce insulin.[22] Insulin makes it possible for glucose, our bodies' fuel, to enter our bodies' cells for energy production.

OUR ENZYME BANK ACCOUNT

Edward Howell writes in his book *Enzyme Nutrition* that each person has a fixed potential for manufacturing enzymes, which he calls our "Enzyme Potential" or "Enzyme Bank Account." If the food we eat has few or no enzymes, then the pancreas must borrow or steal enzymes in order to digest the food we eat, possibly creating a shortage of enzymes in other parts of the body—too much spending and not enough deposits.

Howell writes, "The remarkable thing about the eventual bankruptcy of the enzyme bank account is that it can proceed quite painlessly, without immediate symptoms. Digestion of food takes a high priority and acts as a powerful stimulus in the demand for enzymes. If this function takes more than its rightful share, the other organs and tissues must try to get along with the remaining capacity. The only warning may be a belated malfunction or breakdown in some organ far removed from the digestive tract. But the diagnostician unaware of the importance of enzyme nutrition would have difficulty in connecting such a referred process to the true, underlying cause. This is how an assortment of human ailments may get started."[23]

While there are other experts who may not agree with Howell's concept of the enzyme bank account, it should motivate us to learn about the importance of eating fresh fruits and vegetables. The U.S. Department of Agriculture recommends eating a minimum amount of 2 to 4 servings of fruit and 3 to 5 servings of vegetables per day—some fresh, some cooked.[24] Some foods require heating or cooking as a matter of safety, practicality, and also to increase the bioavailibility of some nutrients. A pure vegetarian diet is not recommended unless under the direct care of a health care provider or nutrition professional.

More details about food enzymes are given later in this chapter, but, for now, let's look at other ways to get more enzymes.

Digestive Enzyme Supplements and Oral Enzyme Therapy

Digestive enzyme supplements are inexpensive, readily available in capsules and tablets, and are taken with a meal to break down foods in the stomach for better digestion. Enzyme therapy, on the other hand, is a recommended or prescribed program for treating a particular condition, illness or disease, often under the direction of a specialist.

Oral enzyme therapy (commonly called "systemic enzyme therapy" because it involves the whole body) requires taking large amounts of enzyme supplements between meals along with a strict diet and detoxification program. Enzyme therapy is also effective when combined with conventional medical therapies.[25] Oral enzyme tablets used for therapy have an enteric coating which prevents the enzymes from being used up in the stomach so their full strength can be released in the small intestine and into the bloodstream. (Enteric means *in the intestine*). These oral enzyme tablets are taken between meals on an empty stomach otherwise the enzymes will be used up just for breaking down food. You can learn more about these enzymes at the Web site www.buywobenzym.com and other Web sites listed later in this chapter.

Enzyme Supplements and the E-F-G Approach

Several experts recommend taking enzyme supplements to promote healing of leaky gut syndrome[26] and *Candida* overgrowth.[27] According to Anthony Cichoke, author of *The Complete Book of Enzyme Therapy*, enzyme supplements are able to stimulate the beneficial bacteria in the digestive tract and help clean and detoxify the colon.[28]

How Important is Enzyme Therapy?

In his book, Dr. Cichoke lists over 150 illnesses, diseases, and conditions for which oral enzyme therapy is helpful.[29] His book is a practical how-to approach and lists many enzymes, vitamins, minerals, cofactors, and other therapies helpful for each illness.

A growing number of physicians who understand the importance of enzyme therapy are prescribing oral enzymes (often combined with conventional medicine) for major illnesses, including multiple sclerosis, arthritis and rheumatic disorders, injuries involving inflammation, circulatory disorders, and age-related illnesses, according to Dr. D. A. Lopez, physician, researcher, and author of *Enzymes—The Fountain of Life*.[30] Lopez gives very clear explanations for some of the theories and research behind the amazing therapeutic actions of enzyme therapy.

Enzyme therapy is a common treatment in Europe and Japan, where it is combined with conventional medical treatments. In the United States, specialized enzyme medications are approved by the FDA for several health conditions, including cardiovascular disorders (enzymes are injected into the bloodstream), cleaning of wounds and burns (enzymes are applied to the skin), and treatment of various diseases such as cystic fibrosis and certain types of cancer.[31] Beginning in April 2010, the FDA is requiring that pancreatic enzyme products (enzyme supplements made from animal sources) become approved as medications.

In Europe, it is very common for physicians to give oral enzyme supplements to cancer patients in addition to using conventional cancer therapies (surgery, chemotherapy, and radiation). Enzyme therapy helps support the patient's immune system and improves his or her quality of life. The results have been very encouraging.[32]

A FASCINATING HISTORY LESSON

In the early 1900s, Dr. John Beard, embryology professor at the University of Edinburgh, observed that a placenta behaves much like a tumor. A placenta attaches to the uterus, grows rapidly, and develops blood vessels in a very similar way that a tumor attaches to tissue and grows. Interestingly, Beard further observed that placenta cells are in fact, very similar to tumor cells in structure and function but somehow, the placenta knows when to stop growing. Beard theorized that if he knew the exact mechanism that halted the growth of the placenta, he might use it to halt the growth of tumors. Continuing his research, he discovered the placenta stopped growing on the very day the baby's liver and pancreas started pouring out enzymes! The mechanism that halted the placenta's growth, to his amazement, was the proteolytic enzyme trypsin—the same enzyme produced by the pancreas that breaks down food proteins in the small intestine! With this knowledge, Beard further demonstrated that the growth of tumors could also be halted and even reversed by injecting pancreatic enzymes in and around the tumor.[33] Beard published his results in major medical journals and in his monologue *The Enzyme Treatment of Cancer* (London: Chatto and Windus, 1911).

Another new age had dawned however, with the experimentation of radiactivity by another talented scientist, polish-born Madame Curie. The media's fixation on this captivating new frontier and its potential applications in science and medicine overshadowed most other scientific work during the early 1900s. Dr. Curie was the first person to receive two Nobel prizes, one for physics and one for chemistry. The potential danger of ionizing radiation was realized in the 1920s and by her untimely death in 1934 at the age of 66 from aplastic anemia, a disease of the blood as a result of excessive exposure to radiation.[34]

It would be some 50 years after the publication of Dr. Beard's book that his brilliant discoveries were again proven an amazing blow against cancer, not by injections of enzymes this time, but by oral enzyme therapy. As long as the quality and proper strength of enzyme products could be assured, proteolytic enzymes proved to be an effective, non-toxic treatment for treating cancer and shrinking tumors.[35]

A Very Successful Protocol for Treating Cancer

Dr. Nicholas Gonzalez, MD PC and Dr. Linda Isaacs, MD have achieved amazing success in their practice in New York City for treating various advanced cancers, allergies and fatigue. Their approach consists of oral enzyme therapy, strict diet and detoxification. Dr. Gonzalez trained under Robert A. Good MD, Ph.D, a former director of Memorial Sloan-Kettering Cancer Center in New York. (Dr. Good is regarded as "the most published author in the history of medicine" and described as the "Founder of Modern Immunology" by *The New York Times.* Sloan-Kettering is the largest and oldest cancer center in the world).

In his book, *The Trophoblast and the Origins of Cancer* (New York: New Spring Press, 2009), Dr. Gonzalez and Dr. Isaacs meticulously describe the history, theory and success of systemic enzyme therapy. See www.dr-gonzalez.com and www.newspringpress.com. to view more information.

ATHLETES AND ENZYMES

Oral enzymes are also used in sports medicine (in relatively large amounts) for more rapid healing of injuries, especially when inflammation is involved. One study of a university football team showed that players who were given oral enzymes prior to injury recovered *twice* as fast as those who were not given enzymes.[36] Another study showed superior recovery from muscle soreness from downhill running.[37] Well over 20 studies have confirmed the effectiveness of oral enzymes for speeding the healing of injuries from boxing, karate, soccer, ice hockey, and other sports. Many studies used the enzyme tablets Wobenzyme N, manufactured by the German company Mucos Pharma.[38] More information is available at www.buywobenzym.com.

Enzyme supplements were used extensively in the training camps of the East German athletes who competed in the 1984 Olympics at Sarajevo, Yugoslavia. The team won 9 gold metals—more first places than any other country.[39]

Oral enzymes may also be helpful for reducing mild knee joint pain from injury,[40] reducing inflammation from arthritis,[41] and providing faster recovery from certain surgeries.[42] Researchers postulate that oral enzymes help activate and regulate inflammation and also help promote the mechanisms that limit damage and promote the formation of new, healthy tissue, according to Lopez.[43]

CAUTIONS WHEN TAKING
ENZYME SUPPLEMENTS

1. Do not take enzyme supplements if you are at high risk of bleeding. Consult with your physician when taking enzymes before or after surgeries.[44] Stop taking enzymes 2 or 3 days before undergoing operative surgery, as enzyme supplements could increase the risk of bleeding.[45]

2. Do not take enzyme supplements if you are taking blood-thinning medications because enzymes can significantly increase the effectiveness of certain medications,[46] especially blood-thinning medications.[47] Enzyme users must work with their physicians to reduce dosages of blood-thinning medications. Enzymes can also increase the effectiveness of certain antibiotics, chemotherapy medications, and the steroid cortisone.[48]

3. Since there are insufficient studies of enzyme supplements for pregnant or nursing mothers, enzyme supplements should not be used during pregnancy or nursing unless under the direction of a physician.[49]

4. For young children with cystic fibrosis, special caution is advised. Several studies show that damage to the large intestine (fibrosing colonopathy) resulted from either the use of extremely large amounts of the enzyme lipase[50] or some unknown interaction between the enteric coating and the enzymes themselves.[51]

5. People who are allergic to pork or other animal foods should not take pancreatic enzymes. Likewise, people who are allergic to pineapple or papaya should not take these enzyme supplements, which contain bromelain or papain.

THE AMAZING WORLD OF PHYTOCHEMICALS

Phytochemicals are plant chemicals that provide some very special benefits to our body. Plant enzymes are just one example of phytochemicals. We learned that the phytochemicals in ginger, garlic, and turmeric have multiple actions that can greatly benefit our health. We also learned that cilantro and chlorella can help remove heavy metals from our bodies. Before we get back to enzymes, let's focus on a vegetable with a potent supply of phytochemicals—kale.

KALE—A CASE STUDY IN PHYTOCHEMICALS

Kale is a dark green, leafy vegetable that grows quickly and can be added to garden salads and soups or, if you don't have a lot of time, simply eaten by itself. Note that kale, like beans, contains the plant sugar raffinose, which can produce some abdominal discomfort (and gas) because it is difficult to digest. Try taking 2 or 3 Beano supplements or other enzyme supplements before eating kale. Cooking or sautéing kale can minimize problems with gas and abdominal discomfort. Eat small servings—even small amounts of kale can provide some extremely important phytochemicals. Actually, the technique that works best for me is to chew on a leaf, swallow the juices then spit out the chewy fibers. It works!

Like ginger, kale is a superfood because it is inexpensive, readily available, and has multiple characteristics that can improve our health. Kale can be harvested in spring, summer, fall, and even into winter in some climates. Outdoor kale plants seem to come back to life very quickly after the winter season and provide salad greens in the early spring. Kale is also available in grocery stores. The main varieties include curly kale, which is the most common; Russian kale, which has purple stems; and ornamental kale, which is grown for its pretty colors. Ornamental kale is edible but is difficult to chew.

Even more impressive is what we get when we eat kale. It contains some amazing phytochemicals along with a rich supply of vitamins, minerals, calcium, fiber, and a bit of omega-3 EFAs. It is also one of the biggest suppliers of antioxidants of all vegetables.[52]

ANTICANCER ACTIONS

Kale is a member of the *Brassica* group of vegetables, which appear to have some very important health benefits. This group of vegetables also includes broccoli, Brussels sprouts, cabbage, cauliflower, collards, bok choy, kohlrabi, mustard greens, rutabaga, and turnips.[53]

A lot of exciting research is targeted at the phytochemicals in the *Brassica* group of vegetables because of their anticancer actions,[54] including defense against breast cancer,[55] colon cancer,[56] prostate cancer,[57] bladder cancer,[58] and lung cancer.[59] The *Brassica* vegetables also appear to have some cholesterol-lowering properties[60] and may work against non-Hodgkin's lymphoma.[61] The phytochemicals in these vegetables also have some antibiotic actions and can inhibit some antibiotic-resistant strains of *Helicobacter pylori* bacteria. Remember that this common bacteria is known to cause stomach ulcers and also increases the risk of stomach cancer (also called gastric cancer).[62] It is estimated that *Helicobacter pylori* causes 80% of stomach ulcers. Approximately two-thirds of the world's population is infected with this bacteria.[63]

Currently, broccoli is the most researched of the *Brassica* vegetables because of the high concentration of phytochemicals in broccoli sprouts.[64] Broccoli, kale, cabbage, and the other *Brassica* vegetables contain disease-fighting phytochemicals called glucosinolates,[65] which change into another chemical in our body called sulforaphane, one of the most intensely studied phytochemicals because of its anticancer actions.[66] Broccoli is a great food; however, it is also one of the most perishable foods and must be replaced in the grocery store every 2 to 3 days so it will remain usable in your refrigerator for another 3 to 5 days.

The *Brassica* vegetables are also called "cruciferous" (or *Cruciferae*),[67] which means cross bearing. If the plants are allowed to mature, their flowers will have 4 petals in a cross pattern. The cruciferous family of vegetables also includes radishes, horseradishes, wasabi, and watercress,[68] all of which also contain glucosinolates.[69]

You may want to know that the glucosinolates in kale increase with age, reaching maximum levels just as flower buds begin to appear. As the buds appear, the glucosinolates in the leaves rapidly decline and go into the buds.[70] It is also important to know that when kale and other *Brassica* vegetables are eaten raw, a special enzyme is released from the plant called myrosinase, which converts the glucosinolates to various disease-fighting chemicals. However, if these vegetables are cooked, the enzyme myrosinase is destroyed. Amazingly, the beneficial bacteria of a healthy digestive tract can convert the glucosinolates into these other disease-fighting chemicals. The bad news is that if the beneficial bacteria have been destroyed by antibiotics or other means, then very few of the glucosinolates in cooked kale or broccoli will be converted, and, in turn, some of the disease-fighting actions will probably be reduced or lost.[71]

KALE'S RICH SUPPLY OF VITAMINS

Kale has extremely high amounts of vitamins K, A, C, and beta-carotene. Just 1 cup of chopped kale (about 67 grams) provides over 600% of the recommended daily value of vitamin K, over 200% of the daily value of vitamin A, and over 130% of the daily value of vitamin C. Spinach, which is also very high in these vitamins, has about one-third the amounts of kale.[72] It is interesting that spinach has high amounts of these vitamins but is not in the *Brassica* group of vegetables. As most of us know, spinach is another great food.

THE BENEFITS OF VITAMIN K

Vitamin K is important for building strong bones in younger people[73] and for keeping bones strong in older people by helping resist fractures and breaks.[74] Exactly how vitamin K works is not completely understood, but it appears to make calcium stick in our bones, helping maintain their structural integrity. Other nutrients required for strong bones in addition to calcium include vitamin D, magnesium,[75] and zinc.[76] It is good to know that the bioavailability of kale's calcium is excellent, even a bit higher than milk, meaning that its calcium is efficiently absorbed into the body.[77]

Vitamin K is also required for proper clotting of blood and was given its name after the Danish word *Koagulations Vitamin* upon its discovery in 1929 by Danish researcher Henrik Dam. Dam observed that diseased chicks with an excessive bleeding disorder had deficiencies in this newly discovered vitamin. It is important that people who are taking blood-thinning medications consult their physician before eating large amounts of kale or spinach and discuss any possible interactions.[78]

KALE'S POTENT ANTIOXIDANTS

Kale contains very high amounts of antioxidants. Only a handful of common plant foods score higher in antioxidants. These foods include various berries, raisins, and prunes. Spinach contains about 70% of the antioxidant level of kale.[79] Animal studies show that a diet of foods with high levels of antioxidants may slow certain age-related inflammatory reactions.[80]

Both vitamins A and C are important antioxidants and also have anti-inflammatory properties, which compliments the E-F-G approach. Since many of these antioxidants and phytochemicals exist in the bright-colored pigments of fruits and vegetables, it is important to include a "rainbow of antioxidants" in our diet.[81]

Kale contains an abundant supply of vitamin A, which is essential to the eyes for good vision[82] and may also help repair a leaky gut (which fits nicely into the theme of the E-F-G approach). While it is generally believed there are no major deficiencies of vitamin A in industrialized countries, vitamin A's effectiveness for improving vision and leaky gut and also for restoring proper growth rate have been well demonstrated in infants with deficiencies in developing countries.[83]

Vitamin A from vegetables is mostly in the form of beta-carotene, a yellow antioxidant that is very important to our eyes and our overall health. The yellow pigment is not visible in kale, spinach, and other green vegetables because it is masked by the large amounts of chlorophyll.

Two Amazing Phytochemicals for the Eyes

Kale (and spinach) contains two phytochemicals that are especially important to the eyes: lutein and zeaxanthin (pronounced loo-teen and ze-uh-zan-thin). It was discovered that the macula in the eye has a rich concentration of these two chemicals.[84] The macula and retina are thin membranes at the back of the eye that pick up light and images, converts them to electrical signals, then transmits the information to the brain. The macula is the most highly sensitive area of the retina and gives us our central vision—our most focused vision that we use for such tasks as reading and driving a car. Eating kale and other dark green leafy vegetables like spinach and collard greens can add lutein and zeaxanthin to the macula. This can help prevent a disease called age-related macular degeneration (AMD).[85] AMD is the medical term for the gradual loss of vision and is the leading cause of blindness in the United States and other industrialized countries.[86]

Sufficient levels of lutein and zeaxanthin in the macula and retina help protect the eyes against damage by helping filter out harmful ultraviolet light,[87] like wearing an invisible set of sunglasses. Lutein and zeaxanthin in the diet can also reduce the risk of developing cataracts.[88] Raw kale is one of nature's richest sources of lutein and zeaxanthin, having over 3 times more than spinach, 4 times more than collards, 15 times more than broccoli and romaine lettuce, and over 20 times more than corn, peas, Brussels sprouts, eggs, and most other fruits and vegetables.[89]

Chlorophyll—Nature's Detoxifier

Kale and other dark green vegetables have rich supplies of chlorophyll. Chlorophyll is the "green blood" in plants, which absorbs light to carry on photosynthesis—the miracle process that sustains plant life (and most other life on earth). It is interesting that chlorophyll is similar in chemical structure to hemoglobin in our blood. Our red blood cells contain hemoglobin, a protein that carries oxygen to all cells in our body. Chlorophyll absorbs light; hemoglobin absorbs oxygen—what an amazing miracle of similarity!

In our bodies, chlorophyll can help neutralize certain harmful toxins such as those found in cooked red meats,[90] cigarette smoke,[91] and other toxins.[92] Chlorophyll also has antioxidant,[93] anti-inflammatory, and antitumor properties,[94] which again adds to the synergy of the E-F-G approach.

When buying kale or any other leafy green vegetables, note that if some leaves appear yellow, much of the nutrients have been lost. If you cook kale or other *Brassica* vegetables, don't throw away the cooking water because up to 90% of the phytochemicals may leach out of the vegetable and into the cooking water. Lightly cooking, stir frying, and steaming vegetables will help retain more phytochemicals than fully cooking them. Vegetables that are finely shredded can also lose up to 75% of their glucosinolates after 6 hours.[95]

Oh yeah, I almost forgot to mention that because kale grows quickly into a small bush, it is very effective at keeping weeds under control—not many superfoods can do that, too!

Now, let's get back to enzymes …

BACK TO ENZYMES

If enzyme therapy offers so many benefits with very few (if any) side effects, then why isn't enzyme therapy widely used in the United States?

Lopez cites several reasons why enzyme therapy has not gained popularity. First, older medical textbooks wrongly state that enzyme molecules are too big to be absorbed by the digestive tract. Research has proven that enzyme molecules are absorbed, although the amount of enzymes reaching a specific site in the body depends on a number of factors (that are beyond the scope of this book). Second, their effects on the body are broad, or systemic. Conventional medical treatment in the United States prefers specific actions by specialized drugs. Preconceived negative attitudes and a lack of understanding are other reasons for the lack of enzyme therapy in the United States even though systemic enzyme therapy has proven successful in other countries. Other reasons for skepticism include the fact that enzyme mixtures and their activities vary from manufacturer to manufacturer and have not been regulated by the FDA. The FDA requires testing as of April, 2010 to verify safety, effectiveness and manufacturing standards. Additionally, the FDA has been slow to accept research done outside the United States. Yet another reason might be that enzyme therapy uses a mixture of enzymes and other nutrients and may appear to be an alternative treatment rather than the preferred magic bullet single-substance medication.[96] It should be noted that some patients may not be willing to put forth the effort and discipline for an effective enzyme therapy program.

MORE DETAILS ABOUT ENZYME THERAPY

1. Proteolytic enzymes help support the immune system,[97] in part by helping to break down and destroy "immune complexes" in our bodies. Immune complexes are typically composed of an antigen (such as bacteria, viruses, poison, or degenerated cells) and an antibody. (Antibodies are Y-shaped protein markers produced by our immune system that attach to antigens.) If these immune complexes become too plentiful, they jam up the immune system, interrupting disease fighting and healing. The immune complexes must be removed from the body in order for healing to proceed.[98] Enteric-coated enzyme supplements can do just that—help remove excess immune complexes from the body.[99] Excess immune complexes are also seen in diabetes and atherosclerosis.[100]

   Researchers postulate that our immune systems build a fibrin (protein) coating around the immune complex in an attempt to isolate the problem, but unfortunately, this coating also disguises the immune complex from the body's immune system. Researchers further postulate that proteolytic enzymes can help degrade this fibrin coating so the body's defenses can recognize and destroy the immune complex.

Enzymes can also help remove excess fibrin from the body. Fibrin is the glue that allows proper clotting of blood; however, too much fibrin can cause blood clots and other problems. Excess fibrin is related to various diseases of the cardiovascular system.[101] Fibrin is also involved in age-related wrinkling of skin caused by the forming of protein "cross-links," which cause the skin to lose its elasticity.[102]

2. Many studies indicate that proteolytic enzymes have anti-tumor and anticancer actions.[103] Researchers point out that proteolytic enzymes may also help to degrade the fibrin coating around cancer cells so the immune system can recognize and destroy the cancer cells. (Cancer cells can have a fibrin coating up to 15 times thicker than normal cells.)[104] One major advantage of enzyme therapy when it is combined with conventional cancer treatments is that lower doses of radiation and chemotherapy can be used to achieve the same effect, according to European scientists.[105]

    Experts believe that enzyme therapy can help reduce the side effects from chemotherapy and radiotherapy during treatment of colorectal cancer.[106] Oral enzyme therapy is currently used in Germany, Italy, and France for cancer patients.

3. Enzyme therapy has helped produce some amazing results. Anthony Cichoke, in his book *The Complete Book of Enzyme Therapy,* tells of the amazing recovery of his son, David, who at the age of 3 fell down the stairway of their house and was diagnosed with brain damage as a result of the fall. It was thought that David might never walk again, as he could not control the movement of his head, arms, and legs. After much physical therapy, combined with nutrition therapy and enzyme therapy, David not only recovered to walk and run, but as he grew older he excelled in athletics to become a nationally ranked

swimmer and runner. He even was up for draft in the National Football League.[108]

4. Enzyme therapy has been shown helpful for disorders of the veins. It is estimated that 1 in 8 adults suffer from some form of chronic problems with veins.[109]

5. Enzyme therapy offers hope for treating children with autism.[110]

MORE DETAILS ABOUT ENZYME SUPPLEMENTS

1. Enzyme supplements are absorbed,[111] are well tolerated, and are quite safe for most people with no significant side effects;[112] however, there are some special cases in which enzyme supplements should not be taken as noted in the previous cautions.

2. Enzymes break down food for proper digestion so our bodies can get the nutrients we need. If nutrients are not broken down, our bodies may not absorb them and our health will suffer.

3. As early as 1935, it was suggested that certain food-related allergies may be linked to undigested food proteins that enter the bloodstream.[113] Later studies support this theory. Enzyme supplements taken with meals can improve digestion.

4. The common proteolytic enzyme bromelain (from pineapple) has some antibacterial and antiviral properties. One study shows bromelain can inhibit certain bacteria including *Salmonella*[114] and *E. coli*.[115] *Salmonella* and *E. coli* are associated with food poisoning.

5. Gingerols (abundant in fresh ginger) inhibit the growth of *H. pylori* bacteria.[116] Remember that *H. pylori* is the bacteria responsible for causing the majority of stomach ulcers and has been linked to certain cancers.[117] Studies show proteolytic enzymes can also help fight against certain viruses.[118]

6. Most enzyme supplements are obtained from plant and animal sources. The protease bromelain comes from the stems of

pineapple. Papain is made from unripe papayas. Pancreatin is a mixture of lipase, amylase, and proteases and is extracted from the pancreas, stomach, and liver of pigs, ox, or beef. Plant enzymes can be many times more potent than the pancreatic enzymes from animal sources.[119] In addition, plant enzymes are effective over a wide pH range, which means they are effective even in the acidic conditions in the stomach.[120]

7. Enzyme supplements are usually labeled by amount (grams or milligrams) and potency (activity units, also called international units). Because amounts, potency, and units of measurement vary among manufacturers, be sure to read label instructions for recommended dose. A USP activity unit rating of 1X means an enzyme supplement can digest 25 grams of casein (milk protein). A rating of 2X can digest 50 grams of casein, 3X can digest 75 grams and so on.

8. One interesting study showed that the pancreas readily absorbs any extra enzymes, adopts them as its own, then recirculates the enzymes throughout the lymphatic circulatory system.[121] This is evidence that the body places a very high priority on keeping and conserving enzymes.

9. Numerous vitamins, minerals, and other substances called cofactors and coenzymes are required for enzymes to work. For example, copper, calcium, magnesium, and zinc are required by hundreds of enzymes.[122] Zinc is also an antioxidant[123] and helps with healing leaky gut syndrome[124] You may want to consider taking a multivitamin supplement from time to time to help avoid shortages. Be careful when taking supplements. For example, taking too much zinc has been known to create a shortage of copper.[125]

10. Another helpful supplement is coenzyme Q10 (abbreviated CoQ10), which occurs in high concentrations in the heart, liver, and immune system. Unfortunately, as we age, our bodies produce less and less CoQ10. CoQ10 is especially important for proper heart function and blood circulation. Foods

that contain CoQ10 include whole grains, oily fish (such as sardines), organ meats, nuts, and seeds.[126] CoQ10 is also available as a supplement. The relationship between low levels of CoQ10 and heart disease was established in the 1970s,[127] and later studies proved CoQ10's effectiveness at improving heart function.[128]

MORE DETAILS ABOUT FOOD ENZYMES

Eating more fresh fruits and vegetables is a difficult challenge for most of us, including myself. Today's rushed lifestyle makes it difficult to buy, keep, and prepare fresh fruits and vegetables, although all of us need to start somewhere. The enzyme concept teaches us that the food we eat can do far more than just fill our stomach—it can be our medicine to help guard our health. When viewed this way, it makes the additional expense and effort all the more worthwhile. You must decide—it's your health! Here are some important points about food enzymes:

1. Fresh, raw fruits and vegetables come prepackaged with the enzymes needed to digest that fruit or vegetable. Enzymes occur naturally in raw, uncooked fruits and vegetables and sprouted nuts and grains. However, enzymes are destroyed when food is heated above 140°F (60°C) and possibly as low as 107°F (42°C) for some foods.[129] Hence, cooked food does not contain enzymes, nor does canned food. Frozen vegetables are usually blanched (heated above 140°F) and then frozen. It is the heating that destroys the enzymes, not the freezing. Be sure to add raw fruits and vegetables gradually to your diet so your body can adjust.

2. Chewing the fruit or vegetable releases the plant's enzymes, which help digest the food as it rests in the upper portion of the stomach for about 1/2 to 1 hour. Food enzymes perform their work in the upper stomach during this resting stage, starting the digestion process. The upper and lower stomach

in humans function similar to multiple stomachs in animals. In the upper stomach food enzymes and enzymes from saliva begin the digestion process. After a period of time, food enters the lower stomach (which is normally squeezed together when empty) where it is mixed with pepsin, the protein-digesting enzyme secreted by the stomach. Hydrochloric acid is also secreted by the stomach and creates the acidic environment required to activate the pepsin.[130] You can see the importance of having adequate levels of hydrochloric acid for proper digestion of food proteins. Refer to chapter 6.

3. Long-term food storage and pesticides decrease enzyme levels in food. Freezing slows the enzyme activity of fruits and vegetables;[131] however, some enzymes should become active again upon thawing. This needs more research.

4. Some experts and researchers equate adequate enzymes in our bodies with the ability to resist illness and disease.[132] A nursing baby receives many enzymes from human milk that are readily absorbed by the baby's immature digestive tract. It is well-known that breast-fed babies have less sickness than babies who were only partially breast-fed or were bottle-fed.[133]

5. Active enzymes enable native Eskimos to eat several pounds of raw animal fat per day yet have clean arteries and no obesity.[134] Raw animal fat contains the enzyme lipase, which breaks down fats. Raw animal meat contains enzymes that break down the proteins after the animal is dead. (However, eating raw meat and raw animal fat is not recommended.)

6. Raw tree nuts, raw seeds, raw beans, and raw grains have natural enzyme inhibitors that keep the seed dormant until water is added. Upon sprouting, the enzyme inhibitors become deactivated and the enzymes become active. It was quickly learned that feeding raw soybeans to cattle resulted in underweight livestock because the cow's pancreas had to supply extra digestive enzymes to overcome the enzyme inhibitors. In addition, the pancreas of each cow was enlarged because it had

to work extra hard to produce this extra supply of digestive enzymes (in a similar way that muscles grow larger when exercised rigorously). When the soybeans were roasted or cooked, the cattle gained normal weight because the heat destroyed the enzyme inhibitors. (Unfortunately, heating also destroys active enzymes.) Edward Howell, pioneer in enzyme research and author of *Enzyme Nutrition*, noted that he experienced some nausea and discomfort in his abdomen after eating too many raw tree nuts and raw wheat germ because of the natural enzyme inhibitors.[135] My suggestion is to eat a slice of fresh ginger or take an enzyme supplement when eating nuts.

7. Sprouts are an excellent source of enzymes and other phytochemicals. Alfalfa sprouts and bean sprouts taste good on salads. Many people enjoy making their own seed sprouts using an inexpensive sprouting kit. I enjoy sprouting mung beans, which are the quickest and easiest that I've found. Howell's studies show that the enzymes in seeds and nuts are at their highest potency when the sprout is 1/4 inch (6 millimeters) long. He notes that squirrels bury nuts in the ground then later dig them up after they have sprouted. Squirrels thrive on the enzyme-rich nut.[136]

8. Salt is an enzyme inhibitor and should be used sparingly.[137]

9. Fermented foods are easier to digest because the food has already undergone partial digestion by the application of enzymes during fermentation. Fermented foods include yogurt, cheese, tofu, and certain ethnic foods including miso, tempeh, natto, and kimchi.[138] Uncooked sauerkraut and naturally fermented soy sauce also contain enzymes.[139]

10. Other ways to get more enzymes are to lightly steam vegetables (instead of fully cooking them) and to eat more fresh salads, which is easy to do in the summer when our bodies don't need as many calories. Juicing vegetables is also a good idea if you have the time and equipment.

11. Common foods with high concentrations of proteolytic

enzymes include fresh ginger, fresh pineapple, kiwi, figs, papaya, and, in lesser amounts, cantaloupe and other melons.[140] Figs are often mentioned in the Bible and were a highly valued food source and also used for payments, gifts, and even healing.[141] Figs and pineapple may be hard on the teeth—figs because of their high sugar content and pineapple because of its high acidic content. Frequently eating acidic foods and beverages may dissolve tooth enamel. Other foods that are highly acidic include lemons (or juice), oranges (or juice), coffee, black tea, wine, beer, soda pop, vinegar, and sauerkraut.[142] Try rinsing your mouth with water mixed with a little baking soda to neutralize the acid after consuming acidic foods and drinks.

12. Enzymes are generally named with the suffix -ase following the substance the enzyme acts on. (Examples: Protease breaks down proteins. Lipase breaks down fat. Amylase breaks down carbohydrates. Lactase breaks down lactose, the sugar in milk). Some proteolytic enzymes such as pepsin, trypsin, and others were already named before this convention was adopted.

13. Lipase is another important enzyme that breaks down and digests fat. Howell reported that lower levels of lipase are found in patients with fatty tumors, obesity, and atherosclerosis.[143] Flaxseeds and sprouted seeds and grains such as malt (sprouted barley seeds) can be excellent sources of lipase.[144] More research is needed to determine the benefits of lipase-containing foods and supplements.

14. Raw foods that contain the enzyme lipase include flaxseeds, germinating seeds, coconuts, and olives (but not olive oil, cottonseed oil, or coconut oil). Raw (unpasteurized) milk and butter made from raw milk also contain lipase.[145] Lipase works to break down fats while resting in the upper stomach. Howell wrote of the danger of eating fats without the enzyme lipase.[146]

15. Amylase is another important food enzyme that breaks down carbohydrates. Amylase is also present in saliva. Common

foods containing amylase include bananas and unprocessed (and unheated) honey.[147] Honey from the comb has active enzymes. Anthony Cichoke writes that fresh ginger increases the concentration of amylase in saliva and also stimulates the flow of saliva and amylase.[148]

16. Missionary pilot Steve Saint reports in his book *End of the Spear* how the Waodoni tribal people of Ecuador produced an energy food made from boiled manioc roots (similar to mashed potatoes). The women would put a ball of the mashed root into their mouths, mix it with their saliva, and then spit it back into the mixing bowl, only to take another mouthful and repeat the process.[149] The amylase in their saliva worked to partially digest the starch so it could be easily digested when eaten, giving the men a quick energy food.

    The Mayan Indians knew papaya was a natural treatment for indigestion and stomach pains (because of its proteolytic enzymes) and offered papaya to distressed Spanish soldiers who ate too much unfamiliar food.[150]

    Fermented soy sauce is probably one of the oldest uses of enzyme supplements. It is interesting that some very old cultures realized the value of food enzymes—and we should, too!

17. Lastly, it is important to know that enzymes require water to carry out their life-giving functions. If you do additional reading about enzymes, you will see the terms *hydrolyze*, *hydrolysis*, or *hydrolytic*, which simply mean enzymes require water to carry out their actions. So remember—drink plenty of good water. If you have public drinking water, be sure to use a filter to take out most of the chlorine.

OTHER REFERENCES FOR ENZYMES

Books:

The Complete Book of Enzyme Therapy, by Anthony J. Cichoke (New York: Avery Publishing, 1999).

Enzymes: The Foundation of Life, by D. A. Lopez, R. M. Williams, and M. Miehlke (Charleston, SC: Neville Press, 1994).

The Trophoblast and the Origins of Cancer, by Nicholas J. Gonzalez, MD and Linda L. Issacs, MD (New York: New Spring Press, 2009) available at www.newspringpress.com

Web sites:

* www.dr-gonzalez.com
* www.buywobenzym.com
* www.dr-murray.com
* www.enzymestuff.com
* www.vitacost.com
* www.askwaltstollmd.com

REFERENCES FOR CHAPTER 15

1.   Howell E. *Enzyme Nutrition.* Garden City Park, New York: Avery Publishing Group, Inc., 1985. p.25.

2a.   Nakamura T, Takebe K, Imamura K, et al. "Fat-soluble vitamins in patients with chronic pancreatitis (pancreatic insufficiency)." *Acta Gastroenterol Belg.* 1996;59:10-4.

2b.   Bang Jorgensen B, Thorsgaard Pedersen N, Worning H. "Short report: lipid and vitamin B12 malassimilation in pancreatic insuffiency." *Aliment Pharmacol Ther.* 1991;5:207-10.

2c.   Harms HK, Kennel O, Bertele RM, Bidlingmeier F, Bohne A. "Vitamin B12 absorption and exocrine pancreatic insufficiency in childhood." Eur J Pediatr. 1981 Mar;136(1):75-9.

2d.   Cichoke A. *The Complete Book of Enzyme Therapy.* New York, Avery, 1999. pp.13-14.

3.   Cichoke A. *The Complete Book of Enzyme Therapy.* New York, Avery, 1999. p.5.

4a.   Howell E. *Enzyme Nutrition.* Garden City Park, New York: Avery Publishing Group, Inc., 1985. pp.12, 27-29, 147-148.

4b.   Cichoke A. *The Complete Book of Enzyme Therapy.* New York:Avery, 1999. p.102.

5.   Howell E. *Enzyme Nutrition.* Garden City Park, New York: Avery Publishing Group, Inc., 1985. p.24-26.

6a.   Howell E. *Enzyme Nutrition.* Garden City Park, New York: Avery Publishing Group, Inc., 1985. pp.4-5, 29.

6b.   Cichoke A. *The Complete Book of Enzyme Therapy.* New York:Avery, 1999. p.17.

7a.   Lopez DA, Williams RM, Miehlke K. *Enzymes - The Fountain of Life.* The Neville Press, Inc. 1994, Germany. pp.129-137.

7b.   Cichoke A. *The Complete Book of Enzyme Therapy.* New York:Avery, 1999. p.44.

8.   Hunt M. "Fresh ginger makes better meat tenderizer." *TwinCities.com* Pioneer Press. Posted on Mon, Feb. 16, 2004; Accessed 6/1/2004. <http://www.realcities.com/mld/twincities/living/7949674.htm>.

9.   Thompson, EH, Wolf ID, Allen CE. "Ginger rhizome: A new source of proteolytic enzyme." *Journal of Food Science* 38, no. 4 (1973): pp.652-55.

10.   Heinicke RM, Gortner WA. "Stem bromelain - A new protease preparation from pineapple plants." 1957. *Econ. Bot.* 11: 225.

11a.   Whitaker JR. "Assay and properties of commercial ficin." 1957a. *Food Res.* 22: p.468.

11b.   Whitaker JR. "Properties of the proteolytic enzymes of commercial ficin." 1957b. *Food Res.* 22: p.483.

12.   Cichoke A. *The Complete Book of Enzyme Therapy.* New York, Avery, 1999. p.37.

13.   Confucius (551 to 479 BC). His writings in his book: *Analects.*

14.   Cichoke A. *The Complete Book of Enzyme Therapy.* New York, Avery, 1999. p.44.

15.   Thompson, EH, Wolf ID, Allen CE. "Ginger rhizome: A new source of proteolytic enzyme." *Journal of Food Science* 38, no. 4 (1973): pp.652-55.

16.   Goto C, Kasuya S, Koga K, Ohtomo H, Kagei N. "Lethal efficacy of extract from Zingiber officinale (traditional Chinese medicine) or [6]-shogaol and [6]-gingerol in Anisakis larvae in vitro." *Parasitol Res* 1990;76(8):653-6.

17.   Thompson, EH, Wolf ID, Allen CE. "Ginger rhizome: A new source of proteolytic enzyme." *Journal of Food Science* 38, no. 4 (1973): pp.652-55.

18.   A. Tiselius. "The Nobel Prize in Chemistry 1946 - Presentation Speech". Web site: Nobelprize.org. Accessed 6/14/2009. <http://nobelprize.org/nobel_prizes/chemistry/laureates/1946/press.html>.

19a.   "Research on the Major Killers of Americans" Physicians Committee for Responsible Medicine. Web site: www.pcrm.org. Citing from "Cancer Rates and Risks". National Cancer Institute (Washington, DC: 1985), and R. Doll and R. Peto, Journal of the National Cancer Institute, 1981, 66(6):1191-1308.

19b.   Vay Liang W. Go, Debra A. Wong and Ritva Butrum. "Diet, Nutrition and
       Cancer Prevention: Where Are We Going from Here?" American Institute for
       Cancer Research 11th Annual Research Conference on Diet, Nutrition and
       Cancer. 3121S-3126S.

20a.   Howell E. *Enzyme Nutrition.* Garden City Park, New York, Avery Publishing
       Group, Inc., 1985. p.x.

20b.   Cichoke A. *The Complete Book of Enzyme Therapy.* New York:Avery, 1999.
       pp.1, 5, 6, 9, 17.

21a.   Lopez DA, Williams RM, Miehlke K. *Enzymes - The Fountain of Life.* The
       Neville Press, Inc. 1994, Germany. pp.7-10.

21b.   Howell E. *Enzyme Nutrition.* Garden City Park, New York, Avery Publishing
       Group, Inc., 1985. pp.x-xi, 73.

22.   Lopez DA, Williams RM, Miehlke K. *Enzymes - The Fountain of Life.* The
       Neville Press, Inc. 1994, Germany. p.106.

23.   Howell E. *Enzyme Nutrition.* Garden City Park, New York: Avery Publishing
       Group, Inc., 1985. p.73.

24.   "Dietary Guidelines for Americans" Web site: U.S. Department of Agriculture.
       Accessed 3/25/2007. <http://www.nal.usda.gov/fnic/dga/dga95/cover.html>.

25.   Dr. Michael T. Murray. "What are Proteolytic Enzymes?" "Proteolytic
       Enzymes in Cancer Therapy" Accessed 3/25/2007. <http://doctormurray.
       com>.

26a.   Hale LP. "Proteolytic activity and immunogenicity of oral bromelain
       within the gastrointestinal tract of mice." Int Immunopharmacol. 2004
       Feb;4(2):255-64.

26b.   Lipski, E. *Leaky Gut Syndrome.* Keats Publishing, Inc., New Canaan, CT.
       1998. p.38.

26c.   Cichoke A. *The Complete Book of Enzyme Therapy.* New York:Avery, 1999.
       pp.288-290.

27.   Cichoke A. *The Complete Book of Enzyme Therapy.* New York:Avery, 1999.
       pp.225-226.

28.   Cichoke A. *The Complete Book of Enzyme Therapy.* New York:Avery, 1999.
       p.39.

29.   Cichoke A. *The Complete Book of Enzyme Therapy.* New York:Avery, 1999.

30.   Lopez DA MD, Williams RM MD Ph.D, Miehlke MD. *Enzymes - The
       Fountain of Life.* The Neville Press, Inc. 1994, Germany.

31.   "Search Results for 'ase'. Web site: U.S. Food and Drug Administration,
       Drugs@FDA Accessed 9/19/2004. <http://www.accessdata.fda.gov/scripts/
       cder/drugsatfda/index.cfm>.

32a.   Cichoke A. *The Complete Book of Enzyme Therapy.* New York:Avery, 1999.
       pp.157-158.

32b.   Wrba, H. & Pecher, O. *Enzymes: A Drug of the Future.* Ecomed
       Verlagsgesellschaft AG& Co. 1993.

32c.   Steinman D. "Fighting Cancer with Proteolytic Enzymes". *The doctor's Prescription for Healthy Living*. Volume 7, Number 3, p.29.

32d.   Hubarieva HO, Kindzel's'kyi LP, Ponomar'ova OV, Udatova TV, Shpil'ova SI, Smolanka II, Korovin SI, Ivankin VS. "[Systemic enzymotherapy as a method of prophylaxis of postradiation complications in oncological patients]" *Lik Sprava*. 2000 Oct-Dec;(7-8):94-100.

32e.   Sakalova A, Mikulecky M, Holomanova D, Langner D, Ransberger K, Stauder G, Mistrik M, Gazova S, Chabronova I, Benzova M, Et al. "[The favorable effect of hydrolytic enzymes in the treatment of immunocytomas and plasmacytomas]" *Vnitr Lek*. 1992 Sep;38(9):921-9.

33.   Nicholas J. Gonzalez, MD, Linda L. Isaacs, MD. *The Trophoblast and the Origins of Cancer*. New Spring Press, PO Box 200, New York, NY 10156, USA. pp.111-122.

34.   "Marie Curie". <http://en.wikipedia.org/wiki/Marie_Curie>. Accessed 3/23/2010.

35.   Nicholas J. Gonzalez, MD, Linda L. Isaacs, MD. *The Trophoblast and the Origins of Cancer*. New Spring Press, PO Box 200, New York, NY 10156, USA. pp.128-130.

36.   Cichoke A. *The Complete Book of Enzyme Therapy*. New York:Avery, 1999. pp.380-381.

37.   Miller PC, Baily SP, et al. "The effects of protease supplementation on skeletal muscle function and DOMS following downhill running." *J Sports Sci*. 2004 Apr;22(4):365-72.

38.   Michael Loes, MD, MD(H) and David Steinan MA. The Aspirin Alternative - The Natural Way to Overcome Chronic Pain, Reduce Inflammation and Enhance the Healing Response. Freedom Press. 2001. pp.139-144.

39.   "The Non-drug European Secret to Healing Sports Injuries Naturally." Web site: The Wobenzym Place. (AGNC, Inc., Las Vegas, NV Accessed 7/8/2004) pp.3-4 of 21. <http://www.buywobenzym.com/the_non-drug_european_ secret_to_healing_sports_ injuries_...>

40.   Walker AF, Bundy R, Hicks SM, Middleton RW. "Bromelain reduces mild acute knee pain and improves well-being in a dose-dependent fashion in an open study of otherwise healthy adults." *Phytomedicine*. Dec. 2002;9(8):681-6.

41.   Loes, Michael, MD, MD(H) and David Steinan MA. The Aspirin Alternative - The Natural Way to Overcome Chronic Pain, Reduce Inflammation and Enhance the Healing Response. Freedom Press. 2001. pp.71-86.

42a.   Orsini RA. Plastic Surgery Educational Foundation Technology Assessment Committee. "Bromelain." *Plast Reconstr Surg*. 2006 Dec;118(7):1640-4.

42b.   Duskova M, Wald M. "Orally administered proteases in aesthetic surgery." *Aesthetic Plast Surg*. 1999 Jan-Feb;23(1):41-4.

42c.   Adamek J, Prausova J, Wald M. "Enzyme therapy in the treatment of lymphedema in the arm after breast carcinoma surgery." *Rozhl Chir.* 1997 Apr;75(4):203-4.

42d. Hoernecke R, Doenicke A. "Perioperative enzyme therapy. A significant supplement to postoperative pain therapy?" *Anaesthesist.* 1993 Dec;42(12):856-61.

42e. Esch PM, Gerngross H, Gabian A. "Reduction of postoperative swelling. Objective measurement of swelling of the upper ankle joint in treatment with serrapeptase - a prospective study (German). *Fortschr Med.* 1989;107(4):67-8, 71-2.

43. Lopez DA, Williams RM, Miehlke K. *Enzymes - The Fountain of Life.* The Neville Press, Inc. 1994, Germany. p.195-196.

44. Lopez DA, Williams RM, Miehlke K. *Enzymes - The Fountain of Life.* The Neville Press, Inc. 1994, Germany. p.133-134.

45. Dr. Michael T. Murray. "What are Proteolytic Enzymes?" "Proteolytic Enzymes in Cancer Therapy" Accessed 3/25/2007. <http://doctormurray.com>.

46a. Lopez DA, Williams RM, Miehlke K. *Enzymes - The Fountain of Life.* The Neville Press, Inc. 1994, Germany. pp.133-137.

46b. Michael Loes MD, MD(H) and David Steinan MA. The Aspirin Alternative - The Natural Way to Overcome Chronic Pain, Reduce Inflammation and Enhance the Healing Response. Freedom Press. 2001. pp.198-199.

47. Grabovac V, Bernkop-Schnurch A. "Improvement of the intestinal membrane permeability of low molecular weight heparin by complexation with stem bromelain." *Int J Pharm.* 2006 Dec 1;326(1-2):153-9. Epub 2006 Jul 4.

48. Lopez DA, Williams RM, Miehlke K. *Enzymes - The Fountain of Life.* The Neville Press, Inc. 1994, Germany. pp.134-135.

49. Lopez DA, Williams RM, Miehlke K. *Enzymes - The Fountain of Life.* The Neville Press, Inc. 1994, Germany. p.134.

50a. Stevens JC, Maguiness KM, Hollingsworth J, et al. "Pancreatic enzyme supplementation in cystic fibrosis patients before and after fibrosing colonopathy." *J Pediatr Gastroenterol Nutr.* 1998;26:80-4.

50b. FitzSimmons SC, Burkhart GA, Borowitz D, Grand RJ, Hammerstrom T, Durie PR, Lloyd-Still JD, Lowenfels AB. "High-dose pancreatic-enzyme supplements and fibrosing colonopathy in children with cystic fibrosis." *N Engl J Med.* 1997 May 1;336(18):1283-9.

51. Pawel BR, de Chadarevian JP, Franco ME. "The pathology of fibrosing colonopathy of cystic fibrosis: a study of 12 cases and review of the literature." *Hum Pathol.* 1997 Apr;28(4):395-9.

KALE

52. Judy McBride "High-ORAC Foods May Slow Aging." February 8, 1999. Web

site: U.S. Department of Agriculture. Agricultural Research Service. Accessed 1/25/2008. <http://www.ars.usda.gov/is/pr/1999/990208.htm?pf=1>.

53.   "Taxon: *Brassica oleracea* L." Web site: U.S. Department of Agriculture. Agricultural Research Service. Accessed 1/5/2008. <http://www.ars-grin.gov/cgi-bin.npgs/html/taxon.p1?7668>.

54a.   Gates MA, Tworoger SS, Hect JL, De Vivo I, Rosner B, Hankinson SE. "A prospective study of dietary flavonoid intake and incidence of epithelial ovarian cancer." *Int J Cancer*. 2007 Nov 15;121(10):2225-32.

54b.   Moreno DA, Carvahal M, Lopez-Berenguer C, Garcia-Viguera C. "Chemical and biological characterization of nutraceutical compounds of broccoli." *J Pharm Biomed Anal*. 2006 Aug 28;41(5):1508-22. Epub 2006 May 19.

54c.   Verhoeven DT, Verhagen H, Goldbohm RA, van den Brandt PA, van Poppel G. "A review of mechanisms underlying anticarcinogenecity by brassica vegetables." *Chem Biol Interact*. 1997 Feb 28;103(2):79-129.

54d.   Verhoeven DT, Goldbohm RA, van Poppel G, Verhagen H, vanden Brandt PA. "Epidemiological studies on brassica vegetables and cancer risk." *Cancer Epidemiol Biomarkers Prev*. 1996 Sep;5(9):733-48.

54e.   Stoewsand GS. "Bioactive organosulfur phytochemicals in Brassica oleracea vegetables--a review." *Food Chem Toxicol*. 1995 Jun;33(6):537-43.

55a.   Cornblatt BS, Ye L, Dinkova-Kostova AT, Erb M, Fahey JW, Singh NK, Chen MA, Stierer T, Garrett-Meyer E, Argani P, Davidson NE, Talalay P, Kensler TW, Visvanathan K. "Preclinical and Clinical Evaluation of Sulforaphane for Chemoprevention in the Breast." *Carcinogenesis*. 2007.

55b.   Ambrosone CB, McCann SE, Freudenheim JL, Marshall JR, Zhang Y, Shields PG. "Breast cancer risk in premenopausal women is inversely associated with consumption of broccoli, a source of isothiocyanates, but is not modified by GST genotype." *J Nutr*. 2004 May;134(5):1134-8.

55c.   Jackson SJT, Singletary KW. "Sulforaphane Inhibits Human MCF-7 Mammary Cancer Cell Mitotic Progression and Tubulin Polymerization." *J Nutr*. 134:2229-36., 2004.

50d.   Fowke JH, Chung FL, Jin F, Qii D, Cai Q, Conaway C, Cheng JR, Shu SO, Gao YT, Zheng W. "Urinary isothiocyanate levels, brassica, and human breast cancer." *Cancer Res*. 2003 Jul 15;63(14):3980-6.

56a.   Kwon D, Yoon S, Carter O, Bailey GS, Dashwood RH. "Antioxidant and antigenotoxic activities of Angelica keiskei, Oenanthe javanica and Brassica oleracea in the Salmonella mutagenicity assay and in HCT116 human colon cancer cells." *BioFactors*. 2006 Vol. 26 No. 4 pp.231-244.

56b.   Seow A, Yaun JM, Sun CL, Van Den Berg D, Lee HP, Yu MC. "Dietary isothiocyanates, glutathione S-transferase polymorphisms and colorectal cancer risk in the Singapore Chinese Health Study." *Carcinogenesis*. 2002 Dec;23(12):2055-61.

56c.   Bonnesen C, Eggleston IM, Hayes JD. "Dietary indoles and isothiocyanates that are generated from cruciferous vegetables can both stimulate apoptosis and confer protection against DNA damage in human colon cell lines." *Cancer Res.* 2001 Aug 15;61(16):6120-30.

56d.   Chung FL, Conaway CC, Rao CV, Reddy BS. "Chemoprevention of colonic aberrant crypt foci in Fischer rats by sulforaphane and phenethyl isothiocyanate." *Carcinogenesis.* 2000 Dec;21(12):2287-91.

57a.   Singh SV, Srivastava SK, Choi S, Lew KL, Antosiewicz J, Xiao D, Zeng Y, Watkins SC, Johnson CS, Trump DL, Lee YJ, Xiao H, Herman-Antosiewicz A. "Sulforaphane-induced Cell Death in Human Prostate Cancer Cells Is Initiated by Reactive Oxygen Species." *J. Biol. Chem.* Vol 280, Issue 20, 19911-19924, May 20, 2005.

57b.   Joseph MA, Moysich KB, Freudenheim JL, Shields PG, Bowman ED, Zhang Y, Marshall JR, Ambrosone CB. "Cruciferous vegetables, genetic polymorphisms in glutathione S-transferases M1 and T1, and prostate cancer risk." *Nutr Cancer.* 2004;50(2):206-13.

57c.   Kristal AR, Lampe JW. "Brassica vegetables and prostate cancer risk: a review of the epidemiological evidence." *Nutr Cancer.* 2002;42(1):1-9.

57d.   Kolonel LN, Hankin JH, Whittemore AS, Wu AH, Gallagher RP, Wilkens LR, John EM, Howe GR, Dreon DM, West DW, Paffengarger RS Jr. "Vegetables, fruits, legumes and prostate cancer: a multiethnic case-control study." *Cancer Epidemiol Biomarkers Prev.* 2000 Aug;9(8):795-804.

57e.   Cohen JH, Kristal AR, Stanford JL. "Fruit and vegetable intakes and prostate cancer risk." *J Natl Cancer Inst.* 2000 Jan 5;92(1):61-8.

57f.   Kolonel LN, Hankin JH, Whittemore AS, Wu AH, Gallagher RP, Wilkens LR, John EM, Howe GR, Dreon DM, West DW, Paffengarger RS Jr. "Vegetables, fruits, legumes and prostate cancer: a multiethnic case-control study." *Cancer Epidemiol Biomarkers Prev.* 2000 Aug;9(8):795-804.

58.   Michaud DS, Spiegelman D, Clinton SK, Rimm EB, Willett WC, Giovannucci EL. "Fruit and vegetable intake and incidence of bladder cancer in a male prospective cohort." *J Natl Cancer Inst.* 1999 Apr 7;91(7):605-13.

59.   Wang LI, Giovannucci EL, Hunter D, Neuberg D, Su L, Christiani DC. "Dietary intake of Cruciferous vegetables, Glutathione S-transferase (GST) polymorphisms and lung cancer risk in a Caucasian population." *Cancer Causes Control.* 2004 Dec;15(10):977-85.

60a.   Maiyoh GK, Kuh JE, Casaschi A, Theriault AG. "Cruciferous indole-3-carbinol inhibits apolipoprotein B secretion in HepG2 cells." *J Nutr.* 2007 Oct;137(10):2185-9.

60b.   Kahlon TS, Chapman MH, Smith GE. 2007. "In vitro binding of bile acids by spinach, kale, Brussels sprouts, broccoli, mustard greens, green bell pepper, cabbage and collards. *Food Chemistry.* 100:1531-1536.

61.   Zhang SM, Hunter DJ, Rosner BA, Giovannucci EL, Colditz GA, Speizer FE, Willett WC. "Intakes of fruits, vegetables, and related nutrients and the risk of

non-Hodgkin's lymphoma among women." *Cancer Epidemiol Biomarkers Prev.* 2000 May;9(5):477-85.

62. Fahey JW, Haristoy X, Dolan PM, Kensler TW, Sholtus I, Stephenson KK, Talalay P, Lozniewski A. "Sulforaphane inhibits extracellular, intracellular, and antibiotic-resistant strains of Helicobacter pylori and prevents benzo[a]pyrene-induced stomach tumors." PNAS May 28, 2002 Vol. 99, no. 11, 7610-7615.

63. "*Helicobacter pylori* and Peptic Ulcer Disease". "The Key to Cure". Web site: Centers for Disease Control and Prevention, Department of Health & Human Services, USA, Accessed 1/17/2008. <http://www.cdc.gov/ulcer/keytocure.htm>.

64. Shapiro TA, Fahey JW, Wade KL, Stephenson KK, Talalay P. "Chemoprotective glucosinolates and isothiocyanates of broccoli sprouts: metabolism and excretion in humans." *Cancer Epidemiol Biomarkers Prev.* 2001 May;10(5):501-8.

65a. Cartea ME, Velasco P, Obregon S, Padilla G, de Haro A. "Seasonal variation in glucosinolate content in Brassica oleracea crops grown in northwestern Spain." *Phytochemistry.* 2007 Sep 21 [Epub ahead of print].

65b. Ciska E, Martyniak-Przbyszewska H. "Content of glucosinolates in cruciferous vegetables grown at the same site for two years under different climatic conditions." *J Agric Food Chem.* 2000 Jul;48(7):2862-7.

66. Farnham MW, Wilson PE, Stephenson KK, Fahey JW. 2004. "Genetic and environmental effects on glucosinolate content and chemoprotective potential of broccoli." *Plant Breeding.* 123:60-65.

67a. "Cruciferous Vegetables." Web site: Linus Pauling Institute at Oregon State University. Accessed 2/3/2008. <http://lpi.oregonstate.edu/infocenter/foods/cruciferous/>.

67b. Kristal AR, Lampe JW. "Brassica vegetables and prostate cancer risk: a review of the epidemiological evidence." *Nutr Cancer.* 2002;42(1):1-9.

68. "Cole Crops Collection" Web site: U.S. Department of Agriculture. Agricultural Research Service. Accessed 1/4/2008. <http://www.ars-usda.gov/Aboutus/docs.htm?docid=6254>.

69. "Cruciferous Vegetables". Web site: Linus Pauling Institute at Oregon State University. Micronutrient Information Center. Accessed 11/10/2008. <http://lpi.oregonstate.edu/infocenter/foods/cruciferous/>.

70. Valesco P, Cartea ME, Gonzalez C, Vilar M, Ordas A. "Factors affecting the glucosinolate content of kale (Brassica oleracea acephala group)." *J Agric Food Chem.* 2007 Feb 7;55(3):955-62.

71a. Shapiro TA, Fahey JW, Wade KL, Stephenson KK, Talalay P. "Human metabolism and excretion of cancer chemoprotective glucosinolates and isothiocyanates of cruciferous vegetables." *Cancer Epidemiol Biomarkers Prev.* 1998 Dec;7(12):1091-100.

71b. Johnson IT. "Glucosinolates: bioavailability and importance to health." *Int J Vitam Nutr Res.* 2002 Jan;72(1):26-31.

72.   "Nutrition Data - Kale, raw." "Nutritional Summary for Spinach, raw." Accessed 1/3/2008. <http://www.nutritiondata.com/facts-C00001-01c20dh. html>.

73a. O'Conner E, Mølgaard C, Michaelson KF, Jakobsen J, Lamberg-Allardt CJ, Cashman KD. "Serum percentage undercarboxylated osteocalcin, a sensitive measure of vitamin K status, and its relationship to bone indices in Danish girls." Br J Nutr. 2007 Apr;97(4):661-6.

73b. van Summeren M, Braam L, Noirt F, Kuis W, Vermeer C. "Pronounced elevation of undercarboxylated osteocalcin in healthy children." Pediatr Res 2007 Mar; 61(3):366-70.

74a. Tsugawa N, Shiraki M, Suhara Y, Kamao M, Ozaki R, Tanaka K, Okano T. "Low plasma phylloquinone concentration is associated with high incidence of vertebral fracture in Japanese women." *J Bone Miner Metab.* 2008;26(1):79-85. Epub 2008 Jan 10.

74b. Bolton-Smith C, McMurdo ME, Paterson CR, Mole PA, Harvey JM, Fenton ST, Prynne CJ, Mishra GD, Sheaer MJ. "Two-year randomized trial of vitamin K1 (phylloquinone) and vitamin D3 plus calcium on the bone health of older women." *J Bone Miner Res.* 2007 Apr;22(4):509-19.

74c. Tsugawa N, Shiraki M, Suhara Y, Kamao M, Ozaki R, Tanaka K, Okano T. "Vitamin K status of healthy Japanese women: age-related vitamin K requirement for gamma-carboxylation of osteocalcin." *Am J Clin Nutr.* 2006;83:380-6.

74d. Luo LZ, Xu L. "[Vitamin K and osteoporosis]." [Article in Chinese]. *Zhongguo Yi Xue Ke Xue Yuan Xue Bao.* 2003 Jun;25(3):346-9.

74e. Booth SL, Broe KE, Gagnon DR, Tucker KL, Hannan MT, MxLean RR, Dawson-Hughes B, Wilson PW, Cupples LA, Kiel DP. "Vitamin K intake and bone mineral density in women and men." *Am J Clin Nutr.* 2003 Feb;77(2):512-6.

74f. Booth SA, Tucker KL, Chen H, Hannan MT, Gagnon DR, Cupples LA, Wilson PWF, Ordovas J, Schaefer EJ, Dawson-Hughes B, Kiel DP. "Dietary vitamin K intakes are associated with hip fracture but not with bone mineral density in elderly men and women." *American Journal of Clinical Nutrition,* Vol. 71, No. 5, 1201-1208, May 2000.

74g. Vermeer C, Knapen MHJ, Schurgers LJ. "Vitamin K and metabolic bone disease." *J Clin Pathol.* 1998;51:424-426.

75a. Kitchin B, Morgan SL. "Not just calcium and vitamin D: other nutritional considerations in osteoporosis." Curr Rheumatol Rep. 2007 Apr;9(1):85-92.

75b. Ryder KM, Shorr RI, Bush AJ, Kritchevsky SB, Harris T, Stone K, Cauley J, Tylavsky FA. "Magnesium intake from food and supplements is associated with bone mineral density in healthy older white subjects." *J Am Geriatr Soc.* 2005 Nov;53(11):1875-80.

76.   Hyun TH, Barrett-Conner E, Milne DB. "Zinc intakes and plasma concentrations in men with osteoporosis: the Rancho Bernardo Study." *Am J Clin Nutr.* 2004 Sep;80(3):715-21.

77.   Heaney RP, Weaver CM, Hinders SN, Martin B, Packard PT. "Absorbability of Calcium from Brassica Vegetables: Broccoli, Bok Choy, and Kale." *Jorurnal of Food Science.* 58 (6), 1378-1380.

78.   "Henrik Dam" Web site: Encyclopedia Britannica online. Accessed 1/23/2008. <http://www.britannica.com/eb/article-9028624/Henrik-Dam>.

79.   Judy McBride. "High-ORAC Foods May Slow Aging." February 8, 1999. Web site: U.S. Department of Agriculture. Agricultural Research Service. Accessed 1/3/2008. <http://www.ars.usda.gov/is/pr/1999/990208.htm?pf=1>.

80.   Gemma C, Mesches MH, Sepesi B. Choo K. Holmes DB, Bickford P. "Diets Enriched in Foods with Antioxidant Activity Reverse Age-Induced Decreases in Cerebellar B-Adrenergic Function and Increases in Proinflammatory Cytokines." *The Journal of Neuroscience*, July 15, 2002, 22(14):6114-6120.

81.   "Plant Pigments Paint a Rainbow of Antioxidants." Web site: U.S. Departmaent of Agriculture. Agricultural Research Service. Published in the November 1996 issue of *Agricultural Research magazine.* Accessed 1/3/2008. <http://www.ars.usda.gov/is/AR/archive/nov96/plant1196.htm?pf=1>.

82.   Underwood BA, Arthur P. "The contribution of vitamin A to public Health." *FASEB J.* 1996 Jul;10(9):1040-8.

83.   Thurnham DI, Nothrop-Clewes CA, McCullough FSW, Das BS, Lunn PG. "Innate Immunity, Gut Integrity, and Vitamin A in Gambian and Indian Infants." The Journal of Infectious Diseases. 2000;182(suppl 1):S23-8.

84.   Bone RA, Landrum JT, Tarsis SL. "Preliminary identification of the human macular pigment." *Vision Res.* 1985;25(11):1531-5.

85a. Seddon JM. "Multivitamin-multimineral supplements and eye disease: age-related macular degeneration and cataract." *Am J Clin Nutr.* 2007;85(suppl):304S-7S.

85b. Seddon JM, Ajani UA, Sperduto RD, Hiller R, Blair N, Burton TC, Farer MD, Gragoudas ES, Haller J, Miller DT, et al. "Dietary carotenoids, vitamins A, C, and E, and advanced age-related macular degeneration. Eye Disease Case-Control Study Group." *JAMA*. 1994 Nov 9;272(18):1413-20.

86.   Jingsheng Tuo, Christine M. Bojanowski, and Chi-Chao Chan. "Genetic factors of age-related macular degeneration." Prog Retin Eye Res. 2004 March; 23(2): 229-249.

87.   Beatty A, Boulton M, Henson D, Koh H-H, Murray IJ. "Macular pigment and age related macular degeneration." *Br J Opthalmol.* 1999;83:867-877.

88a. Brown L, Rimm EB, Seddon JM, Giovannucci EL, Chasen-Taber L, Spiegelman D, Willett WC, Hankinson SE. "A prospective study of carotenoid intake and risk of cataract extraction in US men." *Am J Clin Nutr.* 1999 Oct;70(4):517-24.

88b.   Chasen-Taber L, Willett WC, Seddon JM, Stampfer MJ, Rosner B, Colditz GA, Speizer FE, Hankinson SE. "A prospective study of carotenoid and vitamin A intakes and risk of cataract extraction in US women." *Am J Clin Nutr* 1999;70:509-16.

89.   USDA-NCC Carotenoid Database, 1998. USDA Food Nutrient Database for Standard Release 13. Hart and Scott, 1995.

90a.   de Vogel J, Jonker-Termont DS, van Lieshout EM, Katan MB, van der Meer R. "Green vegetables, red meat and colon cancer: chlorophyll prevents the cytotoxic and hyperproliferative effects of haem in rat colon." *Carcinogenesis.* 2005 Feb;26(2):387-93. Epub 2004 Nov 18.

90b.   Dingley KH, Ubick EA, Chiarappa-Zucca ML, Nowell S, Abel S, Ebeler SE, Mitchell AE, Burns SA, Steinberg FM, Clifford AJ. "Effect of dietary constituents with chemopreventive potential on adduct formation of a low dose of the heterocyclic amines PhIP and IQ and phase II hepatic enzymes." *Nutr Cancer.* 2003;46(2):212-21.

91.   Tachino N, Guo D, Dashwood WM, Yamane S, Larsen R, Dashwood R. "Mechanisms of the in vitro antimutagenic action of chlorophyllin against benzo[a]pyreneL studies of enzyme inhibition, molecular complex formation and degeneration of the ultimate carcinogen." *Mutat Res.* 1994 Jul 16;308(2):191-203.

92a.   Egner PA, Munoz A, Kensler TW. "Chemoprevention with chlorophyllin in individuals exposed to dietary aflatoxin." *Mutat Res.* 2003 Feb-Mar;523-524:209-16.

92b.   Yun CH, Jeong HG, Jhoun JW, Guengerich FP. "Non-specific inhibition of cytochrome P450 activities by chlorophyllin in human and rat liver microsomes." *Carcinogenesis.* 1995 Jun;16(6):1437-40.

93a.   Kumar SS, Devasagayam TP, Bhushan B, Verma NC. "Scavenging of reactive oxygen species by chlorophyllin: an ESR study." *Free Radic Res.* 2001 Nov,35(5):563-74.

93b.   Kama JP, Boloor KK, Devasagayam TP. "Chlorophyllin as an effective antioxidant against membrane damage in vitro and ex vivo." *Biochim Biophys Acta.* 2000 Sep 27;1487(2-3):113-270.

94.   Park KK, Park JH, Jung YJ, Chung WY. "Inhibitory effects of chlorophyllin, hemin and tetrakis(4-benzoic acid) porphyrin on oxidative DNA damage and mouse skin inflammation induced by 12-O-tetradecaanoylphorbol-13-acetate as a possible anti-tumor promoting mechanism." *Mutat Res.* 2003 Dec 9;542(1-2):89-97.

95.   Song L, Thornalley PJ. "Effect of storage, processing and cooking on glucosinolate content of Brassica vegetables." *Food Chem Toxicol.* 2007 Feb;45(2):216-24. Epub 2003 Aug 30.

BACK TO ENZYMES

96. Lopez DA, Williams RM, Miehlke K. *Enzymes - The Fountain of Life.* The Neville Press, Inc. 1994, Germany. pp.110-115, 129-141.

97a. David Steinman, MA. "Fighting Cancer with Proteolytic Enzymes" *The Doctors' Prescription for Healthy Living.* Volume 7, Number 3.

97b. Engwerda CR, Andrew D, Ladhams A, Mynott TL. "Bromelain modulates T cell and B cell immune responses in vitro and in vivo." *Cell Immunol.* May 2001;210(1):66-75.

97c. Engwerda CR, Andrew D, Murphy M, Mynott TL. "Bromelain activates murine macrophages and natural killer cells in vitro." *Cell Immunol.* May 2001;210(1):5-10.

97d. Mynott TL, Ladhams A, Scarmato P, Engwerda CR. "Bromelain, from pineapple stems, proteolytically blocks activation of extracellular regulated kinase-2 in T cells." *J Immunol.* 1999. Sep 1;163(5):2568-75.

97e. Nouza K. "[Systemic enzyme therapy in diseases of the vascular system]." *Bratisi Lek Listy.* 1995 Oct;96(10):566-9.

97f. Ransberger K. "Enzyme treatment of immune complex diseases." Arthritis Rheuma. 1986;8:16-9.

97g. Cichoke A. *The Complete Book of Enzyme Therapy.* New York:Avery, 1999. pp.402-403.

98. Kullich W, Schwann H. "[Circulating immune complexes and complement fragment iC3b in chronic polyarthritis during 12 months therapy with oral enzymes in comparison with oral gold]." *Wien Med Wochenschr.* 1992;142(22):493-7.

99a. Desser L, Holomanova D, Zavadova E, Pavelka K, Mohr T, Herbacek I. "Oral therapy with proteolytic enzymes decreases excessive TGF-beta levels in human blood." *Cancer Chemother Pharmacol.* 2001 Jul;47 Suppl:S10-5.

99b. Steffen C, Menzel J. "[In vivo degradation of immune complexes in the kidney by orally administered enzymes]" *Wien Klin Wochenschr.* 1987 Aug 7;99(15):525-31.

100. David Steinman, MA. "Fighting Cancer with Proteolytic Enzymes" *The Doctors' Prescription for Healthy Living.* Volume 7, Number 3.

101a. Nouza K. "[Systemic enzyme therapy in diseases of the vascular system]." *Bratisi Lek Listy.* 1995 Oct;96(10):566-9.

101b. Lopez DA, Williams RM, Miehlke K. *Enzymes - The Fountain of Life.* The Neville Press, Inc. 1994, Germany. pp.209-211.

102. Lopez DA, Williams RM, Miehlke K. *Enzymes - The Fountain of Life.* The Neville Press, Inc. 1994, Germany. pp.268-270.

103a. Desser L, Holomanova D, Zavadova E, et al. "Oral therapy with proteolytic enzymes decreases excessive TGF-beta levels in human blood." *Cancer Chemother Pharmacol,* 2001:47 Suppl:S10-15.

103b.   Leipner J, Saller R. "Systemic enzyme therapy in oncology: effect and mode of action. *Drugs*. 2000;59:769-80.

103c.   Gonzalez NJ, Isaacs LL. "Evaluation of pancreatic proteolytic enzyme treatment of adenocarcinoma of the pancreas, with nutrition and detoxification support." *Nutr Cancer*. 1999;33:117-24.

103d.   Cichoke A. *The Complete Book of Enzyme Therapy*. New York:Avery, 1999. pp.157-8.

103e.   Cohen LA, Aliaga C, Pitman B, Wynder EL. "Oral enzyme therapy and experimental rat mammary tumor metastasis." *Life Sci*. 1999;65(24):2603-14.

103f.   Wald M, Zavadova E, et al. "Polyenzyme preparation WobeMugos inhibits growth of solid tumors and development of experimental metastases in mice." *Life Sc.*, 1998;62:PL43-PL48.

103g.   Gubareva AA. "The use of enzymes in treating patients with malignant lymphoma with a large tumor mass." *Lik Sprava*. 1998 Aug;(6):141-3.

103h.   Desser L, Rehberger A, Paukovits W. "Proteolytic enzymes and amaylase induce cytokine production in human peripheral blood mononuclear cells in vitro." *Cancer Biother*. 1994;9:253-263.

103i.   Desser L, et al. "Cytokine synthesis in human peripheral blood mononuclear cells after oral administration of polyenzyme preparations." *Oncology*. Nov 1993;50(6):403:7.

103j.   Batkin S, Taussig SJ, Szekerezes J. "Antimetastatic effect of bromelain with or without its proteolytic and anticoagulant activity." *J Cancer Res Clin Oncol*. 1988;114:507-508.

103k.   Desser L, Sakalova A, Zavadova E, et al. "Concentrations of soluble tumor necrosis factor receptors, beta-2-microglogulin, IL-6 and TNF in serum of multiple myeloma patients after chemotherapy and after combined enzyme-chemotherapy." *International Journal of Immunotherapy*, 1997;13:121-130.

103l.   Cichoke AJ. "The effect systemic enzyme therapy on cancer cells and the immune system. *Townsend Letter for Doctors and Patients*. 1995;Nov:30-2 [review].

103m.   Sakalova A, Kunze R, Holomanova D, Hapalova J, Chorvath B, Mistrik M, Sedlak J. "Density of adhesive proteins after oral administration of proteolytic enzymes in multiple myeloma." *Vnitr Lek*. 1995 Dec;41(12):822-6.

103n.   Gerard G. "Anti-cancer therapy with bromelain." *Agressologie*. 1972;13:261-274.

104.   Lopez DA, Williams RM, Miehlke K. *Enzymes - The Fountain of Life*. The Neville Press, Inc. 1994, Germany. p.233.

105.   Lopez DA, Williams RM, Miehlke K. *Enzymes - The Fountain of Life*. The Neville Press, Inc. 1994, Germany. pp.241-243.

106a.   Cichoke A. *The Complete Book of Enzyme Therapy*. New York:Avery, 1999. pp.157-158.

106b.   Tadeuz Popiela, Jan Kulig, Jurgen Hanisch, Paul R. Bock. "Influence of a complementary treatment with oral enzymes on patients with colorectal cancers - an epidemiological retrolective cohort study." *Cancer Chemotherapy and Pharmacology.* Springer-Verlag Heidelberg. Volume 47, Number 7, June 2001. pp.S55-S63.

107. Not used.

108. Cichoke A. *The Complete Book of Enzyme Therapy.* New York:Avery, 1999, pp.xii-xiv.

109. Lopez DA MD, Williams RM MD Ph.D, Miehlke MD. *Enzymes - The Fountain of Life.* The Neville Press, Inc. 1994, Germany. pp.222-226.

110. Jonathan Tommy Reports. "Immune complexes & systemic enzyme therapy." Web site: The Autism File. Accessed 11/9/2008. <http://www.autismfile.com/ Previous/pdf/issue5/5_immune_complexes.pdf>.

111a. Castell JV, Friedrich G, Kuhn CS, Poppe GE. "Intestinal absorption of undegraded proteins in men: presence of bromelain in plasma after oral intake." *Am J Physiol.* 1997 Jul;273(1 Pt 1):G139-46.

111b. Nouza K. "Outlooks of systemic enzyme therapy in rheumatoid arthritis and other immunopathological diseases." *Acta Univ Carol* [Med] (Praha). 1994;40(1-4):101-4.

111c. Lopez DA, Williams RM, Miehlke K. *Enzymes - The Fountain of Life.* The Neville Press, Inc. 1994, Germany. pp.137-140.

112. Lopez DA, Williams RM, Miehlke K. *Enzymes - The Fountain of Life.* The Neville Press, Inc. 1994, Germany. pp.113, 129-137.

113. Oelgoetz AW, Oelgoetz PA, Wittenkind J. "The treatment of food allergy and indigestion of pancreatic origin with pancreatic enzymes." *Am J Dig Dis Nutr.* 1935;2:422-6.

114. Mynott TL, Crossett B, Prathalingam SR. "Proteolytic inhibition of Salmonella enterica serovar typhimurium-induced activation of the mitogen-activated protein kinases ERK and JNK in cultured human intestinal cells." *Infect Immun.* 2002 Jan;70(1):86-95.

115a. Malamud A, Wilson KT. "Treatment of gastrointestinal infections." *Curr Opin Gastroenterol.* 2000 Jan;16(1):51-5.

115b. Mynott TL, Guandalini S, Raimondi F, Fasano A. "Bromelain prevents secretion caused by Vibrio cholerae and Escherichia coli enterotoxins in rabbit ileum in vitro." *Gastroenterology.* 1997 Jul;113(1):175-84.

116. Mahady GB, Pendland SL, Yun GS, Lu ZZ, Stoia A. "Ginger (Zingiber officinale Roscoe) and the gingerols inhibit the growth of Cag A+ strains of Helicobacter pylori." *Anticancer Res.* 2003 Sep-Oct;23(5A):3699-702.

117. "*H. pylori* and Cancer: Questions and Answers" Web site: National Cancer Institute. U.S. National Institutes of Health. Accessed 1/26/2007. <http:// www.cancer.gov/cancertopics/factsheet/HPylori/print?page=&keyword=>.

118a. Billingmann VP. "Enzyme therapy-an alternative in treatment of herpes zoster.

A controlled study of 192 patients [translated from German]. *Fortschr Med.* 1995;113:43-48.

118b. Klein MW, Stauder GM, Beese EW. "The intestinal absorption of orally administered hydrolytic enzymes and their effects in the treatment of acute herpes zoster as compared with those of oral acyclovir therapy." *Phytomedicine.* 1995;2:7-15.

118c. Kleine Michael-W. "Comparison between an oral hydrolytic enzyme combination and oral acyclovir in the treatment of acute zoster:a double-blind, controlled multicentre trial." *Journal of the European Academy of Dermatology and Venereology.* 2 (4), 296-307.

119. McPerson J, et al. *Proceedings of the Society of Experimental Biology and Med.* v. 115, pp.514-17, 1964.

120. Thompson, EH, Wolf ID, Allen CE. "Ginger rhizome: A new source of proteolytic enzyme." *Journal of Food Science* 38, no. 4 (1973): pp.652-55.

121a. Rothman S, Liebow C, Isenman L. "Conservation of digestive enzymes." *Physiol Rev.* 2002 Jan;82(1):1-18.

121b. Liebow C, Rothman SS. "Enteropancreatic circulation of digestive enzymes." *Science.* 1975 Aug 8;189(4201):472-4.

122. Cichoke A. *The Complete Book of Enzyme Therapy.* New York, Avery, 1999. p.4.

123a. Rostan EF, DeBuys HV, Madey DL, Pinnell SR. "Evidence supporting zinc as an important antioxidant for skin." *Int J Dermatol.* 2002 Sep;41(9):606-110.

123b. Saul R. Powell. "The Antioxidant Properties of Zinc." *Journal of Nutrition.* 2000;130:1447S-1454S.

123c. Ebadi M, Leuschen MP, el Refaey H, Hamada FM, Rojas P. "The antioxidant properties of zinc and metallothionein." *Neurochem Int.* 1996 Aug;29(2):159-66.

124a. Roy SK, Behrens RH, Haider R, Akramuzzaman SM, Mahalanabis D, Wahed MA, Tomkins AM. "Impact of zinc supplementation on intestinal permeability in Bangladeshi children with acute diarrhoea and persistent diarrhoea syndrome." *J Pediatr Gastroenterol Nutr.* 1992 Oct;15(3):289-96.

124b. Lipski, E. *Leaky Gut Syndrome.* Keats Publishing, Inc., New Canaan, CT 06840. 1998 p.52.

124c. Cichoke A. *The Complete Book of Enzyme Therapy.* New York, Avery, 1999. p.290.

125. Dollemore, Doug. *New Choices in Natural Healing.* Rodale Press, Inc. 1995. p.135.

126. Cichoke A. *The Complete Book of Enzyme Therapy.* New York, Avery, 1999. p.64.

127a. Littarru GP, Ho L, Folkers K. "Deficiency of coenzyme Q 10 in human heart disease. II. *Int J Vitam Nutr Res.* 1972;42(3):413-34.

127b. Folkers K, Littarru GP, Ho L Runge TM, Havanonda S, Cooley D.

"Evidence for a deficiency of coenzyme Q10 in human heart disease." *Int Z Vitaminforsch.* 1970;40(3):380-90.

128a. Kamikawa T, Kobayashi A, Yamashita T, Hayashi H, Yamazaki N. "Effects of coenzyme Q10 on exercise tolerance in chronic stable angina pectoris." *Am J Cardiol.* 1985 Aug 1;56(4):247-51.

128b. PH Langsjoen, S Vadhanavikit, and K Folkers. "Response of patients in classes III and IV of cardiomyopathy to therapy in a blind and crossover trial with coenzyme Q10. Proc Natl Acad Sci USA. 1985 June; 82(12): 4240-4244.

129. Cichoke A. *The Complete Book of Enzyme Therapy.* New York:Avery, 1999. p.17.

130. Howell E. *Enzyme Nutrition.* Garden City Park, New York: Avery Publishing Group, Inc., 1985. pp.51-57.

131. Cichoke A. *The Complete Book of Enzyme Therapy.* New York:Avery, 1999. pp.1, 21-22.

132a. Howell E. *Enzyme Nutrition.* Garden City Park, New York: Avery Publishing Group, Inc., 1985. p.26, 138-139.

132b. Lopez DA, Williams RM, Miehlke K. *Enzymes - The Fountain of Life.* The Neville Press, Inc. 1994, Germany. pp.1-5.

132c. Cichoke A. *The Complete Book of Enzyme Therapy.* New York, Avery, 1999. pp.1, 5-6.

133. Howell E. *Enzyme Nutrition.* Garden City Park, New York: Avery Publishing Group, Inc., 1985. pp.36-39.

134. Howell E. *Enzyme Nutrition.* Garden City Park, New York: Avery Publishing Group, Inc., 1985. p.xii.

135. Howell E. *Enzyme Nutrition.* Garden City Park, New York: Avery Publishing Group, Inc., 1985. pp.119-127.

136. Howell E. *Enzyme Nutrition.* Garden City Park, New York: Avery Publishing Group, Inc., 1985. p.120.

137. Lopez DA, Williams RM, Miehlke K. *Enzymes - The Fountain of Life.* The Neville Press, Inc. 1994, Germany. p.109.

138. Cichoke A. *The Complete Book of Enzyme Therapy.* New York:Avery, 1999. p.437.

139. Lopez DA MD, Williams RM MD Ph.D, Miehlke MD. *Enzymes - The Fountain of Life.* The Neville Press, Inc. 1994, Germany. p.109.

140. Cichoke A. *The Complete Book of Enzyme Therapy.* New York:Avery, 1999. pp.27, 37.

141. Bible: I Samuel 25:18, 30:12, 2 Samuel 16:1, 2 Kings 20:7, Isaiah 38:21.

142. "Acid Erosion" Web site: Doon South Dental. Accessed 3/26/2007. <http://www.drhendry.ca/InfoAnd Links/Erosion/Erosion.html>.

143. Howell E. *Enzyme Nutrition.* Garden City Park, New York: Avery Publishing Group, Inc., 1985. pp.147, 154-155.

144.   Cichoke A. *The Complete Book of Enzyme Therapy.* New York:Avery, 1999. p.27.

145.   Howell E. *Enzyme Nutrition.* Garden City Park, New York: Avery Publishing Group, Inc., 1985. p.147.

146.   Howell E. *Enzyme Nutrition.* Garden City Park, New York: Avery Publishing Group, Inc., 1985. p.149-150.

147.   Cichoke A. *The Complete Book of Enzyme Therapy.* New York:Avery, 1999. p.45.

148.   Cichoke A. *The Complete Book of Enzyme Therapy.* New York:Avery, 1999. p.75.

149.   Saint S. *End of the Spear.* Tyndale House Publishers, Inc. Carol Stream, IL 60188. 2005 p.113.

150.   "Papaya FAQ's. Web site: Guapa. Accessed 11/11/2008. <http://www.gaupa-fuits.com/papayaFAQ's.htm>.

PART IV

More Amazing Actions

A DEEPER LOOK UNDER THE HOOD

CHAPTER 16

Fighting Inflammation
With the E-F-G Approach

INFLAMMATION (commonly known as swelling) is our body's
natural response to injury. Following an injury, white blood cells
and clear liquid from the blood are allowed to pass through the blood
vessel wall and accumulate at the site of injury. This is the body's defense
mechanism to limit movement and fight infection as evidenced by
warmth, redness, inflammation, and pain. This is called acute or short-
term inflammation.

On the other hand, bad things happen when inflammation occurs
for no reason at all over a long period of time—our body can become its
own enemy and attack its own tissues.[1] This long-term inflammation is
destructive to our bodies and is called chronic inflammation. More and
more research shows that chronic inflammation can increase the risk of
certain diseases, such as atherosclerosis (hardening of the arteries),[2] heart
attack,[3] stroke,[4] and cancer.[5]

DID YOU KNOW ...

- The suffix "itis" generally means a condition resulting from
  inflammation.
- Sinusitis is inflammation of the membranes in the sinuses and
  nasal passages, often caused by an infection. Sinusitis can make
  us feel stuffy, *groggy, tired* and *spacey*. A deviated (crooked)

septum in the nose can block passage ways, cause inflammation and lead to stuffy nose and sinus infections.

- Inflammation can generate large amounts of free radicals which can damage tissues.[6] Free radicals are discussed in the next chapter.
- Arthritis is inflammation of the joints, often resulting in pain and stiffness. Long term arthritis can damage the smooth, slippery cartilage that cushions our joints.[7]
- Chronic inflammation can promote the development of many types of cancer.
- Generally, the longer chronic inflammation persists, the higher the risk of developing cancer.
- Tumors develop at sites of inflammation.
- Tumors can be induced in laboratory animals by injections with chemicals that cause inflammation.
- Chronic inflammation can be caused by infections from bacteria, viruses, parasites, chemicals, and nondigestible particles (such as asbestos and silica dust).[8]

Some inflammation is necessary in our bodies just as a car engine produces some heat in order to run properly. Think of chronic inflammation as a car engine that overheats. Engines do not run well when they overheat. Continuous overheating will cause major engine damage. Likewise, chronic inflammation will eventually damage our bodies.

- Inflammation is *directly related* to the following conditions:[9]
- **Asthma:** inflammation of the air passage to the lungs
- **Allergies:** reactions to foods or chemicals, molds, pollens, or other contaminants in the air
- **Rheumatoid arthritis:** inflammation of the joints resulting in pain and limited movement and thought to be an immune reaction against joint tissues
- **Eczema, also called dermatitis:** skin becomes itchy, red, inflamed, swollen, cracked, crusted, or develops scales

- **Gout:** inflammation of the joints caused by excessive uric acid (eating cherries every day is known to prevent gout)
- **Lupus:** chronic inflammation of the joints; may also involve inflammation of the skin, nervous system, heart, kidney, and lungs
- **Leaky gut syndrome**
- **Ulcerative colitis:** excessive inflammation of the small intestine, primarily in the upper part
- **Crohn's disease:** excessive inflammation of the small intestine, primarily in the lower part
- **Celiac disease:** an allergic reaction caused by gluten, a protein found in wheat and many other grains, that can damage the small intestine and produce other symptoms such as irritability, diarrhea, cramping, and weight loss
- **Psoriasis:** silvery gray scales that form a covering over red patches of skin caused by increased rate of growth of skin cells; occurs mainly at knees, elbows, or scalp
- **Scleroderma:** hardening of the skin or other tissues or organs

Inflammation is a *suspected* cause of these conditions:[10]

- **Alzheimer's disease**
- **Atherosclerosis**
- **Cancer**
- **Diabetes:** inadequate production or utilization of insulin resulting in blood sugar not being properly used for energy or tissue repair
- **Obesity**[11]
- **Alopecia:** Hair loss due to inflammation of hair follicles[12]

One expert estimates that approximately half of all Americans have some type of inflammatory disorder.[13] Being overweight or obese increases the risk of inflammatory diseases because fat cells produce pro-inflammatory chemical transmitters.[14]

GINGER'S ANTI-INFLAMMATORY ACTIONS

Ginger has over 100 compounds with anti-inflammatory actions.[15]

Both fresh and dried ginger help inhibit (fight against) inflammation. How do ginger and certain other foods, drugs, and supplements accomplish this? One way is by regulating a very complex group of chemical transmitters. These chemical transmitters are produced by special groups of enzymes. (Remember from chapter 15 that there are over 3,000 types of enzymes that either start up or speed up the billions of chemical reactions in our bodies.) Two groups of these enzymes are cyclooxygenase (abbreviated COX) and lipoxygenase (abbreviated LOX).

Guess what these enzymes act on? Essential fatty acids! And the chemical transmitters produced are either pro- or anti-inflammatory, depending on whether the enzymes act on omega-6 or omega-3 EFAs.

Generally, anti-inflammatory chemical transmitters are produced when the COX and LOX enzymes act on omega-3 EFAs such as fish and flaxseed oil. That is why eating more foods with omega-3 EFAs can reduce inflammation. On the other hand, pro-inflammatory chemical transmitters are produced when these enzymes act on omega-6 EFAs, which are so abundant in our Western diet.

Anti-inflammatory drugs also reduce inflammation in our bodies by blocking the actions of COX and LOX enzymes. Blocking these enzymes blocks the production of pro-inflammatory chemical transmitters. *Over 30 studies show ginger's actions can alter the balance of these chemical transmitters and thus help reduce inflammation.*[16]

Stated another way, the delicate balance of enzymes and chemical transmitters in our bodies can be manipulated by foods, drugs, and supplements. If we do the right things, we can reduce unnecessary inflammation in our bodies. Some other things that can help reduce inflammation include exercising and eating less refined sugar.

BALANCE, BALANCE, BALANCE

Two groups of chemical transmitters produced by the COX and LOX enzymes—called prostaglandins and leukotrienes (pronounced loo-ko-try-enes)—are largely responsible for regulating inflammation in our bodies.[17] These chemical transmitters also run the immune system, control blood clotting, and regulate the size and permeability (leakiness) of blood vessels. These chemical transmitters represent one of the most complex signaling systems in the body and their *balance with each other* has a direct effect on our bodies' ability to function normally and resist chronic inflammation and disease.[18]

DRUGS

One of the most well-known ways to block inflammation is the use of aspirin and other NSAIDs (nonsteroidal anti-inflammatory drugs), which block the COX enzymes from producing pro-inflammatory prostaglandins and leukotrienes. A natural form of aspirin (from the bark of the willow tree) has been used for thousands of years to reduce pain and inflammation. How aspirin worked was largely a mystery until its mode of action was discovered in 1971 by Sir John Vane of London, England. He and his colleagues were later awarded a Nobel Prize in Medicine in 1982 for discovering how aspirin acts on these chemical transmitters to decrease inflammation and pain.[19] Commonly used NSAIDs include aspirin, ibuprofen, naproxen, and indomethacin. The disadvantage of these NSAIDs is that they also block some protective actions of the COX enzymes, and, as a result, their frequent use can lead to an increased risk of stomach bleeding and ulcers.[20]

Attempting to avoid these side effects, newer NSAIDs were developed that block only a specific group of COX enzymes. These drugs included Celebrex (celecoxib), Vioxx (rofecoxib), and Bextra (valdecoxib). First seen as wonderfully engineered anti-inflammatory medications that gave relief to thousands of people suffering from pain and inflammation, it later became apparent that two of these drugs could significantly increase the risk of heart attack and stroke. Vioxx was voluntarily removed from the market in 2004 and Bextra was removed in 2005. The FDA ordered the relabeling of all remaining NSAIDs to address the increased risk of heart attack and gastrointestinal bleeding with frequent use.[21]

Other medications such as corticosteroids (cortisone, prednisone, prednisolone, and others) are extremely potent anti-inflammatory drugs but carry many risks with long-term use. Efforts are being made in the search for safe new ways to manipulate the delicate balance of these chemical transmitters.

FISH AND FLAXSEED OIL CAN REDUCE INFLAMMATION

We can help our bodies produce more anti-inflammatory transmitters by giving our bodies sufficient amounts of the right materials for the COX and LOX enzymes to act upon. As Dr. Johanna Budwig first discovered during the 1950s (and many other researchers later confirmed), these right materials are omega-3 EFAs! *Since there is a major shortage of omega-3 EFAs in our modern diet, we must make a conscious effort to put them back in.*

As discussed in chapter 13, fish and flaxseed oil have the highest amounts of omega-3 EFAs among foods and supplements. I like to make fruit flax smoothies several times a week, and I also take fish oil supplements. You can also combine flax oil or freshly ground flaxseeds with cottage cheese or yogurt in accordance with the program developed by Dr. Budwig, who developed a successful dietary program for treating arthritis, heart disease, and cancer.[22]

Wild-caught cold water fish are rich sources of omega-3 EFAs. Other foods that contain some omega-3 EFAs include canola oil, walnuts, walnut oil, and soybean oil.[23] Many vegetables, especially the green leafy ones, also contain some omega-3 EFAs. These include spinach, kale, lettuce,[24] and purslane.[25]

Equally important, we must also *reduce* omega-6s in our diet. Reduce foods that contain corn oil, peanut oil, safflower oil and cottonseed oil. Be aware that most animal meats and eggs have high amounts of omega-6 EFAs.[26]

Because saturated animal fats such as butter have received such a bad rap from some well-meaning organizations, food manufacturers have replaced butter with refined vegetable oils, most of which contain large amounts of omega-6 EFAs. This is a serious problem, as our modern diet has become overloaded with omega-6 EFAs.

The typical Western diet has a ratio of more than 15 to 1 omega-6 to omega-3 EFAs, which is way out of balance. Currently, the FDA has no recommendations on the ratio of omega-6 to omega-3 EFAs; however, Canadian guidelines recommend a ratio of 6 to 1 (omega-6 to omega-3 EFAs).[27]

Here are some health benefits of low omega-6 to omega-3 EFA ratios:

- A ratio of 4 to 1 aided in the prevention of cardiovascular disease and reduced mortality by 70%.
- A ratio of 5 to 1 significantly helped patients with asthma while a ratio of 10 to 1 made asthma worse.
- A ratio of 2 or 3 to 1 was shown to reduce inflammation in patients with rheumatoid arthritis.
- A ratio of 2.5 to 1 reduced spread of colon cancer while a ratio of 4 to 1 had no effect.[28]

Remember from chapter 13 that sufficient omega-3 EFAs are required for proper brain function. Omega-3s give our cells' membranes the flexibility and fluidity they need to function properly and at optimum levels.[29]

Enzymes Can Reduce Inflammation

Remember from chapter 15 that certain foods that are high in proteolytic (protein-digesting) enzymes also have anti-inflammatory actions. These foods include the following:

- **Ginger:** fresh ginger is nature's richest source of proteolytic enzymes, over 180 times more concentrated than those in papaya[30]
- **Fresh papaya:** papaya contains the proteolytic enzyme papain
- **Fresh pineapple:** pineapple contains the proteolytic enzyme bromelain
- **Figs**
- **Kiwi**
- **Guava**

The proteolytic enzymes in these foods can help fight inflammation directly by breaking down food proteins and improving digestion. Proteolytic enzymes also help fight inflammation indirectly by helping to fight off bacteria, viruses, parasites, and other infections that are known to cause inflammation.[31]

Oral enzyme supplements have anti-inflammatory actions and help promote healing. Immune complexes in our bodies are formed as our immune systems fight off harmful bacteria, viruses, and parasites. If these immune complexes become too plentiful, they "jam up our immune system" and interrupt healing. Oral enzyme supplements can help remove these immune complexes.[32] Special oral enzymes produced for therapeutic purposes have an enteric coating, which allows the enzymes to be released in the small intestine for better absorption into the bloodstream. Refer back to chapter 15 for more information on enzymes.

DR. FLOYD CHILTON'S ANTI-INFLAMMATORY DIETARY PROGRAM[33]

Floyd Chilton, Ph.D., prominent researcher, physician, and author of *Fighting the War Within* and *Inflammation Nation*, details a complete dietary program to dramatically reduce chronic inflammation. His program is backed by 6 clinical studies. (Dr. Chilton writes that no other dietary program for reducing inflammation has been backed by this many studies.) He developed his program with his sister in mind; she was diagnosed with juvenile rheumatoid arthritis at the age of 13. In her 30s, she underwent 2 knee replacements and 5 surgeries on her hands. After 6 months on his program, she had gained remarkable hand movement. Also, Chilton's son could not participate in football practice from time to time due to his asthma, but after 6 months on the diet did not miss a practice for the next year. Chilton and his team of researchers note reductions in inflammatory markers in as few as 7 days after beginning his special diet.

Chilton's dietary program consists of several steps:

Step 1: Limit intake of foods that contain arachidonic acid, a very pro-inflammatory type of omega-6 EFA.

Arachidonic acid is readily converted to pro-inflammatory chemical transmitters. Foods high in arachidonic acid that must be avoided in his program are farmed-raised Atlantic salmon, pork fat, bacon, turkey fat, dark turkey meat, bear meat, egg yolks, and animal organ foods such as heart, liver, brain, and kidneys.

Step 2: Block the production of pro-inflammatory chemical transmitters.

Chilton's program makes use of omega-3 EFAs by eating wild

caught fish and a very special type of omega-6 EFA called gamma-linolenic acid (GLA), which is present in borage oil, evening primrose oil, black currant oil, and pine nuts. Chilton and his research team found that GLA can actually block certain enzymes from producing pro-inflammatory transmitters. Detailed research by Chilton's team showed that GLA must be TAKEN TOGETHER with omega-3 EFAs from cold-water fish (herring, mackerel, salmon, anchovies, and canned white tuna or their oils). Chilton requires wild-caught salmon and other oily fish in his program because some farm-raised salmon contains too much arachidonic acid and may do more harm than good. (Some farm-raised fish are fed grains that contain mostly omega-6 EFAs.)

On the other hand, fish in the wild eat large amounts of algae, which contains omega-3 EFAs and in turn, increases the omega-3 content of the fish. As discussed in chapter 13, these cold-water fish and their oils contain a special omega-3 EFA called eicosapentaenoic acid (EPA) that, taken with GLA at mealtime, results in the most efficient blocking of pro-inflammatory prostaglandins and leukotrienes. His studies show that at least 600 milligrams of GLA is required each day to produce significant effects for the average adult. (One capsule of borage oil typically contains about 200 milligrams of GLA; therefore, 3 capsules per day are necessary to feel results.) He and his colleagues warn *not* to take just GLA by itself because it will take another chemical path and end up producing pro-inflammatory prostaglandins and leukotrienes, which can be dangerous.

Step 3: Eat foods that have a low-to-moderate glycemic index.

The glycemic index measures how rapidly carbohydrates break down and send sugar into the bloodstream. High levels of blood sugar and insulin produce pro-inflammatory chemical transmitters. The foods with highest glycemic indexes are those with refined white sugar and refined white flour, such as cookies, cakes, doughnuts, and pastries. White potatoes, white bread, cereals (if not whole grain), instant oatmeal, and ice cream also have a high glycemic index. Foods with a low-to-moderate glycemic index include fruits, vegetables, whole grains, beans, cooked cereals, whole grain breads, whole grain pasta, brown rice, lentils, chickpeas, barley, nuts, milk, low-fat yogurt, sweet potatoes, corn, and slow-cooking oatmeal. Low glycemic foods contain complex carbohydrates, which are digested slowly so the sugar is released gradually into the bloodstream.

In general, dietary programs and nutritional supplements take a longer time to work than drugs. For this reason, some medical practitioners use a combination of drugs, diet, and nutritional supplements while encouraging their patients to eventually reduce the use of strong drugs.

GINGER CAN HELP REDUCE INFLAMMATION AND ARTHRITIS

A landmark study of 46 patients with arthritis reported that three-quarters experienced some degree of relief from pain and swelling from rheumatoid arthritis and osteoarthritis. Ten additional patients who had muscular discomfort also experienced some degree of relief.[34]

One interesting animal study showed that shogaol (abundant in dried ginger) protected knee cartilage from the damaging effects of inflammation.[35] It is believed that immune complexes contribute to irreversible damage to cartilage and decreased joint function.[36] Remember form chapter 15 that enteric-coated enzyme supplements can help remove immune complexes.

GINGER HAS SOME ANTICANCER ACTIONS

In the 1970s, researchers suspected a link between chronic inflammation and the development and progression of cancer.[37] It is now known that inflammation is involved in all 3 stages of tumor development: initiation, progression, and metastasis (spreading).[38] It is also known that anti-inflammatory medications such as aspirin and celecoxib, which inhibit COX enzymes, can also help inhibit the growth and reproduction of cancerous tumor cells.[39]

Because ginger also inhibits COX enzymes, it is not surprising some studies indicate ginger also has some interesting anticancer actions[40] against the following conditions:

- **Breast cancer (animal study):**[41] Also remember from chapter 13 that the lignans from flaxseeds contain phytoestrogens (plant estrogens), which also have anticancer actions against breast cancer.

- **Colon cancer (animal study)**[42] Also, a human study is currently in place to study ginger's potential actions against colon cancer;[43] the University of Minnesota has filed a patent application for gingerol, abundant in fresh ginger, as an anticancer agent.[44]

- **Leukemia:** A synthetic form of a chemical in ginger caused human leukemia cells to die.[45]

- **Ovarian cancer (human and animal cells were studied)**[46]
- **Skin cancer (gingerol was applied to skin of animals)**[47]

It appears that the gingerols abundant in fresh ginger are mostly responsible for ginger's anticancer and antitumor actions, although the shogaols in dried ginger may also have some anticancer actions.[48] It is interesting to note that the shogaols in dried ginger can be transformed back into gingerols upon rehydrating—just add water—although the process appears to take several hours.[49] Remember from chapter 4 that ginger's cousin, turmeric, also has some anti-tumor actions.[50]

I should also mention that ginger's anti-inflammatory actions have some actions against Alzheimer's disease[51]—and, likewise, so does turmeric/curcumin as was discussed in chapter 4.

It is known that inflammation generates free radicals, which can cause oxidative damage to cells and tissues, which, in turn, could increase the risk of certain types of cancers.[52] Antioxidants, which are found in many foods, especially ginger, garlic, turmeric, and bright-colored fruits and vegetables, contribute to the health benefits of these foods. We will gain a better understanding of free radicals as we lead into the next chapter.

REFERENCES FOR CHAPTER 16

1.   Floyd H. Chilton, Ph.D., Laura Tucker. *Win the War Within*. Rodale Inc. 2006. pp.4-5, 33-40.

2a. Boncler M, Luzak B, Watala C. "[Role of C-reactive protein in atherogenesis]" *Posteply Hig Med Dosw (Online)*. 2006;60:538-46.

2b. Weintraub WS, Harrison DG. "C-reactive protein, inflammation and atherosclerosis: do we really understand it yet? *Eur Heart J*. 2000 Jun;21(12):958-960.

3a. Ursella S, Mazzone M, Portale G, Testa A, Pignataro G, Covino M, Fenici P, Gasbarrini GB, Gentiloni Silveri N. "How to use C-reactive protein in cardiac disease?" *Minerva Cardioangiol*. 2005 Feb;53(1):59-68.

3b. Morrow DA, Ridker PM. "C-reactive protein, inflammation, and coronary risk." *Med Clin North Am*. 2000 Jan;84(1):149-61, ix.

3c. Haverkate F, Thompson SG, Pyke SD, Gallimore JR, Pepys MB. "Production of C-reactive protein and risk of coronary events in stable and unstable angina. European Concerted Action on Thrombosis and Disabilities Angina Pectoris Study Group." *Lancet*. 1997 Feb 15;349(9050):462-6.

4.   Di Napoli M. Editorial comment - "C-reactive protein and vascular risk on stroke patients: potential use for the future." *Stroke*. 2003 Oct;34(10):2468-70. Epub 2003 Sep 18.

5a. Schacter E, Weitzman SA. "Chronic Inflammation and Cancer." *Oncology*. Vol 16, No 2 (February 2002).

5b. Hofseth LJ, Ying L. "Identifying and diffusing weapons of mass inflammation in carcinogenesis." *Biochim Biophys Acta*. 2006 Jan;1765(1):74-84. Epub 2005 Sep 8.

6a. Federico A, Morgillo F, Tuccillo C, Ciardiello F, Loguercio C. "Chronic inflammation and oxidative stress in human carcinogenesis." *Int J Cancer*. 2007 Dec 1;121(11):2381-6.

6b. Bartsch H, Nair J. "Chronic inflammation and oxidative stress in the genesis and perpetuation of cancer: role of lipid peroxidation, DNA damage, and repair." *Langenbecks Arch Surg.* 2006 Sep;391(5):499-510. Epub 2006 Aug 15.

7. Web site: WebMD.com. "Most Common Arthritis Types" Accessed 2/10/2010. <http://www.webmd.com/rheumatoid-arthritis/guide/...>

8. Schacter E, Weitzman SA. "Chronic Inflammation and Cancer." *Oncology* (Williston Park). 2002 Feb;16(2):217-26, 229; discussion 230-2.

9. Floyd H. Chilton, Ph.D., Laura Tucker. *Win the War Within.* Rodale Inc. 2006. pp.46-49.

10. Floyd H. Chilton, Ph.D., Laura Tucker. *Win the War Within.* Rodale Inc. 2006. pp.49-52, 55-58.

11. Isabelle Aeberli, Luciano Molinari, Giatgen Spinas, Roger Lehmann, Dagmar l'Allemand and Michael B Zimmermann. "Dietary intakes of fat and antioxidant vitamins are predictors of subclinical inflammation in overweight Swiss children" *American Journal of Clinical Nutrition*, Vol. 84, No. 4, 748-755, October 2006.

12. Chittur S, Parr B. Marcovici G. "Inhibition of Inflammatory Gene Expression in Keratinocytes Using a Composition containing Carnitine, Thioctic Acid and Saw Palmetto Extract." *Evid Based Complement Alternat Med.* 2009 Aug 19 [Epub ahead of print].

13. Floyd H. Chilton, Ph.D., Laura Tucker. *Win the War Within.* Rodale Inc. 2006. p.5.

14. Floyd H. Chilton, Ph.D., Laura Tucker. *Win the War Within.* Rodale Inc. 2006. p.25.

15. Jolad SD, Lantz RC, Chen GJ, Chen GJ, Bates RB, Timmermann BN. "Commercially processed dry ginger (Zingiber officinale): composition and effects on LPS-stimulated PGE2 production." Phytochemistry. 2005 Jul;66(13):1614-35.

16a. Lantz RC Chen GJ, Sarihan M, Solyom AM, Jolad SD, Timmerman BN. "The effect of extracts from ginger rhizome on inflammatory mediator production." *Phytomedicine.* 2007 Feb;14(2-3):123-8. Epub 2006 May 18.

16b. Jolad SD, Lantz RC, Chen GJ, Chen GJ, Bates RB, Timmermann BN. "Commercially processed dry ginger (Zingiber officinale): composition and effects on LPS-stimulated PGE2 production." *Phytochemistry.* 2005 Jul;66(13):1614-35.

16c. Setty AR, Sigal LH. "Herbal medications commonly used in the practice of rheumatology: mechanisms of action, efficacy, and side effects." *Semin Arthritis Rheum.* 2005 Jun;34(6):773-84.

16d. Levy A, Simon O, Shelly J, Gardener M. "6-Shogaol reduced chronic inflammatory response in the knees of rats treated with complete Freund's adjuvant." *BC Pharmacol.* 2006; 6: 12.

16e. Kim SO, Kundu Jk, Shin YK, Park JH, Cho MH, Kim TY, Surh YJ.

"[6]-Gingerol inhibits COX-2 expression by blocking the activation of p38 MAP kinase and NF-kappaB in phorbol ester-stimulated mouse skin." *Oncogene.* 2005 Apr 7;24(15):2558-67.

16f.   Phan PV, Sohrabi A, Polotsky A, Hungerford DS, Lindmark L, Frondoza CG. "Ginger extract components suppress induction of chemokine expression in human synoviocytes." *J Altern Complement Med.* 2005 Feb;11(1):149-54.

16g.   Young HY, Luo YL, Cheng HY, Hsieh WC, Liao JC, Peng WH. "Analgesic and anti-inflammatory activities of [6]-gingerol." *J Ethnopharmacol.* 2005 Jan 4;96(1-2):207-10.

16h.   Grzanna R, Lindmark L, Frondoza CG. "Ginger--an herbal medicinal product with broad anti-inflammatory actions." *J Med Food.* 2005 Summer;8(2):125-32.

16i.   Kim SO, Chun KS, Kundu JK, Surh YJ. "Inhibitory effects of [6]-gingerol on PMA-induced COX-2 expression and activation of NF-kappaB and p38 MAPK in mouse skin." *Biofactors.* 2004;21(1-4):27-31.

16j.   Frondoza CG, Sohrabi A, Polotsky A, Phan PV, Hungerford DS, Lindmark L. "An in vitro screening assay for inhibitors of proinflammatory mediators in herbal extracts using human synoviocyte cultures." *In Vitro Cell Dev Biol Anim.* 2004 Mar-Apr;40(3-4):95-101.

16k.   Jolad SD, Lantz RC, Solyom AM, Chen GJ, Bates RB, Timmermann BN. "Fresh organically grown ginger (Zingiber officinale): composition and effects on LPS-induced PGE2 production." *Phytochemistry.* 2004 Jul;65(13):1937-54.

16l.   Gonlachanvit S, Chen YH, Hasler WL, Sun WM, Owyang C. "Ginger reduces hyperglycemia-evoked gastric dysrhythmias in healthy humans: possible role of endogenous prostaglandins." *J Pharmacol Exp Ther.* 2003 Dec;307(3):1098-103. Epub 2003 Oct.

16m.   Wigler I, Grotto I, Caspi D, Yaron M. "The effects of Zintona EC (a ginger extract) on symptomatic gonarthritis." *Osteoarthritis Cartilage.* 2003 Nov;11(11):783-9.

16n.   Shen CL, Hong KJ, Kim SW. "Effects of ginger (Zingiber officinale Ros.) on decreasing the production of inflammatory mediators in sow osteoarthrotic cartilage explants." *J Med Food.* 2003 Winter;6(4):323-8.

16o.   Penna SC, Medeiros MV, Aimbire FS, Faria-Neto HC, Sertie JA, Lopes-Martins RA. "Anti-inflammatory effect of the hydralcoholic extract of Zingiber officinale rhizomes on rat paw and skin edema." *Phytomedicine.* 2003;10(5):381-5.

16p.   Thomson M, Al-Qattan KK, Al-Sawan SM, Alnaqeeb MA, Khan I, Ali M. "The use of ginger (Zingiber officinale Rosc.) as a potential anti-inflammatory and antithrombotic agent." *Prosataglandins Leukot Essent Fatty Acids.* 2002 Dec;67(6):475-8.

16q.   Surh YJ. "Anti-tumor promoting potential of selected spice ingredients with antioxidative and anti-inflammatory activities: a short review." *Food Chem Toxicol.* 2002 Aug;40(8):1091-7.

16r.   Altman RD, Marcussen KC. "Effects of a ginger extract on knee pain in patients with osteoarthritis." *Arthritis Rheum.* 2001 Nov Nov;44(11):2531-8.

16s.   Tjendraputra E, Tran VH, Liu-Brennan D, Roufogalis BD, Duke CC. "Effect of ginger constituents and synthetic analogues on cyclooxygenase-2 enzyme in intact cells." *Bioorg Chem.* 2001 Jun:29(3):156-63.

16t.   Koo KL, Ammit AJ, Tran VH, Roufogalis BD. "Gingerols and related analogues inhibit arachidonic acid-induced human platelet serotonin release and aggregation." *Thromb Res.* 2001 Sep 1;103(5):387-97.

16u.   Surh Y. "Molecular mechanisms of chemopreventive effects of selected dietary and medicinal phenolic substances." *Mutat Res.* 1999 Jul 16;428(1-2):305-27.

16v.   Surh YJ, Park KK, Chun KS, Lee LJ, Lee E, Lee SS. "Anti-tumor-promoting activities of selected pungent phenolic substances present in ginger." *J Environ Pathol Tocicol Oncol.* 1999;18(2):131-9.

16w.   Park KK, Chun KS, Lee JM, Lee SS, Surh YJ. "Inhibitory effects of [6]-gingerol, a major pungent principle of ginger, on phorbol ester-induced inflammation, epidermal ornithine decarboxylase activity and skin tumor promotion in ICR mice." Cancer Lett 1998 Sep 25;131(2):231.

16x.   Katiyar SK, Agarwal R, Mukhtar H. "Inhibition of tumor promotion in SENCAR mouse skin by ethanol extract of Zingiber officinale rhizome." *Cancer Res.* 1996 Mar 1;56(5):1023-30.

16y.   Wu H, Shu W, Qiu L, Ye D. "[The experiment research of ginger detoxification to Rhizoma Pinelliae]" [Article in Chinese]. *Zhong Yao Cai.* 1998 Mar;21(3):137-40.

16z.   Srivastava KC, Mustafa T. "Ginger (Zingiber officinale) in rheumatism and musculoskeletal disorders." *Med Hypotheses.* 1992 Dec;39(4):342-8.

16aa.   Kiuchi F, Ieakami S, Shibuya M, Hanaoka F, Sankawa U. "Inhibition of prostaglandin and leukotriene biosynthesis by gingerols and diarylheptanoids." *Chem Pharm Bull* (Tokyo). 1992 Feb;40(2):387-91.

16ab.   Mascolo N, Jain R, Jain SC, Capasso F. "Ethnopharmacologic investigation of ginger (Zingiber officinale). *J Ethnopharmacol.* 1989 Nov;27(1-2):129-40.

16ac.   Srivastava KC, Mustafa T. "Ginger (Zingiber officinale) and rheumatic disorders." *Med Hypotheses.* 1989 May;29(1):25-8.

16ad.   Backon J. "Ginger: inhibition of thromboxane synthetase and stimulation of prostacyclin: relevance for medicine and psychiatry." *Med Hypotheses.* 1986 Jul;20(3):271-8.

16ae.   Umeda M, Amagaya S, Ogihara Y. "Effects of certain herbal medicines on the biotransformation of arachidonic acid: a new pharmacological testing method using serum." *J Ethnopharmacol.* 1988 May-Jun;23(1):91-8.

17.   Floyd H. Chilton, Ph.D., Laura Tucker. *Win the War Within.* Rodale Inc. 2006. pp.32-33.

18. Percival M. "Understanding The Natural Management of Pain and Inflammation." *Clinical Nutrition Insights*. Advanced Nutrition Publications, Inc. Rev. 1999.

19. "The Nobel Prize in Physiology or Medicince 1982." The Nobel Assembly at the Karolinska Institute. Press Release 11 October 1982. Web site: Nobelprize. org. Accessed 4/16/2007. <http://nobelprize.org>.

20a. Floyd H. Chilton, Ph.D., Laura Tucker. *Win the War Within*. Rodale Inc. 2006 p.67.

20b. "Ibuprofen" Web site: Medline Plus. Accessed 3/29/2009. <http://www.nlm. nih.gov/medlineplus/druginfo/meds/a682159.html>.

21. "COX-2 Selective (includes Bextra, Celebrex, and Vioxx) and Non-Selective Non-Steroidal Anti-Inflammatory Drugs (NSAIDs)." Web site: U.S. Food and Drug Administration. Accessed 4/16/2007. <http://www.fda.gov/cder/drug/ infopage/cox2/>.

22. Budwig, Johanna. *Flax Oil as a True Aid Against Arthritis, Heart Infarction, Cancer and Other Diseases*. Apple Publishing Co. Ltd. 1994.

23. Dr. Diane H. Morris. "Omega-3 fats in flax and fish are similar in many ways." Web site: Flax Council of Canada. Accessed 5/2/2007. <www.flax-council.ca>.

24. "Kale". "The world's healthiest foods." George Mateljan Foundation. Web site: whfoods.org. Accessed 5/4/2007. <http://www.whfoods.com/genpage.php?pfri endly=1&tname=foodspice&dbid=38>.

25. Simopoulos AP, Normann HA, Gillaspy JE, Duke JA. "Common purslane: a source of omega-3 fatty acids and antioxidants." *J Am Coll Nutr*. 1992 Aug;11(4):374-82.

26. Percival M. "Understanding The Natural Management of Pain and Inflammation." *Clinical Nutrition Insights*. Advanced Nutrition Publications, Inc. Rev. 1999.

27. "Clarifying omega-3 fatty acid recommendations." CFP MFC. Official Publication of The College of Family Physicians of Canada. *Can Fam Physician*. 2006 September 10; 52(9): 1061-1062.

28. Simopoulus AP. "The importance of the ratio of omega-6/omega-3 essential fatty acids." *Biomed Pharmacother*. 2002 Oct;56(8):365-79.

29a. Haag M. "Essential Fatty Acids and the brain." *Can J Psychiatry*. 2003 Apr;48(3):195-203.

26b. Young G, Conquer J. "Omega-3 fatty acids and neuropsychiatric disorders." *Reprod Nutr Dev*. 2005 Jan-Feb;45(1):1-28.

29c. Simopoulos AP. "Omega-3 fatty acids in health and disease and in growth and development." *Am J Clin Nutr*. 1991 Sep;54(3):438-63.

30. Thompson, EH, Wolf ID, Allen CE. "Ginger rhizome: A new source of proteolytic enzyme." *Journal of Food Science* 38, no. 4 (1973): pp.652-55.

31.   Lopez DA, Williams RM, Miehlke K. *Enzymes - The Fountain of Life.* The
       Neville Press, Inc. 1994, Germany. pp.8, 21-25, 149-152.
32a.   Desser L, Holomanova D, Zavadova E, Pavelka K, Mohr T, Herbacek I.
       "Oral therapy with proteolytic enzymes decreases excessive TGF-beta levels in
       human blood." *Cancer Chemother Pharmacol.* 2001 Jul;47 Suppl:S10-5.
32b.   Lopez DA, Williams RM, Miehlke K. *Enzymes - The Fountain of Life.* The
       Neville Press, Inc. 1994, Germany. pp.22, 156, 181.
33.   Floyd H. Chilton, Ph.D., Laura Tucker. *Win the War Within.* Rodale Inc.
       2006. pp.8-12, 101-105, 114-127, 129, 140-141, 135-136, 193-199.
34.   Srivastava KC, Mustafa T. "Ginger (Zingiber officinale) in rheumatism and
       musculoskeletal disorders." *Med Hypotheses.* 1992 Dec;39(4):342-8.
35.   Levy A, Simon O, Shelly J, Gardener M. "6-Shogaol reduced chronic inflam-
       matory response in the knees of rats treated with complete Freund's adjuvant."
       BC Pharmacol. 2006; 6: 12.
36.   Jasin HE. "Immune mediated cartilage destruction." *Scand J Rheumatol Suppl.*
       1988;76:111-6.
37.   Jaffe BM. "Prostaglandins and cancer: an update." *Prostaglandins.* 1974 Jun
       25;6(6):453-61.
38.   "Executive Summary of Inflammation and Cancer Think Tank". Web site:
       National Cancer Institute, Division of Cancer Biology. Accessed 12/28/2008.
       <http://dcb.nci.nih.gov/thinktank/Executive_Summary_of_Inflammation_
       and_Cancer_Think_Tank.cfm>.
39a.   D. Mazhar, R. Gillmore and J. Waxman. "COX and cancer: *Q J Med.* 2005;
       98:711-718.
39b.   Asano TK, McLeod TS. "Non steroidal anti-inflammatory drugs (NSAID)
       and Aspirin for preventing colorectal adenomas and carcinomas." *Cochrane
       Database Syst Rev.* 2004;(2):CD004079.
39c.   Arun B, Goss P. "The role of COX-2 inhibition in breast cancer treatment and
       prevention." *Semin Oncol.* 2004 Apr;31(2 Suppl 7):22-9.
39d.   Baron JA, Cole BF, Sandler RS, et al. "A randomized trial of aspirin to prevent
       colorectal adenomas." *N Engl Med.* 2003 Mar 6;348(10):891-9.
39e.   Grösh S, Tegeder I, Niederberger E, Bräutigam L, Geisslinger G. "COX-2
       independent induction of cell cycle arrest and apoptosis in colon cancer
       cells by the selective COX-2 inhibitor celecoxib." *FASEB J.* 2001
       Dec;15(14):2742-4. Epub 2001 Oct 15.
39f.   Williams CS, Watson AJ, Sheng H, Helou R, Shao J, DuBois RN. "Celecoxib
       prevents tumor growth in vivo without toxicity to normal gut: lack of
       correlation between in vitro and in vivo models." *Cancer Res.* 2000 Nov
       1;60(21):6045-51.
40.   Shukla Y, Singh M. "Cancer preventive properties of ginger: a brief review."
       Food Chem Toxicol. 2007 May;45(5):683-90. Epub 2006 Nov 12.
41.   Nagasawa H, Watanabe K, Inatomi H. "Effects of bitter melon

(Momordica charantia l.) or ginger rhizome (Zingiber officinale rosc) on spontaneous mammary tumorigenesis in /SHN mice." *Am J Chin Med.* 2002;30(2-3):195-205.

42. Manju V, Nalini N. "Chemopreventive efficacy of ginger, a naturally occurring anticarcinogen during the initiation, post-initiation stages of 1,2 dimethylhydrazine-induced colon cancer." *Clin Chim Acta.* 2005 Aug;358(1-2):60-7.

43. Suzanna M. Zick, ND, MPH. "A Phase II Study of the Effect of Ginger Root on Markers of Inflammation in Gut Mucosa" NCI 1 K07 CA102592-01A1. University of Michigan Health Systems, Ann Arbor, MI.02/12/07 V4.

44. "Dietary Ginger May Work Against Cancer Growth". Source: University of Minnesota. October 29, 2003. Web site: ScienceDaily Accessed: 5/21/2007. <http://www.sciencedaily.com/releases/2003/10/031029064357.htm>.

45a. Hsu MH, Kuo SC, Chen CJ, Chung JG, Lai YY, Huang LJ. 1-(3,4-dimethoxyphenyl)-3,5-dodecenedione (I6) induces G1 arrest and apoptosis in human promyelocytic leukemia HL-60 cells. Leuk Res. 2005 Dec;29(12):1399-406. Epub 2005 May 31.

45b. Wei QY, Ma JP, Cai YJ, Yang L, Liu ZL. "Cytotoxic and apoptotic activities of diarylheptanoids and gingerol-related compounds from the rhizome of Chinese ginger." *J Ethnopharmacol.* 2005 Nov 14;102(2):177-84. Epub 2005 Jul 15.

45c. Wang CC, Chen LG, Lee LT, Yang LL. "Effects of 6-gingerol, an antioxidant from ginger, on inducing apoptosis in human leukemic HL-60 cells. *In Vivo.* 2003 Nov-Dec;17(6):641-5.

45d. Miyoshi N, Nakamura Y, Ueda Y, Abe M, Ozawa Y, Uchida K, Osawa T. "Dietary ginger constituents, galanals A and B, are potent apoptosis inducers in Human T Lymphoma Jurkat cells." *Cancer Lett.* 2003 Sep 25;199(2):113-9.

46a. Jennifer Rhode, Sarah Fogoros, Suzanna Zick, Heather Wahl, Kent A Griffith, Jennifer Huang, and J Rebecca Liu. "Ginger inhibits cell growth and modulates angiogenic factors in ovarian cancer cells." *BMC Complement Altern Med.* 2007; 7: 44

46b. Unnikrishnan MC, Kuttan R. "Cytotoxicity of extracts of spices to cultured cells." *Nutr Cancer.* 1988;11(4):251-7.

47a. Kim SO, Chun KS, Kundu JK, Surh YJ. "Inhibitory effects of [6]-gingerol on PMA-induced COX-2 expression and activation of NF-kappaB and p38 MAPK in mouse skin." *Biofactors.* 2004;21(1-4):27-31.

47b. Surh Y. "Molecular mechanisms of chemopreventive effects of selected dietary and medicinal phenolic substances." *Mutat Res.* 1999 Jul 16;428(1-2):305-27.

47c. Park KK, Chun KS, Lee JM, Lee SS, Surh YJ. "Inhibitory effects of [6]-gingerol, a major pungent principle of ginger, on phorbol ester-induced inflammation, epidermal ornithine decarboxylase activity and skin tumor promotion in ICR mice." Cancer Lett 1998 Sep 25;131(2):231.

47d. Katiyar SK, Agarwal R, Mukhtar H. "Inhibition of tumor promotion in

SENCAR mouse skin by ethanol extract of Zingiber officinale rhizome."
Cancer Res. 1996 Mar 1;56(5):1023-30.

48a.   Shukla Y, Singh M. "Cancer preventive properties of ginger: a brief review."
Food Chem Toxicol. 2007 May;45(5):683-90. Epub 2006. Nov 12.

48b.   Leal PF, Braga ME, Sato DN, Carvalho JE, Marques MO, Meireles MA.
"Functional properties of spice extracts obtained via supercritical fluid extraction." *J Agric Food Chem.* 2003 Apr 23;51(9):2520-5.

48c.   Bode AM, Ma WY, Surh YJ, Dong Z. "Inhibition of epidermal growth factor-induced cell transformation and activator protein 1 activation by [6]-gingerol."
Cancer Res. 2001 Feb 1;61(3):850-3.

48d.   Vimala S, Norhanom AW, Yadav M. "Anti-tumour promoter activity in
Malaysian ginger rhizobia used in traditional medicine." *Br J Cancer.* 1999
Apr;80(1-2):110-6.

48e.   Surh YJ, Park KK, Chun KS, Lee LJ, Lee E, Lee SS. "Anti-tumor-promoting
activities of selected pungent phenolic substances present in ginger." *J Environ
Pathol Tocicol Oncol.* 1999;18(2):131-9.

49.   Bhattarai S, Tran VH, Duke CC. "The stability of gingerol and shogaol in
aqueous solutions." J Pharm Sci. 2001 Oct;90(10):1658-64.

50.   Leal PF, Braga ME, Sato DN, Carvalho JE, Marques MO, Meireles MA.
"Functional properties of spice extracts obtained via supercritical fluid extraction." *J Agric Food Chem.* 2003 Apr 23;51(9):2520-5.

51.   Grzanna R, Phan P, Polotsky A, Lindmark L, Frondoza CG. "Ginger extract
inhibits beta-amyloid peptide-induced cytokine and chemokine expression in cultured THP-1 monocytes." *J Altern Complement Med.* 2004
Dec;10(6):1009-13.

52a.   Kondu JK, Surh YJ. "Inflammation: gearing the journey to cancer." *Mutat Res.*
2008 Jul-Aug;659(1-2):15-30. Epub 2008 Mar 16.

52b.   Di Giacomo C, Acquaviva R, Lanteri R, Licata F, Licata A, Vanella A.
"Nonproteic antioxidant status in plasma of subjects with colon cancer." *Exp
Biol Med (Maywood).* 2003 May;228(5):525-8.

52c.   Okada F. "Inflammation and free radicals in tumor development and progression." *Redox Rep.* 2002;7(6):357-68.

52d.   Krystyna Frenkel, PhD. "Chronic Inflammation and Cancer." *Oncology.* Vol.
16 No. 2. February 1, 2002.

CHAPTER 17

Antioxidants to the Rescue!

IN addition to controlling inflammation, another key to staying healthy is to limit the damage caused by an overload of free radicals. Free radicals are atoms or molecules that are missing an electron, typically oxygen or nitrogen. This makes free radicals very reactive because they want to steal electrons from the cells around them.

Free radicals are both good and bad. Free radicals are helpful in limited amounts and are essential for fighting off disease. The body's immune system uses free radicals to destroy harmful bacteria, viruses, and diseased cells. However, free radicals become harmful when they damage healthy cells around them, which then release even more free radicals. This sets off a chain reaction that can overload our bodies' ability to repair the damaged cells and tissues.

Another name for the damaging effects of free radicals is oxidation, which is similar to the process that causes steel to rust. When the chain reaction produces far more free radicals than our bodies' antioxidants can manage, it is termed "oxidative stress."[1] In addition, other harmful toxins are produced by oxidation that further stress our immune system.[2]

DID YOU KNOW ...

- The average cell receives about 10,000 hits a day from free radicals.[3]

- Inflammation produces large amounts of free radicals; free radicals produce more inflammation.[4]
- Free radicals are involved in the process of aging.[5]
- Overexposure to the sun's ultraviolet rays produces free radicals, which can cause premature aging of our skin.[6]
- Free radicals erode the cartilage in arthritic joints.[7]
- Free radicals can convert harmless tumors into cancerous tumors.[8]
- Heavy metals in our bodies can produce large amounts of free radicals[9]; heavy metals include arsenic (from food and drinking water), lead (from food, water, air, paint and other sources), mercury (from food, water, air, fish, and mercury dental fillings), and cadmium (from cigarette smoke, environmental pollution, and food contamination).[10]
- Other things that increase oxidative chain reactions are radiation,[11] certain pesticides,[12] bacterial and viral infections,[13] and high blood sugar.[14]

It is known that free radicals are involved in the occurrence of the following illnesses:

- Alzheimer's[15]
- Arthritis[16]
- Atherosclerosis (hardening and narrowing of the arteries)[17]
- Diabetes[18]
- Gastrointestinal disorders[19]
- Multiple sclerosis[20]
- Pancreatic disease[21]
- Parkinson's disease[22]
- Schizophrenia[23]
- Stroke[24]
- Tumors and cancer[25]
- Various other illnesses[26]

It is also important to note that proper balance between oxidant and antioxidant mechanisms is required for the proper function of blood vessels.[27]

Oxidative stress in our bodies can be compared to extra wear and tear on a car's engine from abusive driving and overheating in addition to normal wear and tear. Eventually, problems will develop. (When a car rusts out, it actually is oxidative damage.)

ANTIOXIDANTS—HOW THEY HELP US

Antioxidants help our bodies in many ways by doing the following:

- Giving up their electrons over to free radicals, making the radical satisfied and harmless
- Scavenging free radicals—cleaning up and removing them
- Neutralizing the harmful by-products of the oxidation process
- Blocking certain enzymes needed by free radicals to carry on the chain reaction[28]
- Chelating (combining with) metals and other materials they act upon, taking away their fuel and helping stop the chain reaction[29]

GINGER—A POTENT ANTIOXIDANT

Ginger contains over 50 antioxidant compounds,[30] making it one of nature's most potent antioxidant foods. Over 25 studies affirm ginger's antioxidant actions.[31] One major study analyzed the antioxidant potencies of 120 natural foods. Ginger ranked very high on the list, with only a handful of foods scoring higher in antioxidant potency. The foods scoring higher than ginger were certain types of berries, sour cherries, pomegranates, walnuts, and sunflower seeds.[32] Other common herbs and foods with high amounts of antioxidants include rosemary,[33] allspice, cinnamon, clove, lemon balm, oregano, peppermint, sage, thyme,[34] brewed coffee, grape juice, pecans, and unsweetened baking chocolate.[35]

Considering that ginger is economical and available in many grocery stores all year round, it stands out as a great protector of our heath when we consider its many protective actions in our body. Ginger's antioxidant compounds also contribute to its anticancer actions.[36]

How Free Radicals Damage Our Bodies

Normal processes in our bodies produce free radicals such as eating, breathing, exercising, fighting infection, stress, and inflammation.

Inflammation produces very large amounts of free radicals,[37] and, in turn, free radicals produce more inflammation.[38] You can see how ginger's ability to fight inflammation combined with its potent antioxidants work together to help stop this vicious cycle.

Heavy metals in our bodies can dramatically increase free radical chain reactions. These metals include mercury, arsenic, cadmium, nickel,[39] lead,[40] and aluminum.[41] Arsenic is present in some pesticides and treated wood. Smoking cigarettes gives off cadmium. It is reported that many autism patients have higher concentrations of heavy metals along with leaky gut syndrome and *Candida*.[42]

Free radicals readily attack EFAs in cell membranes.[43] As a result, the membranes become damaged and lose their flexibility and fluidity. This is called lipid peroxidation (lipids are another name for fats and fatty acids). As the cell wall becomes damaged and stiffened, its function is degraded.[44] Lipid peroxidation can harm the villi of the digestive tract,[45] which may offer yet another clue to solving the digestion puzzle. The villi are the millions of microscopic finger-like projections that line the wall of the small intestine. The villi's function is to absorb food nutrients and transport the nutrients into the bloodstream. Dietary antioxidants can help protect the villi and the digestive tract. Probably the most well-known antioxidant supplement is vitamin C. One study showed that vitamin C and the herbs green tea and cat's claw also contain strong antioxidants that have protective properties against oxidative damage to the digestive tract.[46]

Free radicals can stiffen red blood cells. Because lipid peroxidation also affects red blood cells (which are also called platelets or erythrocytes), the membranes become less flexible and less functional, resulting in decreased cell survival rate.[47] (Red blood cells carry oxygen to all parts of our bodies and remove carbon dioxide and other wastes.) One study showed that aged garlic extract helped protect red blood cells from lipid peroxidation. Aged garlic extract was also shown to improve circulation to tiny arteries and help protect red blood cells by acting as a scavenger of free radicals.[48]

Free radicals also damage the DNA in our bodies' cells.[49] DNA is the control center of each cell and controls cell growth and multiplication. Oxidative damage to DNA contributes to the occurrence of cancer.[50] Remember that the DNA in every cell in our bodies receives thousands of oxidative interactions each day from free radicals. Free radicals also contribute to aging and decreased function of the brain.[51] A lab study showed that ginger's antioxidant actions appear to help protect red blood cells against DNA damage.[52]

MORE AMAZING ACTIONS OF GINGER AND OTHER ANTIOXIDANTS

- Antioxidants have been used for several thousand years for preserving foods. Older cultures used spices such as ginger, turmeric, and pepper to help prevent oxidation and, in effect, prevented spoiling of food. Modern technology has provided refrigeration to reduce spoiling as well as newer, synthetic antioxidants such as BHA (butylated hydroxyanisole) and BHT (butylated hydroxytoluene). As a result, the knowledge and use of traditional spices has not been passed down to our generation. Ginger has been shown to be a favorite spice down through history for preserving and flavoring foods.

- An animal study using an extract of fresh ginger showed ginger's antioxidant actions significantly reduced oxidation of LDL cholesterol and slowed development of atherosclerosis in mice.[53]
- Another animal study showed ginger extract helped reduce the effects of high doses of radiation when fed to mice *before* they were subjected to radiation. The mice that received ginger showed reduced radiation sickness, reduced gastrointestinal deaths, and reduced bone marrow deaths.[54] Ginger's radio-protective actions are believed to result from its potent free radical scavenging actions.[55]
- Fresh ginger extract was found to help protect against oxidative damage from the chemicals arsenic[56] and malathion.[57] Arsenic and malathion are present in some pesticides. Arsenic is also used as a preservative in wood for outdoor use. Arsenic-treated wood is commonly used on porches and decks.
- The gingerols in fresh ginger appear to be the most potent of its antioxidant compounds.[58] Ginger's antioxidant properties were shown to be equal to or better than vitamin C (ascorbic acid).[59]
- Some experts believe the natural antioxidant actions of fruits and vegetables are a bigger help in the prevention of colon cancer than their fiber.[60] Remember that many fruits and vegetables are rich in many other disease-fighting phytochemicals in addition to their antioxidant actions.
- The antioxidant actions of combined ginger, garlic, and

vitamin E helped protect the liver against the toxic chemical carbon tetrachloride, according to one animal study in Nigeria. (Carbon tetrachloride is one of the most potent toxins to the liver.) Inflammation of the liver was significantly reduced in the rats that were pretreated with ginger, garlic, and vitamin E.[61]

ANTIOXIDANT SUPPLEMENTS

Popular antioxidant supplements such as vitamins A, C, E, beta-carotene, selenium, zinc, chromium, and many others have proved helpful in hundreds of studies; however, results have not been consistent. Researchers and vitamin producers had high expectations for these well-known supplements in the treatment of cancer and atherosclerosis (hardening and narrowing of the arteries); however, some recent studies have shown disappointing results. Several studies showed that coronary artery disease was not consistently helped by vitamin E[62] or beta-carotene.[63] One study showed that vitamin E and beta-carotene actually worked against the cholesterol-reducing medication simvastatin-niacin (used for coronary heart disease therapy) while selenium enhanced the medication.[64]

Some experts are even disputing the long-held free radical theory of disease and aging because cancer and atherosclerosis were not helped by some of these single antioxidant supplements.[65] Keep in mind that there are 8 different types of vitamin E that act very differently in the body. Two types of vitamin E (that are not antioxidants) are undergoing research for possible treatment for breast cancer.[66]

Selenium has important antioxidant and anticancer actions[67] and several actions against mercury toxicity. Selenium can bind to mercury, preventing it from reaching its target tissue. For this to happen, selenium must already be present in the body at the time of mercury uptake. Secondly, selenium's antioxidant actions can significantly reduce the overload of free radicals produced from mercury. Mercury is currently one of the most widespread pollutants in our environment.[68] James

Duke, author of *The Green Pharmacy*, recommends eating 1 or 2 Brazil nuts per day because of their rich selenium content. He writes that just 1 Brazil nut can have more than the recommended daily value of selenium, which is 70 micrograms.[69] Exactly how selenium exerts its preventive actions is not yet completely understood.[70]

Coenzyme Q10 (CoQ10) is an antioxidant known to help protect the membrane of mitochondria from attack by free radicals.[71] (Mitochondria are the power plants within each cell that produce the cell's chemical energy. Remember also that coenzymes are required to make enzymes work.) CoQ10 is also found in high concentrations in the heart, liver, and immune system. As we age, our bodies make less of this important antioxidant. Foods that contain CoQ10 include whole grains, nuts, seeds, organ meats, and oily fish (i.e., sardines and salmon).[72] Low levels of CoQ10 are found in patients with cancer, diabetes, heart conditions, muscular dystrophies, Parkinson's disease, and HIV/AIDS.[73] CoQ10 is another great supplement to take!

While there are arguments on both sides of the antioxidant supplement debate, keep in mind that the E-F-G approach uses basic foods as much as possible as well as some of these supplements.

FOOD—A GREAT WAY TO GET YOUR ANTIOXIDANTS AND OTHER PHYTOCHEMICALS

Most berries are rich in antioxidants and are great foods to eat if you can grow them or if they fit into your food budget and are available.

Blueberries and ginger have very high amounts of quercetin. Quercetin is an important phytochemical that is also an antioxidant, has anti-inflammatory actions, and helps regulate and strengthen the blood vessels. It is also available as a supplement. Quercetin is also present in onions, spinach, purple beans,[74] onion skins,[75] apples, apple skins,[76] and many other fruits and vegetables including broccoli, squash, grape seeds, grape skins, green tea, and other natural sources.[77]

Remember Rutin! Rutin is an antioxidant similar to quercetin and is also known to strengthen blood vessels. Rutin can help people who bruise or bleed easily. The richest source of rutin, by far, is buckwheat.[78] Buckwheat is also one of nature's richest grain sources of high quality protein.[79] Rutin is also found in citrus fruit (especially the white pulp), apricots, cherries, blackberries, and apple skins.[80] James Duke recommends rutin for varicose veins. He also recommends eating kasha, a type of cereal made from roasted buckwheat.[81] Strangely, buckwheat is not in the wheat or grain family. It is actually a fruit in the same family as rhubarb. Since buckwheat has no gluten, it is a great food for people with celiac disease. It is easy to make buckwheat pancakes by substituting one-quarter to two-thirds of the flour in pancake recipes.

Other foods high in antioxidants are kale, collards, broccoli, Brussels sprouts, cabbage, carrots, cauliflower, garlic, onions, spinach, tomatoes,[82] asparagus, grapefruit, oranges, avocadoes, peaches, watermelon, potatoes, purslane,[83] chili peppers, green and colored bell peppers, parsley, artichokes, and many others. Remember to include a rainbow of fruits and vegetables in your diet as much as possible.

Kale again! Kale ranks second in antioxidant potency out of 32 vegetables studied, behind chili peppers. Kale has approximately 65% of the total antioxidant potency of ginger.[84] The lush green leaves of kale and collards can be eaten as is or used in a salad. These green plants grow quickly and are ready to eat just several weeks after planting—much sooner than most other vegetables. They continually produce leaves all summer long, throughout the fall season, and into winter. Kale and collards, if left in the ground through the winter, should come back to life for a second season.

Olive oil and flaxseeds also have antioxidant actions.[85]

(Remember from chapter 13 that Dr. Budwig wrote about electron clouds in flaxseeds). This is yet another advantage of the E-F-G approach.

Fruits, vegetables, and whole grains have hundreds of phytochemicals, many of which complement each other in our bodies in a complex network of interactions that may never be completely understood. Much recent research is focused on the phytochemicals in berries, garlic, and the *Brassica* vegetables (broccoli, collards, kale, cauliflower, and cabbage) because of their anticancer actions and many other benefits.

REFERENCES FOR CHAPTER 17

1a.   Valko M, Rhodes CJ, Moncol J, Izakovic M, Mazur M. "Free radicals, metals and antioxidants in oxidative stress-induced cancer." *Chem Biol Interact.* 2006 Mar 10;160(1):1-40. Epub 2006 Jan 23.

1b.   Henrotin Y, Kurz B, Aigner T. "Oxygen and reactive oxygen species in cartilage degradation: friends or foes?" *Osteoarthritis Cartilage.* 2005 Aug;13(8):643-54.

1c.   Bonnefoy M, Drai J, Kostka T. "[Antioxidants to slow aging, facts and perspectives]" [Article in French]. *Presse Med.* 2002 Jul 27;31(25):1174-84.

1d.   Droge W. "Free radicals in the physiological control of cell function." *Physiol Rev.* 2002 Jan;82(1):47-95.

1e.   Conner EM, Grisham MB. "Inflammation, free radicals, and antioxidants." *Nutrition.* 1996 Apr;12(4):274-7.

1f.   Winrow VR, Winyard PG, Morris CJ, Blake DR. "Free radicals in inflammation: second messengers and mediators of tissue destruction." *Br Med Bull.* 1993 Jul;49(3):506-22.

2a.   Chen K, Kazachkov M, Yu PH. "Effect of aldehydes derived from oxidative deamination and oxidative stress on beta-amyloid aggregation; pathological implications to Alzheimer's disease." *J Neural Transm.* 2007 Jun;114(6):835-9. Epub 2007 Mar 31.

2b.   Poon HF, Calabrese V, Scapagnini G, Butterfield DA. "Free radicals and brain aging." *Clin Geriatr Med.* 2004 May;20(2):329-59.

2c.   Bonnefoy M, Drai J, Kostka T. "[Antioxidants to slow aging, facts and perspectives]." [Article in French]. *Presse Med.* 2002 Jul 27;31(25):1174-84.

2d.   Maeda H, Akaike T. "Nitric oxide and oxygen radicals in infection, inflammation, and cancer." *Biochemistry (Mosc).* 1998 Jul;63(7):854-65.

2e. Halliwell B. "Reactive oxygen species and the central nervous system." *J Neurochem.* 1992 Nov;59(5):1609-23.

3. Poon HF, Calabrese V, Scapagnini G, Butterfield DA. "Free radicals and brain aging." *Clin Geriatr Med.* 2004 May20(2):329-59.

4. Winrow VR, Winyard PG, Morris CJ, Blake DR. "Free radicals in inflammation: second messengers and mediators of tissue destruction." *Br Med Bull.* 1993 Jul;49(3):506-22.

5a. Filipcik P, Cente M, Ferencik M, Hulin I, Novak M. "The role of oxidative stress in the pathogenesis of Alzheimer's disease." *Bratisl Lek Listy.* 2006;107(9-10):384-94.

5b. Poon HF, Calabrese V, Scapagnini G, Butterfield DA. "Free radicals and brain aging." *Clin Geriatr Med.* 2004 May20(2):329-59.

5c. Harman D. "The free radical theory of aging." *Antioxid Redox Signal.* 2003 Oct;5(5):557-61.

5d. Bonnefoy M, Drai J, Kostka T. "[Antioxidants to slow aging, facts and perspectives]." *Presse Med.* 2002 Jul 27;31(25):1174-84.

5e. Moskovitz J, Yim MB, Chock PB. "Free radicals and disease." *Arch Biochem Biophys.* 2002 Jan 15;397(2):354-9.

5f. Droge W. "Free radicals in the physiological control of cell function." *Physiol Rev.* 2002 Jan;82(1):47-95.

5g. Wei YH, Ma YS, Lee HC, Lee CF, Lu CY. "Mitochondrial theory of aging matures-roles of mtDNA mutation and oxidative stress in human aging." *Zhonghua Yi Xue Za Zhi (Taipei),* 2001 May;64(5):259-70.

5h. Knight JA. " The biochemistry of aging." *Adv Clin Chem.* 2000;35:1-62.

5i. Butterfield DA, Howard B, Yatin S, Koppal T, Drake J, Hensley K, Aksenov M, Aksenova M, Subramaniam R, Varadarajan S, Harris-White ME, Pedigo NW Jr, Carney JM. "Elevated oxidative stress in models of normal brain aging and Alzheimer's disease." *Life Sci.* 1999;65(18-19):1883-92.

5j. Beckman KB, Ames BN. "The free radical theory of aging matures." *Physiol Rev.* 1998 Apr;78(2):547-81.

5k. Harman D. "Free radical theory of aging." *Mutat Res.* 1992 Sep;275(3-6):257-66.

5l. Harman D. "Aging: a theory based on free radical and radiation chemistry." *J Gerontol.* 1956 Jul;11(3):298-300.

6. Alisa Zapp Machalek. "UV Skin Damage in a Different Light" Embargoed by Journal, Monday, August 31, 1998. Web site: United States National Institutes of Health. Accessed 10/10/2009. <http://www.nih.gov/news/pr/aug98/nigms-31.htm>.

7a. Hadjigogos K. "The role of free radicals in the pathogenesis of rheumatoid arthritis." *Panminerva Med.* 2003 Mar;45(1):7-13.

7b. Henrotin Y, Deby-Dupont G, Deby C, Franchimont P, Emerit I. "Active oxygen species, articular inflammation and cartilage damage." *EXS.* 1992;62:308-22.

8.   Okada F. "Inflammation and free radicals in tumor development and progres-
        sion." *Redox Rep.* 2002;7(6):357-68.

9a.   Houston MC. "The role of mercury and cadmium heavy metals in vascular
        disease, hypertension, coronary heart disease, and myocardial infarction." *Altern
        Ther Health Med.* 2007 Mar-Apr;13(2):S128-33.

9b.   Jie XL, Jin GW, Cheng JP, Wang WH, Lu J, Qu LY. "Consumption of mercury-
        contaminated rice induces oxidative stress and free radical aggravation in rats."
        Biomed Environ Sci. 2007 Feb;20(1):84-9.

9c.   Valko M, Morris H, Cronin MT. "Metals, toxicity and oxidative stress." *Curr
        Med Chem.* 2005;12(10):1161-208.

10.   Järup L. "Hazards of heavy metal contamination." *Br Med Bull.*
        2003;68:167-82.

11.   Bonnefoy M, Drai J, Kostka T. "[Antioxidants to slow aging, facts and perspec-
        tives]." [Article in French]. *Presse Med.* 2002 Jul 27;31(25):1174-84.

12.   Ahmed RS, Seth V, Pasha ST, Banerjee BD. "Influence of dietary ginger
        (Zingiber officinale Rosc) on oxidative stress induced by malathion in rats." *Food
        Chem Toxicol.* 2000 May;38(5):443-50.

13.   Maeda H, Akaike T. "Nitric oxide and oxygen radicals in infection, inflamma-
        tion, and cancer." *Biochemistry (Mosc).* 1998 Jul;63(7):854-65.

14.   Vincent AM, Russell JW, Low P, Feldman EL. "Oxidative stress in the pathogen-
        esis of diabetic neuropathy." *Endocr Rev.* 2004 Aug;25(4):612-28.

15a.   Chen K, Kazachkov M, Yu PH. "Effect of aldehydes derived from oxidative
        deamination and oxidative stress on beta-amyloid aggregation: pathological
        implications to Alzheimer's disease." *J Neural Transm.* 2007 Jun;114(6):835-9.
        Epub 2007 Mar 1.

15b.   Reynolds A, Laurie C, Mosley RL, Gendelman HE. "Oxidative stress
        and the pathogenesis of neurodegenerative disorders." Int Rev Neuroviol.
        2007;82:297-325.

15c.   Filipcik P, Cente M, Ferencik M, Hulin I, Novak M. "The role of oxida-
        tive stress in the pathogenesis of Alzheimer's disease." *Bratisl Lek Listy.*
        2006;107(9-10):384-94.

15d.   Perluigi M, Joshi G, Sultana R, Calabrese V, De Marco C, Coccia R, Butterfield
        DA. "Invivo protection by the xanthate tricyclodecan-9-yl-xanthogenate
        against amyloid beta-peptide (1-42)-induced oxidative stress." Neuroscience.
        2006;138(4):1161-70. Epug 2006 Jan 19.

15e.   Kim H, Park BS, Lee KG, Choi CY, Jang SS, Kim YH, Lee SE. "Effects of
        naturally occurring compounds on fibril formation and oxidative stress of beta-
        amyloid." *J Agric Food Chem.* 2005 Nov 2;53(22):8537-41.

15f.   Aslan M, Ozben T. "Reactive oxygen and nitrogen species in Alzheimer's
        disease." *Curr Alzheimer Res.* 2004 May;1(2):111-9.

15g.   Butterfield DA, Howard B, Yatin S, Koppal T, Drake J, Hensley K, Aksenov M,
        Aksenova M, Subramaniam R, Varadarajan S, Harris-White ME, Pedigo NW

Jr, Carney JM. "Elevated oxidative stress in models of normal brain aging and Alzheimer's disease." *Life Sci.* 1999;65(18-19):1883-92.

15h.   Markesbery WR. "Oxidative stress in Alzheimer's disease." *Free Radic Biol Med.* 1997;23(1):134-47.

15i.   Smith MA, Pery G. "Free radical damage, iron, and Alzheimer's disease." *J Neurol Sci.* 1995 Dec;134 Suppl:92-4.

16a.   Azu Seven, Savas Güzel, Mahmure Aslan and Veda Hamuryudan. "Lipid, protein, DNA oxidation and antioxidant status in rheumatoid arthritis." *Clinical Biochemisty.* Volume 41, Issues 7-8, May 2008, Pages 538-543.

16b.   Cuzzocrea S. "Role of nitric oxide and reactive oxygen species in arthritis." *Curr Pharm Des.* 2006;12(27):3551-70.

16c.   Henrotin Y, Kurz B, Aigner T. "Oxygen and reactive oxygen species in cartilage degradation: friends or foes?" *Osteoarthritis Cartilage.* 2005 Aug;13(8):643-54.

16d.   Hajigogos K. "The role of free radicals in the pathogenesis of rheumatoid arthritis." *Panminerva Med.* 2003 Mar;45(1):7-13.

16e.   Droge W. "Free radicals in the physiological control of cell function." *Physiol Rev.* 2002 Jan;82(1):47-95.

16f.   Jasin HE. "Oxidative modification of inflammatory synovial fluid immuno-globulin G." *Inflammation.* 1993 Apr;17(2):167-81.

16g.   Henrotin Y, Deby-Dupont G, Deby C, Franchimont P, Emerit I. "Active oxygen species, articular inflammation and cartilage damage." *EXS.* 1992;62:308-22.

17a.   Rosenblat M, Coleman R, Aviram M. "Increased macrophage glutathione content reduces cell-mediated oxidation of LDL and atherosclerosis in apolipo-protein E-deficient mice." *Atherosclerosis.* 2002 Jul;163(1):17-28.

17b.   Droge W. "Free radicals in the physiological control of cell function." *Physiol Rev.* 2002 Jan;82(1):47-95.

17c.   Aviram M. "Review of human studies on oxidative damage and antioxidant protection related to cardiovascular diseases." *Free Radic Res.* 2000 Nov;33 Suppl:S85-97.

17d.   Dargel R. "Liquid peroxidation-a common pathogenic mechanism?" *Exp Toxicol Pathol.* 1992 Aug;44(4):169-81.

18a.   Yung LM, Leung FP, Yao X, Chen ZY, Huang Y. "Reactive oxygen species in vascular wall." *Cardiovasc Hematol Disord Drug Targets.* 2006 Mar;6(1):1-19.

18b.   Vincent AM, Russell JW, Low P, Feldman EL. "Oxidative stress in the pathogen-esis of diabetic neuropathy." *Endocr Rev.* 2004 Aug;25(4):612-28.

18c.   Maritim AC, Sanders RA, Watkins JB 3rd. "Effects of alpha-lipoic acid on biomarkers of oxidative stress in streptozotocin-induced diabetic rats." *J Nutr Biochem.* 2003 May;14(5):288-94.

18d.   Yorek MA. "The role of oxidative stress in diabetic vascular and neural disease." *Free Radic Res.* 2003 May;37(5):471-80.

18e.   Droge W. "Free radicals in the physiological control of cell function." *Physiol Rev.* 2002 Jan;82(1):47-95.

18f.   Rosen P, Nawroth PP, King G, Moller W, Tritschier HJ, Packer L. "The role of
        oxidative stress in the onset and progression of diabetes and its complications: a
        summary of a Congress Series sponsored by UNESCO_MCBN, the American
        Diabetes Association and the German Diabetes Society." *Diabetes Metab Res Rev.*
        2001 May-Jun;17(3):189-212.

19.   Bulger EM, Helton WS. "Nutrient antioxidants in gastrointestinal diseases."
        Gastroenterol Clin North Am. 1998 Jun;27(2):403-19.

20a.   Smith KJ, Kapoor R, Felts PA. "Demyelination the role of reactive oxygen and
        nitrogen species." *Brain Pathol.* 1999 Jan;9(1):69-92.

20b.   Levine SM. "The role of reactive oxygen species in the pathogenesis of multiple
        sclerosis." *Med Hypothesis.* 1992 Nov;39(3):271-4.

21a.   Tadao M, Yuji O. "[Role of free radicals in the development of severe acute
        pancreatitis]." *Nippon Rinsho.* 2004 Nov;62(11):2015-20.

21b.   Braganza JM. "Pancreatic disease: a casualty of hepatic "detoxification"?" *Lancet.*
        1983 Oct 29;2(8357):1000-3.

21c.   Braganza JM, Wickens DG, Cawood P, Dormandy TL. "Lipid-peroxidation
        (free-radical-oxidation) products in bile from patients with pancreatic disease."
        Lancet. 1983 Aug 13;2(8346):375-9.

22a.   Reynolds A, Laurie C, Mosley RL, Gendelman HE. "Oxidative stress
        and the pathogenesis of neurodegenerative disorders." Int Rev Neuroviol.
        2007;82:297-325.

22b.   Halliwell B. "Reactive oxygen species and the central nervous system." *J
        Neurochem.* 1992 Nov;59(5):1609-23.

23.   Fendri C, Mechri A, Khiari G, Othman A, Kerkeni Am Gaha L. "[Oxidative
        stress involvement in schizophrenia pathophysiology: a review]." *Encephale.*
        2006 Mar-Apr;32(2 Pt 1):244-52.

24.   Yorek MA. "The role of oxidative stress in diabetic vascular and neural disease."
        Free Radic Res. 2003 May;37(5):471-80.

25a.   Valko M, Rhodes CJ, Moncol J, Izakovic M, Mazur. "Free radicals, metals and
        antioxidants in oxidative stress-induced cancer." *Chem Biol Interact.* 2006 Mar
        10;160(1):1-40. Epub 2006 Jan 23.

25b.   Okada F. "Inflammation and free radicals in tumor development and progres-
        sion." *Redox Rep.* 2002;7(6):357-68.

25c.   Droge W. "Free radicals in the physiological control of cell function." *Physiol
        Rev.* 2002 Jan;82(1):47-95.

25d.   Maeda H, Akaike T. "Nitric oxide and oxygen radicals in infection, inflamma-
        tion, and cancer." *Biochemistry (Mosc).* 1998 Jul;63(7):854-65.

25e.   Bulger EM, Helton WS. "Nutrient antioxidants in gastrointestinal diseases."
        Gastroenterol Clin North Am. 1998 Jun;27(2):403-19.

25f.   Dargel R. "Liquid peroxidation-a common pathogenic mechanism?" *Exp Toxicol
        Pathol.* 1992 Aug;44(4):169-81.

26a. Droge W. "Free radicals in the physiological control of cell function." *Physiol Rev.* 2002 Jan;82(1):47-95.

26b. Bulger EM, Helton WS. "Nutrient antioxidants in gastrointestinal diseases." *Gastroenterol Clin North Am.* 1998 Jun;27(2):403-19.

26c. Rao NA. "Role of oxygen free radicals in retinal damage associated with uveitis." *Trans Am Ophthalmol Soc.* 1990; 88: 797-850.

27a. Rojas A, Figueroa H, Morales MA, Re L. "Facing up the ROS labyrinth--Where to go?" *Curr Vasc Pharmacol.* 2006 Jul;4(3):277-89.

27b. Yung LM, Leung FP, Yao X, Chen ZY, Huang Y. "Reactive oxygen species in vascular wall." *Cardiovasc Hematol Disord Drug Targets.* 2006 Mar;6(1):1-19.

27c. Droge W. "Free radicals in the physiological control of cell function." *Physiol Rev.* 2002 Jan;82(1):47-95.

28a. Henrotin Y, Kurz B. "Antioxidant to treat osteoarthritis: dream or reality?" *Curr Drug Targets.* 2007 Feb;8(2):347-57.

28b. Bonnefoy M, Drai J, Kostka T. "[Antioxidants to slow aging, facts and perspectives]." [Article in French]. *Presse Med.* 2002 Jul 27;31(25):1174-84.

28c. Halvorsen BL, Holte K, Myhrstad MC, Barikmo I, Hvattum E, Remberg SF, Wold AB, Haffner K, Baugerod H, Andersen LF, Moskaug Ø, Jacobs DR, Blomhoff R. "A Systematic Screening of Total Antioxidants in Dietary Plants." *J Nutr.* 2002 Mar;132(3):461-71.

28d. Halliwell B. "Reactive oxygen species and the central nervous system." *J Neurochem.* 1992 Nov;59(5):1609-23.

29a. Masuda Y, Kikuzaki H, Hisamoto M, Nakatani N. "Antioxidant properties of gingerol related compounds from ginger." *Biofactors.* 2004;21(1-4):293-6.

29b. Halliwell B. "Reactive oxygen species and the central nervous system." *J Neurochem.* 1992 Nov;59(5):1609-23.

30. Masuda Y, Kikuzaki H, Hisamoto M, Nakatani N. "Antioxidant properties of gingerol related compounds from ginger." *Biofactors.* 2004;21(1-4):293-6.

31a. Patrick-Iwuanyanwu KC, Wegwu MO, Ayalogu EO. "Prevention of CC14-induced liver damage by ginger, garlic and vitamin E." *Pak J Biol Sci.* 2007 Feb 15;10(4):617-21.

31b. Ajith TA, Nivitha V, Usha S. "Zingiber officinale Roscoe alone and in combination with a-tocopherol protect the kidney against cisplatin-induced acute renal failure." *Food and chemical toxicology.* 2007, Vol. 45, pp. 921-927.

31c. Haskar A, Sharma A, Chawla R, Kumar R, Arora R, Singh S, Prasad J, Gupta M, Tripathi RP, Arora MP, Islam F, Sharma RK. "Zingiber officinale exhibits behavioral radioprotection against radiation-induced CTA in a gender-specific manner." *Pharmacol Biochem Behav.* 2006 Jun;84(2):179-88. Epub 2006 Jun 21.

31d. Manju V, Nalini N. "Chemopreventive efficacy of ginger, a naturally occurring anticarcinogen during initiation, post-initiation stages of 1,2 dimethylhydrazine-induced colon cancer." *Clin Chim Acta.* 2005 Aug;358(1-2):60-7.

31e. Kuo PC, Damu AG, Cherng CY, Jeng JF, Teng CMMM, Lee EJ, Wu TS. "Isolation of a natural antioxidant, dehydrozingerone from Zingiber officinale and synthesis of its analogues for recognition of effective antioxidant and antityrosinase agents." *Arch Pharm Res.* 2005 May;28(5):518-28.

31f. Jagetia G, Baliga M, Venkatesh P. "Ginger (Zingiber officinale Rosc.), a dietary supplement, protects mice against radiation-induced lethality: mechanism of action." *Cancer Biother Radiopharm.* 2004 Aug;19(4):422-35.

31g. Masuda Y, Kikuzaki H, Hisamoto M, Nakatani N. "Antioxidant properties of gingerol related compounds from ginger." *Biofactors.* 2004;21(1-4):293-6.

31h. Lako J, Trenerry C, Wahlqvist ML, Wattanapenpaiboon N, Sotheesqaran S, Premier R. "Total antioxidant capacity and selected flavonols and carotenoids of some Australian and Fijian fruits and vegetables." *Asia Pac J Clin Nutr.* 2004;13(Suppl):S127.

31i. Wang CC, Chen LG, Lee LT, Yang LL. "Effects of 6-gingerol, an antioxidant from ginger, on inducing apoptosis in human leukemic HL-60 cells." *In Vivo.* 2003 Nov-Dec;17(6):641-5.

31j. Ippoushi K, Azuma K, Ito H, Higashio H. "[6]-Gingerol inhibits nitric oxide synthesis in activated J774.1 mouse macrophages and prevents peroxynitrite-induced oxidation and nitration reactions." *Life Sci.* 2003 Nov 14;73(26):3427-37.

31k. Lu P, Lai BS, Liang P, Chen ZT, Shun SQ. "[Antioxidation activity and protective effection of ginger oil on DNA damage in vitro]." *Zhongguo Zhong Yao Za Zhi.* 2003 Sep;28(9):873-5.

31l. Baglia MS, Jagetia GC, Rao SK, Babu K. "Evaluation of nitric oxide scavenging activity of certain spices in vitro: a preliminary study." *Nahrung.* 2003 Aug;47(4):261-4.

31m. Leal PF, Braga ME, Sato DN, Carvalho JE, Marques MO, Meireles MA. "Functional properties of spice extracts obtained via supercritical fluid extraction." *J Agric Food Chem.* 2003 Apr 23;51(9):2520-5.

31n. Odunola OA. "Comparative effects of some local food condiments on sodium arsenite-induced clastogenicity." *Afr J Med Sci.* 2003 Mar;32(1):75-80.

31o. Liu N, Hio G, Zhang L, Zhang X. "[Effect of Zingiber Officinale Rosc on lipid peroxidation in hyperlipidemia rats]." *Wei Sheng Yan Jiu.* 2003 Jan;32(1):22-3.

31p. Topic B, Tani E, Tsiakitzis K, Kourounakis PN, Dere E, Hasenohrl RU, Hacker R, Mattern CM, Huston JP. "Enhanced maze performance and reduced oxidative stress by combined extracts of zingiber officinale and ginkgo biloba in the aged rat." *Neurobiol Aging.* 2002 Jan-Feb;23(1):135-43.

31q. Ahmed RS, Seth V, Banerjee BD. "Influence of dietary ginger (Zingiber officinale Rosc) on antioxidant defense system in rat: comparison with ascorbic acid." *Indian J Exp Biol.* 2000 Jun;38(6):604-6.

31r. Ahmed RS, Seth V, Pasha ST, Banerjee BD. "Influence of dietary ginger

(Zingiber officinale Rosc) on oxidative stress induced by malathion in rats." *Food Chem Toxicol.* 2000 May;38(5):443-50.

31s.   Khanom F, Kayahara H, Tadasa K. "Superoxide-scavenging and prolyl endopeptidase inhibitory activities of Bangladeshi indigenous medicinal plants." *Biosci Biotechnol Biochem.* 2000 Apr;64(4):837-40.

31t.   Sekiwa Y, Kubota K, Kobayashi A. "Isolation of novel glucosides related to gingerdiol from ginger and their antioxidative activities." *J Agric Food Chem.* 2000 Feb;48(2):373-7.

31u.   Nakatani N. "Phenolic antioxidants from herbs and spices." *Biofactors.* 2000;13(1-4):141-6.

31v.   Surh YJ, Park KK, Chun KS, Lee LJ, Lee E, Lee SS. "Anti-tumor-promoting activities of selected pungent phenolic substances present in ginger." *J Environ Pathol Toxicol Oncol.* 1999;18(2):131-9.

31w.   Craig W, Beck L. "Phytochemicals: Health Protective Effects." *Can J Diet Pract Res.* 1999 Summer;60(2):78-840.

31x.   Guo P, Su J, Su S, Wang K. "[Inhibition of hydrogen peroxide production on chondrocytes induced by fulvic acid by ginger volatile oil]." *Zhongguo Zhong Yao Za Ahi.* 1997 Sep;22(9):559-61.

31y.   Zhou Y, Xu R. "[Antioxidative effect of Chinese drugs]." *Zhongguo Zhong Yao Za Ahi.* 1992 Jun;17(6):368-9, 373 inside back cover.

32.   Halvorsen BL, Holte K, Myhrstad MC, Barikmo I, Hvattum E, Remberg SF, Wold AB, Haffner K, Baugerod H, Andersen LF, Moskaug O, Jacobs DR, Blomhoff R. "A Systematic Screening of Total Antioxidants in Dietary Plants." *J Nutr.* 2002 Mar;132(3):461-71.

33.   Leal PF, Braga ME, Sato DN, Carvalho JE, Marques MO, Meireles MA. "Functional properties of spice extracts obtained via supercritical fluid extraction." *J Agric Food Chem.* 2003 Apr 23;51(9):2520-5.

34a.   Blomhoff R. "[Antioxidants and oxidative stress]." [Article in Norwegian]. *Tidsskr Nor Laegeforen.* 2004 Jun 17;124(12):1643-5.

34b.   Dragland S, Senoo H, Wake K, Holte K, Blomhoff R. "Several culinary and medicinal herbs are important sources of dietary antioxidants." *J Nutr.* 2003 May;133(5):1286-90.

35.   Halvorsen BL, Carlsen MH, Phillips KM, Bohn SK, Holte K, Jacobs DR, Blomhoff R. "Content of redox-active compounds (ie, antioxidants) in foods consumed in the United States." *Am J Clin Nutr.* 2006 Jul;84(1):95-135.

36a.   Manju V, Nalini N. "Chemopreventive efficacy of ginger, a naturally occurring anticarcinogen during initiation, post-initiation stages of 1,2 dimethylhydrazine-induced colon cancer." *Clin Chim Acta.* 2005 Aug;358(1-2):60-7.

36b.   Wang CC, Chen LG, Lee LT, Yang LL. "Effects of 6-gingerol, an antioxidant from ginger, on inducing apoptosis in human leukemic HL-60 cells." *In Vivo.* 2003 Nov-Dec;17(6):641-5.

36c.   Surh YJ, Park KK, Chun KS, Lee LJ, Lee E, Lee SS. "Anti-tumor-promoting activities of selected pungent phenolic substances present in ginger." *J Environ Pathol Toxicol Oncol.* 1999;18(2):131-9.

37a. Okada F. Inflammation and free radicals in tumor development and progression." *Redox Rep.* 2002;7(6):357-68.

37b. Winrow VR, Winyard PG, Morris CJ, Blake DR. "Free radicals in inflammation: second messengers and mediators of tissue destruction." *Br Med Bull.* 1993 Jul;49(3):506-22.

38a. Cuzzocrea S. "Role of nitric oxide and reactive oxygen species in arthritis." *Curr Pharm Des.* 2006;12(27):3551-70.

38b. Conner EM, Grisham MB. "Inflammation, free radicals, and antioxidants." *Nutrition.* 1996 Apr;12(4):274-7.

38c. Winrow VR, Winyard PG, Morris CJ, Blake DR. "Free radicals in inflammation: second messengers and mediators of tissue destruction." *Br Med Bull.* 1993 Jul;49(3):506-22.

38d. Jasin HE. "Oxidative modification of inflammatory synovial fluid immunoglobulin G." *Inflammation.* 1993 Apr;17(2):167-81.

39. Valko M, Morris H, Cronin MT. "Metals, toxicity and oxidative stress." *Curr Med Chem.* 2005;12(10):1161-208.

40a. Machartová V, Racek J, Kohout J, Senft B, Trefil L. "[Effect of antioxidant therapy on indicators of free radical activity in workers at risk of lead exposure]." *Vnitr Lek.* 2000 Aug;46(8):444-6.

40b. Chaurasia SS, Gupta P, Kar A, Maiti PK. "Free radical mediated membrane perturbation and inhibition of type-I iodothyronine 5'-monodeiodinase activity by lead and cadmium in rat liver homogenate." *Biochem Mol Biol Int.* 1996 Jul;39(4):765-70.

41. Halliwell B. "Reactive oxygen species and the central nervous system." *J Neurochem.* 1992 Nov;59(5):1609-23.

42. Dr. T.E. Gabriel. "Heavy Metal Detoxification in the treatment of autism and the use of metyhlcobalamin." Accessed 7/23/2007. <http://www.chelation-ireland.com/autism.ppt>.

43a. Tadao M, Yuji O. "[Role of free radicals in the development of severe acute pancreatitis]" *Nippon Rinsho.* 2004 Nov;62(11):2015-20.

43b. Bonnefoy M, Drai J, Kostka T. "[Antioxidants to slow aging, facts and perspectives]." *Presse Med.* 2002 Jul 27;31(25):1174-84.

43c. Fujita T. "[Formation and removal of reactive oxygen species, lipid peroxides and free radicals, and heir biological effects]." *Yakygaku Zasshi.* 2002 Mar;122(3):203-18.

43d. Cheeseman KH. "Mechanisms and effects of lipid peroxidation." *Mol Aspects Med.* 1993;14(3):191-7.

43e. Dargel R. "Liquid peroxidation-a common pathogenic mechanism?" *Exp Toxicol Pathol.* 1992 Aug;44(4):169-81.

44a. Jourd'heuil D, Meddings JB. "Oxidative and drug-induced alterations in brush border membrane hemileaflet fluidity, functional consequences for glucose transport." *Biochem Biophys Acta*. 2001 Feb 9;1510(1-2):342-53.

44b.   Jourd'heuil D, Vaananen P, Meddings JB. "Lipid peroxidation of the brush-border membrane: membrane physical properties and glucose transport." *Am J Physiol*. 1993 Jun;264(6 Pt 1):G1009-15.

44c.   Ohyashiki T, Ohtsuka T, Mohri T. "A change in the lipid fluidity of the porcine intestinal brush-border membranes by lipid peroxidation. Studies using pyrene and fluorescent stearic acid derivatives." *Biochim Biophys Acta*. 1986 Oct 9;861(2):311-8.

45a.   Jourd'heuil D, Meddings JB. "Oxidative and drug-induced alterations in brush border membrane hemileaflet fluidity, functional consequences for glucose transport." *Biochem Biophys Acta*. 2001 Feb 9;1510(1-2):342-53.

45b.   Jourd'heuil D, Vaananen P, Meddings JB. "Lipid peroxidation of the brush-border membrane: membrane physical properties and glucose transport." *Am J Physiol*. 1993 Jun;264(6 Pt 1):G1009-15.

45c.   Ohyashiki T, Ohtsuka T, Mohri T. "A change in the lipid fluidity of the porcine intestinal brush-border membranes by lipid peroxidation. Studies using pyrene and fluorescent stearic acid derivatives." *Biochem Biophys Acta*. 1986 Oct p;861(2):311-8.

46.   Miller MJS, Angeles FM, Reuter BK, Bobrowski P, Sandoval M. "Dietary antioxidants protect gut epithelial cells from oxidant-induced apoptosis." *BMC Complement Altern Med*. 2001;1:11. Published online 2001 December 10.

47.   Jain SK, Mohandas N, Clark MR, Shohet SB. "The effect of malonyldialde-hyde, a product of lipid peroxidation on the deformability, dehydration and 51Cr-survival of erythrocytes." *Br J Haematol*. 1983 Feb;53(2):247-55.

48.   Moriguchi T, Takasugi N, Itakura Y. "The Effects of Aged Garlic Extract on Lipid Peroxidation and the Deformability of Erythrocytes." *J Nutr*. 2001;131:1016S-1019S.

49a.   Valko M, Rhodes CJ, Moncol J, Izakovic M, Mazur M. "Free radicals, metals and antioxidants in oxidative stress-induced cancer." *Chem Biol Interact*. 2006 Mar 10;160(1):1-40. Epub 2006 Jan 23.

49b.   Valko M, Morris H, Cronin MT. "Metals, toxicity and oxidative stress." *Curr Med Chem*. 2005;12(10):1161-208.

49c.   Wei YH, Ma YS, Lee HC, Lee CF, Lu CY. "Mitochondrial theory of aging matures-roles of mtDNA mutation and oxidative stress in human aging." *Zhonghua Yi Xue Za Zhi (Taipei)*, 2001 May;64(5):259-70.

49d.   Hruszkewycz AM. "Evidence for mitochondrial DNA damage by lipid peroxida-tion." *Biochem Biophys Res Commun*. 1988 May 31;153(1):191-7.

50.   Thompson HJ. "DNA Oxidation Products, Antioxidant Status, and Cancer Prevention." *J. Nutr*. 134: 3186S-3187S 2004.

51.   Poon HF, Calabrese V, Scapagnini G, Butterfield DA. "Free radicals and brain aging." *Clin Geriatr Med*. 2004 May20(2):329-59.

52a.   Lu P, Lai BS, Liang P, Chen ZT, Shun SQ. "[Antioxidation activity and protec-
        tive effection of ginger oil on DNA damage in vitro]." *Zhongguo Zhong Yao Za
        Zhi.* 2003 Sep;28(9):873-5.

52b.   Mukhopadhyay MJ, Mukherjee A. "Clastogenic effect of ginger rhizome in
        mice." *Phytother Res.* 2000 Nov;14(7):555-7.

53.   Fuhrman B, Rosenblat M, Hayek T, Coleman R, Aviram. "Ginger extract
        consumption reduces cholesterol, inhibits LDL oxidation and attenuates devel-
        opment of atherosclerosis in atherosclerotic, apolipoprotein E-deficient mice." *J
        Nutr.* 2000 May;130(5):1124-31.

54.   Jagetia G, Baliga M, Venkatesh P. "Ginger (Zingiber officinale Rosc.), a dietary
        supplement, protects mice against radiation-induced lethality: mechanism of
        action." *Cancer Biother Radiopharm.* 2004 Aug;19(4):422-35.

55a.   Haskar A, Sharma A, Chawla R, Kumar R, Arora R, Singh S, Prasad J, Gupta
        M, Tripathi RP, Arora MP, Islam F, Sharma RK. "Zingiber officinale exhibits
        behavioral radioprotection against radiation-induced CTA in a gender-specific
        manner." *Pharmacol Biochem Behav.* 2006 Jun;84(2):179-88. Epub 2006 Jun
        21.

55b.   Jagetia G, Baliga M, Venkatesh P. "Ginger (Zingiber officinale Rosc.), a dietary
        supplement, protects mice against radiation-induced lethality: mechanism of
        action." *Cancer Biother Radiopharm.* 2004 Aug;19(4):422-35.

56.   Odunola OA. "Comparative effects of some local food condiments on sodium
        arsenite-induced clastogenicity." *Afr J Med Sci.* 2003 Mar;32(1):75-80.

57.   Ahmed RS, Seth V, Pasha ST, Banerjee BD. "Influence of dietary ginger
        (Zingiber officinale Rosc) on oxidative stress induced by malathion in rats." *Food
        Chem Toxicol.* 2000 May;38(5):443-50.

58.   Ippoushi K, Azuma K, Ito H, Horie H, Higashio H. "[6]-Gingerol inhibits
        nitric oxide synthesis in activated J774.1 mouse macrophages and prevents
        peroxynitrite-induced oxidation and nitration reactions." Life Sci. 2003 Nov
        14;73(26):3427-37.

59.   Ahmed RS, Seth V, Banerjee BD. "Influence of dietary ginger (Zingiber offici-
        nale Rosc) on antioxidant defense system in rat: comparison with ascorbic acid."
        Indian J Exp Biol. 2000 Jun;38(6):604-6.

60.   Roizen MF, Oz MC. "Dangerous Medical Myths, How to protect yourself-and
        those you love." *BottomLine health.* Vol. 19 No. 9, Sept. 2005.

61.   Patrick-Iwuanyanwu KC, Wegwu MO, Ayalogu EO. "Prevention of CC14-
        induced liver damage by ginger, garlic and vitamin E." *Pak J Biol Sci.* 2007 Feb
        15;10(4):617-21.

62a.   Lee IM, Cook NR, Gaziano JM, Gordon D, Ridker PM, Manson JE,
        Hennekens CH, Buring JE. "Vitamin E in the primary prevention of cardiovas-
        cular disease and cancer: the Women's Health Study: a randomized controlled
        trial." *JAMA.* 2005 Jul 6;294(1):56-65.

62b.   Williams KJ, Fisher EA. "Oxidation, lipoproteins, and atherosclerosis: which is wrong, the antioxidants or the theory?" *Curr Opin Clin Nutr Metab Care.* 2005 Mar;8(2):139-46.

62c.　Vivekananthan DP, Penn MS, Sapp SK, Hsu A, Topol EJ. "Use of antioxidant vitamins for the prevention of cardiovascular disease: meta-analysis of randomised trials." *Lancet.* 2003 Jun 14;361(9374):2017-23.

62d.　Blumberg JB. "An update: vitamin E supplementation and heart disease." *Nutr Clin Care.* 2002 Mar-Apr;5(2):50-5.

62e.　Heinecke JW. "Is the emperor wearing clothes? Clinical trials of vitamin E and the LDL oxidation hypothesis." *Arterioscler Thromb Vasc Biol.* 2001 Aug;21(8):1261-4.

62f.　Blumberg JB. "An update: vitamin E supplementation and heart disease." *Nutr Clin Care.* 2002 Mar-Apr;5(2):50-5.

62g.　Upston JM, Kritharides L, Stocker R. "The role of vitamin E in atherosclerosis." *Prog Lipid Res.* 2003 Sep;42(5):405-22.

62h.　Vivekananthan DP, Penn MS, Sapp SK, Hsu A, Topol EJ. "Use of antioxidant vitamins for the prevention of cardiovascular disease: meta-analysis of randomised trials." *Lancet.* 2003 Jun 14;361(9374):2017-23.

63.　Hennekens CH, Buring JE, Manson JE, Stampfer M, Rosner B, Cook NR, Belanger C, LaMotte F, Gaziano JM, Ridker PM, Willett W, Peto R. "Lack of Effect of Long-Term Supplementation with Beta Carotene on the Incidence of Malignant Neoplasms and Cardiovascular Disease." *New Eng J Med.* 1996 May;334(18):1145-9.

64.　Brown BG, Cheung MC, Lee AC, Zhao X-Q, Chait A. "Antioxidant Vitamins and Lipid Therapy." *Arteriosclerosis, Thrombosis, and Vascular Biology.* 2002;22:1535

65.　Randolph Michael Howes M.D., PhD. "Antioxidant Vitamins A, C & E; Death in Small Doses and Legal Liability?" Web site: Philica. Accessed 6/15/2007. <http://www.philica.com/printer_article.php?article_id=9>.

66.　Kline K. "The Promising Future of Vitamin E." University of Texas-Austin. Article published in the *American Institute for Cancer Research NEWSLETTER.* Fall 2004, Issue 85.

67a.　Ryan-Harshman M, Aldoori W. "The relevance of selenium to immunity, cancer, and infectious/inflammatory diseases." Can J Diet Pract Res. 2005 Summer;66(2):98-102.

67b.　Schrauzer G. "Selenium, Your Secret Weapon Against Cancer." BottomLine health. Vol. 19 No. 12 Dec. 2005.

68.　Chunying Chen, Hongwei Yu, Jiujiang Zhao, Bai Li, Liya Qu, Shuiping Liu, Peiqun Zhang, and Zhifang Chai. "The Roles of Serum Selenium and Selenoproteins on Mercury Toxicity in Environmental and Occupational Exposure." *Environmental Health Perspectives.* Vol. 114 No. 2, February 2006.

69.　Duke JA. *The Green Pharmacy.* Rodale Press, Emmaus, Pa.1997, pp.24-25.

70.　Gromadzinska J, Reszka E, Bruzelius K, Wasowicz W, Akesson B. "Selenium and cancer : biomarkers of selenium status and molecular action of selenium supplements." *Eur J Nutr.* 2008 May;47 Suppl 2:29-50.

71. Matthews RT, Yang L, Browne S, et al. "Coenzyme Q10 administration increases brain mitochondrial concentrations and exerts neuroprotective effects." *Proc Natl Acad Sci USA.* 1998 Jul 21; 85(15):8892-7.

72. Cichoke A. *The Complete Book of Enzyme Therapy.* New York:Avery, 1999. p.64.

73. "Coenzyme Q10" Web site: Medline Plus. Accessed 1/21/2009. <http://www.nlm.nih.gov/medlineplus/print/druginfo/natural/patient-coenzymeq10.html>.

74. Lako J, Trenerry C, Wahlqvist ML, Wattanapenpaiboon N, Sotheeswaran S, Premier R. "Total antioxidant capacity and selected flavanols and carotenoids of some Australian and Fijian fruits and vegetables." *Asia Pac J Clin Nutr.* 2004;13(Suppl):S127.

75. James A. Duke, Ph.D. *The Green Pharmacy.* Rodale Press, Emmaus, PA 1997. p.447.

76a. Lee LW, Kim YJ, Kim DO, Lee HJ, Lee CY. "Major phenolics in apple and their contribution to the total antioxidant capacity." *J Agric Food Chem.* 2003 Oct 22;51(22):6516-20.

76b. HW Siegelman. "Quercetin Glycosides of Grimes Golden Apple Skin." Biological Sciences Branch, Agricultural Marketing Service, United States Department of Agriculture, Beltsville, Maryland. September 17, 1954.

77. Cichoke A. *The Complete Book of Enzyme Therapy.* New York:Avery, 1999. p.65.

78. "Rutin". Web site: Phytochemicals. Accessed 1/11/2009. <http://www.phytochemicals.info/phytochemicals/ruin.php>.

79. Salene Yeager and the Editors of Prevention Magazine. *The Doctors Book of Food Remedies.* Rodale Press, Inc. Emmaus, Pa. 1998. pp.94-97.

80. Cichoke A. *The Complete Book of Enzyme Therapy.* New York:Avery, 1999. p.65.

81. Duke JA. *The Green Pharmacy.* Rodale Press, Emmaus, Pa.1997, pp.445-447.

82. Blomhoff R. "Dietary antioxidants and cardiovascular disease." *Curr Opin Lipidol.* 2005 Feb;16(1):47-54.

83. James A. Duke, Ph.D. *The Green Pharmacy.* Rodale Press, Emmaus, PA. 1997. p.60.

84. Halvorsen BL, Holte K, Myhrstad MC, Barikmo I, Hvattum E, Remberg SF, Wold AB, Haffner K, Baugerod H, Andersen LF, Moskaug O, Jacobs DR, Blomhoff R. "A Systematic Screening of Total Antioxidants in Dietary Plants." *J Nutr.* 2002 Mar;132(3):461-71.

85. Kris-Etherton PM, Hecker KD, Bonanome A, Coval SM, Binkoski AE, Hilpert KF, Griel AE, Etherton TD. *Am J Med.* 2002 Dec 30;113 Suppl 9B:71S-88S.

CHAPTER 18

Antibacterial, Antiviral, & Antimicrobial Actions of Ginger, Garlic, & Turmeric

HOW MICROBES CAN AFFECT OUR BRAINS

T is amazing how bacteria, viruses, and other microbes can affect our lives and the lives of those we love—often working in stealth and most times without our knowledge until we realize our mental and physical abilities have been degraded. A whole new world of understanding opens up when we consider that bacteria, viruses, parasites, and other infections can cause behavioral changes and even various forms of mental and physical illnesses.

The November 2006 issue of *Prevention* magazine tells of a healthy 11-year-old boy who suddenly acquired certain obsessive-compulsive behaviors and habits (also called tics), such as repeating phrases 3 or 4 times, taking 4 steps when walking, blinking 4 times, and reading backward every phrase he had just read forward. He also developed several other peculiar habits. Previous to this illness, he had been an ideal son and an honor student, athlete, and musician. His pediatrician's diagnosis: an infection of *Streptococcus* bacteria. Because the boy had contracted strep throat 5 times the previous winter, his health care provider was able to target the infection and begin proper treatment. After 3 rounds of antibiotic treatment, all of the strange behaviors, tics, and language problems disappeared. The article tells of more cases where bacteria, viruses, and other microbes harm mental and physical well-being and in many cases go undiagnosed.[1] *Candida* infections can also cause profound mental and physical problems, as discussed in chapter 14.

It is also known that Lyme disease, a bacterial infection caused by a bite from an infected deer tick, can result in panic attacks, depression, and psychotic symptoms as described by some patients.[2]

After the outbreak of the West Nile virus in New York City in 1999, patients reported light-headedness, loss of concentration, confusion,[3] and depression. West Nile virus is transmitted by infected mosquitoes and is reported to be the most common cause of encephalitis—inflammation of the brain—and resulting mood disorders. One study estimates that more than 1 million people in the United States may have been infected with this virus.[5]

Infections from bacteria, viruses, and parasites can cause chronic inflammation in our bodies, which can damage tissues and lead to other illnesses, including cancer.[6]

Did You Know ...

- One of the ways to study inflammation in lab animals is by inducing a bacterial infection.[7]
- Periodontal disease, a bacterial infection of the gums, appears to increase the risk of atherosclerosis. The link appears to be inflammatory chemicals given off by the immune system in response to the infection.[8] More studies are needed to determine if infections in the mouth can be a predictor of heart disease and atherosclerosis.
- The most common cause of traveler's diarrhea is *E. coli* bacteria in food.[9]
- Certain cases of weight gain and obesity have been linked to a virus[10] and also certain bacteria in the digestive tract.[11] Human studies are underway.

- One study showed ginger to be effective against several types of fruit and vegetable fungi.[12]
- Shogaol, a compound in dried ginger, was found to be a very good antifouling agent.[13] (Antifouling agents are used as coatings on the hulls of ships and other marine equipment to prevent tiny sea creatures from attaching to underwater surfaces.)

WHAT ABOUT GINGER, GARLIC, AND TURMERIC?

Although ginger, garlic, and turmeric have an impressive list of antibacterial, antiviral, antioxidant, and anti-inflammatory actions, in no way am I suggesting that these or other food supplements be used in place of prudent medical treatment by a health care professional.

When medical treatment with strong antibiotics is necessary, it should be followed up with probiotic supplements and frequent eating of yogurt. This follow-up therapy helps repopulate the beneficial bacteria in the digestive tract that broad-spectrum antibiotics may have destroyed. This beneficial bacteria helps us in many ways and also helps protect us from potentially harmful microbes.[14]

The overuse of antibiotics has become a hot issue. Resistant strains of bacterial-related illnesses are increasing at an alarming rate. Ginger, garlic, and turmeric are strong performers and certainly deserve consideration in your wellness program.

WHAT ARE BACTERIA?

Bacteria are single-celled organisms that live, eat, give off wastes, and die. They are all around us—in our air, food, and water; in the soil; in plants and animals; and inside us. Ginger can inhibit the 3 most common bacteria that make us sick from contaminated food and water.

BACTERIA FROM FOOD AND WATER

E. coli (Escherichia coli): Ginger can inhibit a harmful strain of *E.*

coli bacteria.[15] Several strains of *E. coli* are harmless and normally live in the intestines of healthy humans and animals. However, a few strains of *E. coli* are known to produce toxins in our bodies.

E. coli infection is the most common cause of traveler's diarrhea, which can happen during travel to countries where there is poor sanitation and contamination of food and water is likely to occur.[16] In the United States, we have seen major food recalls due to *E. coli* contamination in some commercially sold ground beef products and fresh produce.

It only takes microscopic amounts of human or animal feces to contaminate food or water with *E. coli*. Symptoms of harmful *E. coli* infection include severe cramping (abdominal pain) and diarrhea that is initially watery but becomes bloody. Fever and vomiting may or may not occur. Symptoms normally last a week but can last up to a month.[17] In 3% to 5% of cases, a very serious condition called hemolytic uremic syndrome can occur, which involves kidney failure, reduced red blood cell count (anemia), and severe bleeding.[18]

Other spices that can also inhibit *E. coli* include bay leaves, cinnamon, cloves, lemon grass, oregano, thyme,[19] and raw garlic.[20]

Salmonella: *Salmonella* is another bacteria that can infect food. Raw garlic proved to be very effective at inhibiting *Salmonella* and several other potentially harmful bacteria;[21] however, studies using ginger and turmeric showed mixed results. One study showed an extract of ginger inhibited *Salmonella*,[22] while another study showed that neither ginger nor turmeric extracts offered any protection against *Salmonella*.[23]

Symptoms of *Salmonella* infection include nausea, vomiting, abdominal cramps, diarrhea, fever, and headache. In some severe cases, arthritic symptoms can follow 3 to 4 weeks after infection. *Salmonella* can infect raw meat, eggs, milk and other dairy products, and many other common foods.[24] A certain strain of *Salmonella* is the cause of typhoid fever in some underdeveloped countries where contaminated water is more common. Symptoms of typhoid fever include nausea, vomiting, fever, and, in many cases death. *Salmonella* can infect just about any food; however, chicken and eggs are at a higher risk of carrying the bacteria.[25]

Salmonella infection can be prevented by thoroughly cooking food and washing hands and utensils with soapy water after handling raw meat. Also, keep raw meat separated from cooked meat and other foods.[26]

C. jejuni (Campylobacter jejuni): One lab study showed ginger oil to be more effective at inhibiting *C. jejuni* than essential oils from 96 other plants and herbs.[27]

C. jejuni is the leading cause of bacterial diarrhea in the United States. Other symptoms include fever, abdominal pain, nausea, headaches, and muscle pain. *C. jejuni* is carried by healthy cattle, chickens, birds, flies, and is sometimes in unchlorinated water such as streams and ponds. It is very important to thoroughly cook meat (especially chicken) and to make sure raw meat does not come into contact with cooked meat. Remember to wash utensils and plates that may have touched raw meat.[28]

TWO-THIRDS OF THE WORLD'S POPULATION CARRY THIS ULCER-CAUSING BACTERIA

H. pylori (Helicobacter pylori): *H. pylori* is the bacteria largely responsible for ulcers in the stomach and upper intestine.[29] One study showed that gingerols (abundant in fresh ginger) were able to inhibit the growth of 19 strains of *H. pylori* used in the study.[30] Other studies confirm ginger's effectiveness at inhibiting the *H. pylori* bacteria.[31] Turmeric, with its active compound curcumin, was also found to inhibit 19 strains of *H. pylori*[32] and, like ginger, has other antibiotic and anti-cancer actions.[33] Garlic is also very effective at inhibiting *H. pylori*.[34] *H. pylori* causes damage by producing ammonia, which results in inflammation and free radicals—all of which can damage the stomach and intestine wall.[35]

It is estimated that two-thirds of the world's population carries this bacteria. It is also estimated that up to 20% of people infected with *H. pylori* could develop ulcers. *H. pylori* is transmitted through contaminated food and water and by mouth-to-mouth contact. The ammonia from *H. pylori* also decreases the acidity of the stomach, making it easier for *H. pylori* to survive. If *H. pylori* is untreated, it can result in chronic inflammation of tissues, which can lead to increased risk of cancers of the digestive tract.[36]

Fairly recently, in 1982, researchers linked stomach ulcers to infection with *H. pylori*. Prior to this, the accepted theory was that ulcers were a result of food, acid, and lifestyle. The medical community's acceptance of a bacterial cause was a slow one. The two Australian researchers who first discovered the link between bacteria and ulcers chose to voluntarily infect themselves with the bacteria; they developed ulcers and proved their theory by curing themselves with antibiotic treatment. The researchers were awarded a Nobel Prize in Medicine in 2005 for their discovery.[37]

Ginger helped reduce and prevent ulcers in animal studies.[38]

GINGER INHIBITS RESPIRATORY TRACT BACTERIA

An African study of 333 individuals with runny nose, cough, and inflammation of mucus membranes (stuffy nose and sore throat) showed that ginger inhibited 4 types of bacterial infections of the respiratory tract. The bacteria inhibited were *Staphylococcus aureus, Streptococcus pyogenes, Streptococcus pneumoniae,* and *Haemophilus influenzae.* The herb bitter cola also inhibited this bacteria.[39]

Staphylococcus aureus (S. aureus) normally exists on human hair and skin and in the nose and throat of 50% of healthy people. It also exists in the air, dust, food, milk, water, and sewage. Some strains of *S. aureus* can cause food poisoning that result in nausea, vomiting, and abdominal cramping. More severe cases include headache, muscle cramping, and changes in blood pressure. These bacteria can become harmful in food if the food has not been refrigerated at sufficiently cold temperatures

(45°F, 7.2°C or below) or heated sufficiently (above 140°F, 60°C). It can infect meats; poultry; eggs; milk and other dairy products; cream-filled pastries; and egg salad and other salads, including tuna, chicken, and potato.[40] *S. aureus* infection can also cause skin infections, pneumonia, blood poisoning, and toxic shock syndrome.[41]

There have been recent outbreaks of antibiotic-resistant strains such as methicillin-resistant *Staphylococcus aureus* (MRSA). This bacteria is transmitted by skin-to-skin contact with an infected person or by contact with shared items such as towels, razors, or other surfaces that come in contact with infected skin. MRSA infections appear as boils on the skin and are often red, swollen, painful, and may have some pus drainage. Infections are most likely to occur on areas of the body covered with hair, such as the back of the neck, groin, buttocks, armpits, and the facial area of bearded men.[42] (Methicillin is one of the strongest antibiotics that targets a specific group of bacteria, some of which are resistant to this and other penicillin-type antibiotics.)

Streptococcus pyogenes is a bacteria that can cause strep throat, scarlet fever, impetigo (skin infection causing pimple-like sores), pneumonia, acute kidney inflammation, toxic shock syndrome, blood poisoning, and several other illnesses. This bacteria infects only humans so there are very few animal studies.43

Streptococcus pneumoniae is a bacteria that can cause pneumonia, ear and sinus infections, meningitis (inflammation of the membranes that surround the brain and spinal cord), and several other illnesses.44

Haemophilus influenzae is now prevented by vaccination in many industrialized countries. Before the availability of these vaccines in 1998, it was the leading cause of bacterial meningitis among preschool children.[45]

GARLIC CHASES AWAY MORE THAN VAMPIRES!

Raw garlic appears to be superior among most foods for inhibiting a wide range of bacteria. It is important to know that both ginger and garlic will lose their antibiotic properties after prolonged heating,[46] which may explain why some forms of garlic or ginger were not effective in some studies. Eating raw garlic may produce digestive discomfort and has a risk of potentially harmful side effects for some people. It appears that aged garlic extract has many of the advantages of fresh garlic but without the odor and potential discomfort.[47]

In addition, folklore tells that garlic is supposed to drive away vampires. This tale probably originated because garlic is also a natural mosquito repellant. Since mosquitoes suck blood and spread disease, this was probably the beginnings of the vampire tale.[48] Adding olive oil to crushed garlic and spreading on toasted bread is a nice way to get it into your diet. I like to sprinkle parmesan cheese on top. Remember to eat your garlic in the evening and on weekends and away from the public (unless, of course, you want to scare some people away).

GINGER HAS ANOTHER TRICK FOR FIGHTING OFF BACTERIA

Ginger can help our bodies fight off bacteria another way—by increasing the flow of bile into the digestive tract.[49] Bile acts as a strong detergent that breaks down fats and also aids in killing harmful bacteria.[50] (Bile is produced by the liver, stored in the gall bladder, flows through the bile duct, and is released into the small intestine upon eating fatty foods.)

Several other studies around the world affirm ginger's effectiveness at inhibiting many types of harmful bacteria.[51] Many of these studies used standardized extracts from fresh ginger.

WHAT ARE VIRUSES?

A virus is made up of a strand of genetic material (DNA or RNA) and is encased in a protective protein shell. The DNA and RNA contain the virus's genetic code of instructions for reproducing itself. Viruses are extremely tiny—about 100 times smaller than bacteria and can only be seen using an electron microscope. For example, 16,000 rhinoviruses (this virus causes the common cold) could fit side by side across the head of a pin. Unlike bacteria, a virus is not a living organism and may remain dormant in our bodies for years or even for a lifetime. [52]

When an active virus gets into a living host cell, it takes control of it by writing its own genetic instructions into the host cell. The host cell then becomes a factory for producing new viruses, which go on to attack other cells. In addition to the common cold, viral infections also cause the flu (influenza), hepatitis, mumps, some types of pneumonia, shingles, AIDS and hundreds of variations of other infections and diseases. [53]

Viruses are very difficult to treat because they easily mutate, which means they change their genetic code and may become resistant to a specific vaccine. Strains of bacteria and viruses that are resistant to drugs and vaccines are a big threat to our health.

A virus has a protein shell that can disguise itself from our body's immune system. Zingibain, ginger's potent proteolytic (protein-digesting) enzyme, can help break down this protein coating[54] and by disrupting its protective shell, may allow our immune system to recognize and destroy the virus.

RHINOVIRUS AND THE COMMON COLD

Rhinovirus: "Rhino" means this virus infects the membranes in the nose. Several compounds in ginger were found to help destroy rhinoviruses.[55] More than half of all common colds are caused by various types of rhinoviruses[56] (there are over 100 different types). Ginger and chicken soup have both been used for hundreds of years to help speed recovery from colds. There are even some scientific explanations why chicken soup helps relieve some cold symptoms. Zinc lozenges and sprays can also help shorten the duration of a cold.[57]

It is believed that rhinoviruses can also weaken a person's immune system, making him or her more susceptible to related illnesses, such as lower respiratory tract and bacterial infections.[58]

EPSTEIN-BARR VIRUS - MOST OF US HAVE IT

Epstein-Barr virus: Ginger inhibits the Epstein-Barr virus.[59] The Epstein-Barr virus is the cause of some fevers and most cases of mononucleosis.[60] (Mononucleosis results in fever, sore throat, and swollen lymph glands.) These are the milder illnesses many people experience; however, the virus can be very harmful in some people.

It is common for the Epstein-Barr virus to be picked up during early childhood by the transfer of saliva between people—hence calling it the "kissing disease." It is estimated that 95% of people carry this virus by age 40, although most people are infected by age 20. The virus stays with us for the rest of our lives[61] but remains dormant in most people.

Recent studies show that the Epstein-Barr virus may be linked to multiple sclerosis,[62] tumors,[63] several types of cancers including certain cases of breast cancer,[64] Burkitt's lymphoma,[65] Hodgkin's disease,[66] nasal T cell lymphoma,[67] and several other illnesses.[68] (Lymphoma is a cancer of the tissues of the lymph system—it is seen in the lymph nodes in Burkitt's lymphoma and Hodgkin's disease.[69] The lymph system is made up of tiny vessels and nodes that collect fluid from every part the body and transport it back into the bloodstream. The lymph system helps filter out bacteria and fight off disease. Lymph nodes also remove destroyed microorganisms from the lymph fluid.)

It is interesting that extracts from citrus fruits (from the peels and seeds) can also inhibit the Epstein-Barr virus.[70]

ENZYME THERAPY CAN FIGHT VIRUSES

Two human studies show that enteric-coated proteolytic enzymes were an effective treatment for patients with shingles.[71] Shingles (also known as herpes zoster) is a painful and itchy rash on the skin that is more common in elderly persons. It is caused by the same virus that causes chicken pox in younger people. Enzyme therapy was also helpful in treating some virus-caused illnesses such as hepatitis C[72] and Reiter's disease.[73] Hepatitis is an inflammation of the liver and Reiter's disease is a type of arthritis that can occur after a bacterial infection.[74]

Ironically, one study showed that the enzyme trypsin (which is secreted into our small intestine during digestion) actually caused faster reproduction of the human rotavirus.[75] Rotavirus is a common cause of diarrhea in infants and young children. The virus spreads from one child to another and sometimes gets passed to adults. Treatment consist of drinking lots of water to replace lost fluids along with sugar and mineral supplements.[76]

GINGER, GARLIC, AND TURMERIC— THE FUNGUS FIGHTERS

These amazing foods are also able to kill off certain types of fungi and, in turn, help fight off fungal infections.[77]

CANDIDA—"STEALTH" INFECTION OF THE MODERN AGE

Candida (Candida albicans): Ginger has been shown to be effective at killing *Candida* in several studies[78] and is even effective against a wide variety of fungi, including some strains highly resistant to prescription antifungal medications amphotericin B and ketoconazole.[79]

Candida in its mild form naturally exists as a yeast on everyone's skin and mucus membranes; however, it has the ability to change into 7 different forms. This makes it difficult to detect and diagnose.

Candida's fungal form is very aggressive. It can infect the digestive tract and grow tentacles that poke holes through the wall of the intestines. This can lead to leaky gut syndrome. Making matters worse, *Candida* gives off toxins that enter the bloodstream and cause a wide array of physical and mental problems that can mimic other illnesses. The infection is known as candidiasis. Like other infections, it can grow slowly and stealthily but can eventually suck the life out of your career, your family, and your relationships and can jeopardize your hopes and dreams. Mild forms of *Candida* infection are likely to go undiagnosed, probably because focus is placed on treating symptoms, which can be very different from person to person. The many physical and psychological effects of *Candida* are discussed in chapter 14.

Other studies affirm ginger's antifungal properties.[80] Garlic is also very effective against *Candida*.[81] In fact, one study showed garlic to have greater activity against *Candida* than the prescription antifungal medication Nystatin.[82]

Another interesting note: it is known that *Candida albicans* can cause inflammation in mouth tissues that are underneath dentures (a condition called *stomatitis*).[83] Since ginger can help destroy *Candida* yeast and fungal infections, it strengthens the case for slowly chewing on fresh ginger and possibly using it in dental products. Ginger's anti-inflammatory properties are an added bonus when treating this condition.

STUFFY NOSE AND SINUS INFECTIONS

An interesting study by the Mayo Clinic in 2002 of patients with chronic rhinosinusitis (persistent stuffy nose and sinus infections) determined that 75% reported improvement in their condition after receiving an antifungal medication in their nose.[84]

GINGER KILLS WORMS

Nobody likes to talk about those nasty little parasite creatures (some not so little) that can live inside us. Some worms can deposit thousands of eggs per day in our bodies. Here are some types of worms that ginger can help destroy:

Worms from fish: Ginger kills *Anisakis larvae*.[85] *Anisakis* worms are parasites that live in ocean fish and are transmitted to humans who eat raw or undercooked infected fish. Symptoms of infection include nausea, vomiting, and violent stomach pain within several hours after ingesting the larva. (The larvae are tiny worms approximately 2 centimeters long).[86]

Very few cases of infection have been reported in the United States. Sometimes surgical removal of the worms or their dead remains is required.[87] Now we have a better understanding of the Japanese tradition of serving slices of pickled ginger with sushi, a Japanese delicacy prepared from raw fish.

Warm-climate flatworms: Gingerol (abundant in fresh ginger) completely stopped the infectivity of *Schistosoma mansoni* worms in an animal study.[88] This flatworm lives in water in warm tropical climates and infection can occur when the flatworm penetrates the skin of a human while wading, swimming, or otherwise contacting infected water. The worms make their way into human blood vessels, where they produce their eggs. Symptoms of infection include rash or itchy skin within days of being infected. Fever, chills, cough, and muscle aches can develop 1 or 2 months after infection. These parasites grow and develop in certain types of snails, which discharge the worms into the water.[89]

Dog worms: A ginger extract killed worms (*Dirofilaria immitis*) in dogs when the dogs were given injections under the skin.[90] This round worm typically infects animals but, in rare cases, can also infect humans. The worms infect the heart and can result in chronic heart failure. The worm larvae are carried by mosquitoes.[91]

SYMPTOMS OF INFECTION CAN BE IMMEDIATE

One clue that mental and physical problems may have been brought on by a hidden infection (rather than a purely psychiatric origin) is the sudden development of symptoms in a previously stable individual.

A healthy and energetic psychologist returned from vacation in Bhutan and suddenly developed severe depression, exhaustion, and rheumatoid arthritis. After over 100 treatments by various practitioners, she was later diagnosed as having 3 different parasite infections.[93]

Symptoms of Infection Can Be Delayed

Mothers who are infected with herpes simplex type 2 infection during pregnancy face an increased risk of their offspring developing mental abnormalities (psychoses) as adults.[94]

Childhood infection by the parasite *Toxoplasma gondii* may increase risk of developing symtoms of schizophrenia later in life.[95] This parasite can exist in undercooked, contaminated meats and in the feces of infected cats. (Cats become infected by eating infected rodents, birds, or other small animals. Cats then release millions of cysts in their feces for as long as 3 weeks after infection.) It is estimated that 22.5% of the population 12 years and older in the United States and Europe have been infected with this parasite which typically remains inactive and kept in check by our immune system. In some hot, humid climates, up to 95% of some populations have been infected. Humans can become infected with *Toxoplasma gondii* by several ways including:

• Eating undercooked, infected meat (especially pork, lamb, and venison)
• Eating food that came in contact with contaminated utensils or raw, contaminated meat
• Accidental ingestion of contaminated water, soil, garden foods or anything that came in contact with infected cat feces
• Passed from mother to baby just prior to, or during pregnancy[96]
Various psychological symptoms of childhood infection may not appear until later in life, the 20s and 30s, or when the immune system is compromised.[97] It is interesting that several drugs that are used for the treatment of bipolar disorder and schizophrenia also inhibit the parasite *Toxoplasma gondii*.[98] This infection is not considered dangerous unless infection occurs just prior to, or during pregnancy. It is believed *Toxoplasma gondii* accounts for only a portion of the 1% of people having

symtoms of schizophrenia.[99] This is another example how an infection early in life can lead to dysfunction of the brain in later years.

Candida is a classic example of an infection with slow and delayed symptoms that may not be diagnosed until many years of suffering have passed.

FRESH GINGER KILLS BAD BACTERIA IN OUR MOUTH, HELPS OUR GUMS, TEETH AND MORE!

I like to slowly chew on slices of fresh ginger because it makes a great breath freshener and even helps clean the teeth, especially after eating sugary foods. It's like having a natural tooth brush. (Yes, I still continue brushing and flossing my teeth.) I have a hunch that fresh ginger slices can also help prevent cavities, and here is my reasoning: tooth decay begins with the buildup of plaque, which is formed from many layers of bacteria. This bacteria is of the *Streptococcus* strain.[100] Ginger is known to inhibit the growth of various strains of *Streptococcus* bacteria[101] and, therefore, should help prevent the development of tooth decay. (One of the roles of low levels of fluoride in drinking water is to help inhibit the growth of bacteria on the teeth.)[102]

Inflammation of the gums, also called periodontitis, is a serious condition that can result in tooth loss. Free radicals are one of the causes of inflammation of the gums.[103] It is logical that ginger's potent antioxidants and anti-inflammatory actions should greatly benefit our gums. Anyone out there in dental research who would like to test ginger and/ or its components for preventing tooth decay? If my reasoning is correct, maybe we will someday see ginger products including tooth paste, mouthwash, lozenges … and even candy that fights tooth decay?

Several studies show a relationship between patients with poor dental hygiene (gum disease and tooth loss) and increased risk of rheumatoid arthritis[104] and atherosclerosis.[105] The connection appears to be inflammation in other parts of the body originating from infection in the mouth. Having a healthy mouth is a great start for a healthier mind and body. I believe chewing on fresh ginger can help!

REFERENCES FOR CHAPTER 18

1. Alexis Jetter. *Prevention.* November 2006. pp.150-182.
2. Jonathan R. Strong. "Lyme Disease Newsgroup FAQ. Web site: [sci.med. diseases.lyme] Accessed 11/8/2007. <http://www.faqs.org/faqs/medicine/lyme-disease/ld-faq/>.
3. Klee AL, Maidin B, Edwin B, Poshni I, Mostashari F, Fine A, Layton M, Nash D. "Long-term prognosis for clinical West Nile virus infection." *Emerg Infect Dis.* 2004 Aug;10(8):1405-11.
4. Murray KO, Resnick M, Miller V. "Depression after Infection with West Nile Virus." Web site: U.S. Centers for Disease Control and Prevention, Department of Health and Human Services. Accessed 11/8/2007. <http://www2a.cdc.gov/ncidod/ts/print.asp>.
5. Davis LE, DeBiasi R, Goade DE, Haaland KY, Harrington JA, Harnar JB, Pergam SA, King MK, DeMasters BK, Tyler KL. "West nile virus neuroinvasive disease." *Ann Neurol.* 2006 Sep;60(3): 286-300.
6a. Emily Shacter, Phd, Sigmund A. Weitzman, MD. "Chronic Inflammation and Cancer." *Oncology.* Vol 16,No 2 (February 2002).
6b. Vicki Brower. "Feeding the Flame: New Research Adds to Role of Inflammation in Cancer Development" *Journal of the National Cancer Institute.* Vol. 97, No. 4, February 16, 2005.
7. Arkene SA Levy, Oswald Simon, Janet Shelly, and Michael Gardener. "6-Shogaol reduced chronic inflammatory response in the knees of rats treated with complete Freund's adjuvant." *BMC Pharmacol.* 2006; 6: 12.
8a. Mustapha IZ, Debrey S, Oladubu M, Ugarte R. "Markers of systemic bacterial exposure in periodontal disease and cardiovascular disease risk: a systematic review and meta-analysis." *J Periodontal.* 2007 Dec;78(12):2289-302.
8b. Chun YH, Chun KR, Olguin D, Wang HL. "Biological foundation for periodontitis as a potential risk factor for atherosclerosis." *J Periodontal Res.* 2005 Feb;40(1):87-95.
8c. Jukka H. Meurman, Mariano Sanz, and Sok-Ja Janket. "Oral Health, Atherosclerosis, and Cardiovascular Disease" *Critical Reviews in Oral Biology & Medicine,* Vol. 15, No. 6, 403-413 (2004).
8d. Sok-Ja Janket, DMD, MPH; Markku Qvarnstrom, DDS, MS; Jukka H. Meurman, DDS, MD; et al. "Asymptotic Dental Score and Prevalent Coronary Heart Disease" *Circulation.* 2004;109:1095-1100.

8e.   Beck JD, Offenbacher S, Williams R, Gibbs P, Garcia R. "Periodontitis: a risk factor for coronary heart disease?" *Ann Periodontal.* 1998 Jul;3(1):127-41.

9a.   Goldsmid JM, Leggat PA. "The returned traveler with diarrhoea." *Aust Fam Physician.* 2007 May;36(5):322-7.

9b.   Lima AA. "Tropical diarrhoea: new developments in traveler's diarrhoea." *Curr Opin Infect Dis.* 2001 Oct;14(5):547-52.

9c.   DuPont HL. "Travelers' diarrhoea: contemporary approaches to therapy and prevention." *Drugs.* 2006;66(3):303-14.

10a. Atkinson RL. "Viruses as an etiology of obesity." *Mayo Clinic Proc.* 2007 Oct;82(10):192-8.

10b. Atkinson RL, Dhurandhar NV, Allison DB, Bowen RL, Israel BA, Albu JB, Augustus AS. "Human adenovirus-36 is associated with increased body weight and paradoxical reduction of serum lipids." *Int J Obes (Lond).* 2005 Mar;29(3):281-6.

10c. Whigmam LD, Israel BA, Atkinson RL. "Catching Obesity: Identifying Viruses That May Make Us Fat." The American Physiological Society web site. Accessed 10/10/2007. <http://www.the-aps.org/press/journal/06/4.htm>.

11a. Shanahan F. "Exploring the link between gut microbes and obesity." *Future Microbiol.* 2007 Jun;2:261-3.

11b. Turnbaugh PJ, Ley RE, Mahowald MA, Magrini V, Mardis ER, Gordon JI. "An obesity-associated gut microbiome with increased capacity for energy harvest." *Nature.* 2006 Dec 21;444(7122):1027-10.

12.   Wang H, Ng TB. "An antifungal protein from ginger rhizomes." *Biochem Biophys Res Commun.* 2005 Oct 14;336(1):100-4.

13.   Etoh H, Kondoh T, Noda R, Singh IP, Sekiwa Y, Morimitsu K, Kubota K. "Shogaols from Zingiber officinale as promising antifouling agents." *Biosci Biotechnol Biochem.* 2002 Aug;66(8):1748-50.

14.   Servin AL. "Antagonistic activities of lactobacilli and bifidobacteria against microbial pathogens." *FEMS Microbiol Rev.* 2004 Oct;28(4):405-40.

15a. Gupta S, Ravishankar S. "A comparison of the antimicrobial activity of garlic, ginger, carrot, and turmeric pastes against Escherichia coli O157:H7 in laboratory buffer and ground beef." *Foodborne Pathog Dis.* 2005 Winter;2(4):330-40.

15b. Jagetia GC, Baliga MS, Venkatesh P, Ulloor JN. "Influence of ginger rhizome (Zingiber officinale Rosc) on survival, glutathione and lipid peroxidation in mice after whole-body exposure to gamma radiation." *Radiat Res.* 2003 Nov;160(5):584-92.

15c. Janes ME, Nannapaneni R, Johnson MG. "Identification and characterization of two bacteriocin-producing bacteria isolated from garlic and ginger root." *J Food Prot.* 1999 Aug;62(8):899-904.

16.   "Travelers' Diarrhea" Web site: U.S. Department of Health and Human Services. Centers for Disease Control and Prevention. Accessed 10/10/2007. <http://www.cdc.gov/ncidod/dbmd/diseaseinfo/travelersdiarrhea_g.htm>

17. *"Escherichia coli 0157:H7"*. Bad Bug Book. Web site: U.S. Food and Drug Administration. Accessed 10/23/2007. <http://www.cfsan.fda.gov/~mow/chap15.html>.

18. "Foodborne Illness." "Frequently Asked Questions". Article dated January 10, 2005. Web site: U.S. Centers for Disease Control and Prevention. www.http://www.cdc.gov

19. Friedman M, Henika PR, Mandrell RE. "Bactericidal activities of plant essential oils and some of their isolated constituents against Campylobacter jejuni, Escherichia coli, Listeria monocytogenes, and Salmonella enterica." *J Food Prot.* 2002 Oct;65(10):1545-60.

20. Chen HC, Chang MD, Chang TJ. "[Antibacterial properties of some spice plants before and after heat treatment]." *Zhonghua Min Guo Wei Sheng Wu Ji Mian Yi Xue Za Zhi.* 1985 Aug;18(3):190-5.

21. Chen HC, Chang MD, Chang TJ. "[Antibacterial properties of some spice plants before and after heat treatment]." *Zhonghua Min Guo Wei Sheng Wu Ji Mian Yi Xue Za Zhi.* 1985 Aug;18(3):190-5.

22. Jagetia GC, Baliga MS, Venkatesh P, Ulloor JN. "Influence of ginger rhizome (Zingiber officinale Rosc) on survival, glutathione and lipid peroxidation in mice after whole-body exposure to gamma radiation." *Radiat Res.* 2003 Nov;160(5):584-92.

23. Thongson C, Davidson PM, Mahakarnchanakul W, Vibulsresth P. "Antimicrobial effect of Thai spices against Listeria monocytogenes and Salmonella typhimurium DT104." *J Food Prot.* 2005 Oct;68(10):2054-8.

24. *"Salmonella spp."* Bad Bug Book. Web site: U.S. Food and Drug Administration. Accessed 10/23/2007. <http://www.cfsan.fda.gov/~mow/chap1.html>.

25. "Salmonella information". Web site: Salmonella.org. Accessed 10/15/2007. <http://www.salmonella.org/info.html>.

26. "Foodborne Illness". "Frequently Asked Questions". Web site: U.S. Centers for Disease Control and Prevention. Article dated January 10, 2005. <www.http://www.cdc.gov>.

27. Friedman M, Henika PR, Mandrell RE. "Bactericidal activities of plant essential oils and some of their isolated constituents against Campylobacter jejuni, Escherichia coli, Listeria monocytogenes, and Salmonella enterica." *J Food Prot.* 2002 Oct;65(10):1545-60.

28. *"Campylobacter jejuni"*. Bad Bug Book. Web site: U.S. Food and Drug Administration. Accessed 10/23/2007. <http://www.cfsan.fda.gov/~mow/chap4.html>.

29. *"Helicobacter pylori* and Peptic Ulcer Disease." Web site: U.S. Centers for Disease Control and Prevention, Department of Health and Human Services Accessed 2/10/2006. <http://www.cdc.gov/ulcer/md.htm>.

30. Mahady GB, Pendland SL, Yun GS, Lu ZZ, Stoia A. "Ginger (Zingiber

officinale Roscoe) and the gingerols inhibit the growth of Cag A+ strains of Helicobacter pylori." *Anticancer Res.* 2003 Sep-Oct;23(5A):3699-702.

31. Nostro A, Cellini L, Di Bartolomeo S, Cannatelli MA, Di Campli E, Procopio F, Grande R, Marzio L, Alonzo V. "Effects of combining extracts (from propolis or Zingiber officinale) with clarithromycin on Helicobacter pylori." *Phytother Res.* 2006 Mar;20(3):187-90.

32. Mahady GB, Pendland SL, Yun GS, Lu ZZ. "Turmeric (Curcuma longa) and curcumin inhibit the growth of Helicobacter pylori, a group 1 carcinogen." *Anticancer Res.* 2002 Nov-Dec;22(6C):4179-81.

33. Leal PF, Braga ME, Sato DN, Carvaljo JE, Marques MO, Meireles MA. "Functional properties of spice extracts obtained via supercritical fluid extraction." *J Agric Food Chem.* 2003 Apr 23;51(9):2520-5.

34. Sivam GP, Lampe JW, Ulness B, Swanzy SR, Potter JD. "Helicobacter pylori--invitro susceptibility to garlic (Allium sativum) extract." *Nutr Cancer.* 1997;27(2):118-21.

35a. H Shirin, SF Moss. "*Helicobacter pylori* induced apoptosis" *Gut.* 1998;43:592-594.

35b. Triebling AT, Korsten MA, Dlugosz JW, Paronetto F, Lieber CS. "Severity of Helicobacter-induced gastric injury correlates with gastric juice ammonia." *Dig Dis Sci.* 1991 Aug;36(8):1089-96.

36a. "H. pylori and Cancer: Questions and Answers." National Cancer Institute FactSheet. Web site: National Cancer Institute. Accessed 1/26/2007. <http://www.cancer.gov/cancertopics/factsheet/Hpylori/print?page=&keyword=>.

36b. Vicki Brower V. "Feeding the Flame:New Research Adds to Role of Inflammation in Cancer Development." *Journal of the National Cancer Institute.* Vol. 97, No. 4, February 16, 2005.

37. "H. pylori and Cancer: Questions and Answers." National Cancer Institute FactSheet. Web site: National Cancer Institute. Accessed 1/26/2007. <http://www.cancer.gov/cancertopics/factsheet/Hpylori/print?page=&keyword=>.

38a. al-Yahya MA, Rafatullah S, Mossa JS, Ageel AM, Parmar NS, Tariq M. "Gastroprotective activity of ginger zingiber officinale rosc., in albino rats." *Am J Chin Med.* 1989;17(1-2):51-6.

38b. Yamahara J, Mochizuki M, Rong HQ, Matsuda H, Fujimura H. "The anti-ulcer effect in rats of ginger constituents." *J Ethnopharmacol.* 1988 Jul-Aug;23(2-3):299-304.

39. Akoachere JF, Ndip RN, Chenwi EB, Ndip LM, Njock TE, Anong DN. "Antibacterial effect of Zingiber officinale and Garcinia kola on respiratory tract pathogens." *East Afr Med J.* 2002 Nov;79(11):588-92.

40. "*Staphylococcus aureus*". Bad Bug Book. Web site: U.S. Food and Drug Administration. Accessed 10/23/2007. <http://www.cfsan.fda.gov/~mow/chap3.html>.

41. "Staphylococcal Infections." Web site: Medline Plus. A service of the U.S.

National Library of Medicine and the National Institutes of Health. Accessed 10/15/2007. <http://www.nlm.nih.gov/medlineplus/print/staphylococcalinfections.html>.

42. "Questions and Answers about methicillin-Resistant *Staphylococcus aureus* (MRSA) in Schools." Web site: U.S. Centers for Disease Control and Prevention. Accessed 11/14/2007. <www.http://www.cdc.gov/Features/MRSAinSchools/>.

43. "Scientists Sequence Genome of Strep Throat, Scarlet Fever Bacterium". Web site: National Institutes of Health. National Institute of Allergy and Infectious Diseases. NIH News Release. Monday, April 9, 2001. Accessed 11/15/2007. <http://www.nih.gov/news/pr/apr2001/niaid-09.htm>

44. "Drug-resistant *Streptococcus pneumoniae*." Web site: U.S. Centers for Disease Control and Prevention. Accessed 11/15/2007. <www.http://www.cdc.gov/ncidod/dbmd/diseaseinfo/dugresiststreppneum_t.htm.>

45. "Progress Toward Eliminating Haemophilus influenzae Type b Disease Among Infants and Children – United States, 987-1997" Web site: U.S. Centers for Disease Control and Prevention. Accessed 11/15/2007. <www.http://www.cdc.gov/mmwr/preview/mmwrhtml/00055745.htm>.

46. Chen HC, Chang MD, Chang TJ. "[Antibacterial properties of some spice plants before and after heat treatment]." *Zhonghua Min Guo Wei Sheng Wu Ji Mian Yi Xue Za Zhi*. 1985 Aug;18(3):190-5.

47. "Scientific Literature Review of Aged Garlic Extract: Pharmacological Aspects." Web site: KYOLIC Information. Accessed 10/15/2007. <http://www.kyolic.com./html/linfo/vol3_3.htm>.

48. "Garlic and Vampires". Web site: Garlic Central. Accessed 1/18/2009. <http://www.garlic-central.com/vampires.html>.

49. Yamahara J, Miki K, Chisaka T, Sawada T, Fujimura H, Tomimatsu T, Nakano K, Nohara T. "Cholagogic effect of ginger and its active constituents." *J Ethnopharmacol*. 1985 May;13(2):217-25.

50. Begley M, Gahan CG, Hill C. "The interaction between bacteria and bile." *FEMS Microbiol Rev*. 2005 Sep;29(4):625-51.

51a. Nguefack J, Budde BB, Jakobsen M. "Five essential oils from aromatic plants of Cameroon: their antibacterial activity and ability to permeabilize the cytoplasmic membrane of Listeria innocua examined by flow cytometry." *Lett Appl Microbiol*. 2004;39(5):395-400.

51b. Alzoreky NS, Nakahara K. "Antibacterial activity of extracts from some edible plants commonly consumed in Asia." *Int J Food Microbiol*. 2003 Feb 15;80(3):223-30.

51c. Janes ME, Nannapaneni R, Johnson MG. "Identification and characterization of two bacteriocin-producing bacteria isolated from garlic and ginger root." *J Food Prot*. 1999 Aug;62(8):899-904.

51d. Mascolo N, Jain R, Jain SC, Capasso F. "Ethnopharmacologic investigation of ginger (Zingiber officinale)." *J Ethnopharmacol.* 1989 Nov;27(1-2):129-40.

52a. "Virus" Web site: Wikipedia.org. Accessed 3/30/2010. <http://en.wikipedia.org/wiki/Virus.

52b. "rhinovirus" Medical-Dictionary Web site. Accessed 3/31/2010. <http://medical-dictionary.thefreedictionary.com/p/rhinoviruses>.

53. Bukrinski MI. "What You Need to Know About Avian Flu...and other dangerous viruses." *Bottom Line/Health.* December 2005.

54. International Patent Application No. PCT/AU2006/001717. Pub. No. WO/2007/056811. Publication Date: 24.05.2007. Inventor: Hawkins, Clifford J. Web site Accessed 1/18/2009. <http://www.wipo.int/pctdb/en/wo.jsp?IA=AU2006001717&WO=2007056811&DISPLAY...>.

55. Denyer CV, Jackson P, Loakes DM, Ellis MR, Young DA. "Isolation of anti-rhinoviral sequiterpenes from ginger (Zingiber officinale)." *J Nat Prod.* 1994 May;57(5):658-62.

56. Turner RB. "Rhinovirus: More than Just a Common Cold Virus." *Journal of Infectionus Diseases.* 2007;195:765-6.

57. McCoy L. "Rhinovirus: An Unstoppable Cause of The Common Cold." *The Science Creative Quarterly.* Three Sept 07.

58. Turner RB. "Rhinovirus: More than Just a Common Cold Virus." *Journal of Infectionus Diseases.* 2007;195:765-6.

59a. Vimala S, Norhanom AW, Yadav M. "Anti-tumour promoter activity in Malaysian ginger rhizobia used in traditional medicine." *Br J Cancer.* 1999 Apr;80(1-2):110-6.

59b. Murakami A, Morita H, Safitri R, Ramlan A, Koshimizu K, Ohigashi H. "Screening for In Vitro Anti-Tumor-Promoting Activities of Edible Plants from Indonesia." *Cancer Detection & Prevention.* 22 (6), 516-525.

60. "Medical Encyclopedia: Mononucleosis". Web Site: Medline Plus. Accessed 5/10/2009. <http//www.nlm.nih.gov/medlineplus/print/ency/article/000591.htm>.

61. "Epstein-Barr Virus." Web site: All about Multiple Sclerosis. Accessed 10/18/2007. <http://mult-sclerosis.org/EpsteinBarrvirus.html>.

62a. Alonso A, Egüés Olazábal N, Ayo Martin O. "[Infection by Epstein-Barr virus and multiple sclerosis]." [Article in Spanish]. *Neurologia.* 2006 Jun;21(5):249-55.

62b. Cook SD. "Does epstein-barr virus cause multiple sclerosis?" *Rev Neurol Dis.* 2004 Summer;1(3):115-23.

62c. Ascherio A, Munch M. "Epstein-Barr virus and multiple sclerosis." *Epidemiology.* 2001 Jan;12(1):134-5.

62d. Warner HB, Carp RI. "Multiple sclerosis etiology--an Epstein-Barr virus hypothesis." *Med Hypotheses.* 1988 Feb;25(2):93-7.

63a. Vimala S, Norhanom AW, Yadav M. "Anti-tumour promoter activity in

Malaysian ginger rhizobia used in traditional medicine." *Br J Cancer*. 1999 Apr;80(1-2):110-6.

63b.   "Clue Found To Epstein-Barr Virus Sustain Tumors" Web site: ScienceDaily. Source: University of Wisconsin-Madison. Date of Article: September 6, 2 006. Accessed 9/18/06. <http://www.sciencedaily.com/ releases/2006/09/060905224346.htm>.

63c.   Tathagata Choudhuri, Subhash C. Verma, Ke Lan, Masanao Murakami, and Erle S. Robertson. "The ATM/ATR Signaling Effector Chk2 Is Targeted by Epstein-Barr Virus Nuclear Antigen 3C To Release the G_2/M Cell Cycle Block" *Journal of Virology*. June 2007, p.6718-6730, Vol. 81, No. 12.

64a.   Perkins RA, Sahm K, Marando C, Dickson-Witmer D, Pahnke GR, Mitchell M, Petrilli NJ, Berkowitz IM, Soteropoloulos P, Aris VM, Dunn SP, Krueger LJ. "Analysis of Epstein-Barr virus reservoirs in paired blood and breast cancer primary biopsy specimens by real time PCR." Breast Cancer Research. 2006. Vol. 8, Issue 6, 2006.

64b.   Preciado MV, Chabay PA, De Matteo EN, Gonzalez P, Grinstein S, Actis A, Gass HD. "Epstein-Barr virus in breast carcinoma in Argentina." *Arch Pathol Lab Med*. 2005 Sep;129(3):377-81.

64c.   Glaser SL, Hsu JL, Gully ML. "Epstein-Barr virus and breast cancer: state of the evidence for viral carcinogenesis." *Cancer Epidemiol Biomarkers Prev*. 2004 May;13(5):688-97.

64d.   Bonnet M, Guinebretiere JM, Kremmer E, Grunewald V, Benhamou E, Contesso G, Joab I. "Detection of Epstein-Barr virus in invasive breast cancers." *J Natl Cancer Inst*. 1999 Aug 18;91(16):1376-81.

64e.   Labrecque LG, Barnes DM, Fentiman IS, Griffin BE. "Epstein-Barr virus in epithelial cell tumors: a breast cancer study." *Cancer Res*. 1995 Jan 1;55(1):39-45.

65a.   Hochberg D, Middeldorp JM, Catalina M, Sullivan JL, Luzuriaga K, Thorley-Lawson DA. "Demonstration of the Burkitt's lymphoma Epstein-Barr virus phenotype in dividing latently infected memory cells in vivo." *Proc Natl Acad Sci U S A*. 2004 January 6; 101(1): 239-244.

65b.   Kennedy G, Komano J, Sugden B. "Epstein-Barr virus provides a survival factor to Burkitt's lymphomas." *Proc Natl Acad Sci U S A*. 2003 Nov 25;100(24):14269-74. Epub 2003 Nov 5.

66.   Hammerschmidt W, Sugden B. "Epstein-Barr virus sustains Burkitt's lymphomas and Hodgkin's disease." *Trends Mol Med*. 2004 Jul;10(7):331-6.

67.   van Gorp J, Brink A, Oudejans JJ, van den Brule AJ, van den Tweel JG, Jiwa NM, de Bruin PC, Meijer CJ. "Expression of Epstein-Barr virus encoded latent nasal T cell lymphomas." *J Clin Pathol*. 1996 January; 49(1): 72-76.

68.   Jones JF, Ray CG, Minnich LL, Hicks MJ, Kibler R, Lucas DO. "Evidence for active Epstein-Barr virus infection in patients with persistent, unexplained

illnesses: elevated anti-early antigen antibodies." *Ann Interm Med.* 1985 Jan;102(1):1-7.

69.   "What is Lymphoma?" Web site: Lymphoma Information Network. Accessed 10/18/2007. <http://www.lymphomamaininfo.net/lymphoma/whatis.html>.

70.   Iwase Y, Takemura Y, Ju-ichi M, Kawii S, Yano M, Okuda Y, Mukainaka T, Tsuruta A, Okuda M, Takayasu J, Tokuda H, Nishino H. "Inhibitory effect of Epstein-Barr virus activation by Citrus fruits, a cancer chemopreventor." *Cancer Lett.* 1999 May 24;139(2):227-36.

71a. Billigmann P. "[Enzyme therapy--an alternative in treatment of herpes zoster. A controlled study of 192 patients]. *Fortschr Med.* 1995 Feb 10;113(4):43-8.

71b. Klaus Uffelmann. "Wobe-Mugos® in the therapy of herpes zoster infections" Accessed 11/7/2007. <http://www.mucos.cz/eng/infekt/wmbvzie.html>.

72.   Stauder G, Kabil S. "Oral enzyme therapy in hepatitis C patients." *Journal of Immunotherapy.* 1997 Vol. XIII, No. 3/4, pp 153-158, ISSN 0255-9625.

73a. Mikazans I. "Systemic enzyme therapy in patients with Reiter's syndrome caused by Chlamydia." 7th Congress of the European Academy of Dermatology and Venerology, October 7-11, 1998, Nice, France published in JEAVEQ, 1998, Vol.11, Suppl 2, Abstract P 478, pp.S298 - ISSN 0926-9959.

73b. Mikazans I. "New possibilities for treatment of chlamydial infection with enzyme therapy." 6th Congress of the European Academy of Dermatology and Venerology, September 11-15, 1997, Dublin, Ireland - published in JEAVEQ 9 (Suppl,1), 1997, pp S 227, abstract P320.

74.   "Reactive arthritis." Web site: Medline Plus. A service of the U.S. National Library of Medicine and the National Institutes of Health. Accessed 11/15/2007. <http://www.nlm.nih.gov/medlineplus/ency/article/000440. htm>.

75a. Kitaoka S, Suzuki H, Numazaki Y, Ishida N. "The effect of trypsin on the growth and infectivity of human rotavirus." *Tohoku J Exp Med.* 1986 Aug;149(4):437-47.

75b. Barnett BB, Spendlove RS, Clark ML. "Effect of enzymes on rotavirus infectivity." *J Clin Microbiol.* 1979 Jul;10(1):111-3.

75c. Almeida JD, Hall T, Banatvala JE, Totterdell BM, Chrystie IL. "The effect of trypsin on the growth of rotavirus." *J Gen Virol.* 1978 Jul;40(1):213-8.

75e. Herrmann JE, Cliver DO. "Degradation of Coxsackievirus Type A9 by Proteolytic Enzymes." *Infect Immun.* 1973 April; 7(4):513-517.

75f. Gifford GE, Klapper DG. "Effect of proteolytic enzymes on vaccinia virus replication." *Archives of Virology.* Vol. 26 No. 4, Dec. 1969.

75g. Keller R. "Studies on the mechanism of the enzymatic reactivation of antibody-neutralized poliovirus." *J Immunol.* 1968 May;100(5):1071-99.

76.   "Rotavirus Infections" Web site: MedlinePlus. Accessed 1/23/2009. http://www.nlm.nih.gov/medlineplus/print/rotavirusinfections.html>.

77a. Wuthi-udomlert M, Grisanapan W, Luanratana O, Caichompoo W.

"Antifungal activity of Curcuma longa grown in Thailand." *Southeast Asian J Trop Med Public Health.* 2000;31 Suppl 1:178-82.

77b. Apisariyakul A, Vanittanakom N, Buddhasukh D. "Antifungal activity of turmeric oil extracted from Curcuma longa (Zingiberaceae)." *J Ethnopharmacol.* 1995 Dec 15;49(3):163-9.

77c. Ankri S, Mirelman D. "Antimicrobial properties of allicin from garlic." *Microbes Infect.* 1999 Feb;1(2):125-9.

78a. Jagetia GC, Baliga MS, Venkatesh P, Ulloor JN. "Influence of ginger rhizome (Zingiber officinale Rosc) on survival, glutathione and lipid peroxidation in mice after whole-body exposure to gamma radiation." *Radiat Res.* 2003 Nov;160(5):584-92.

78b. Ficker CE, Arnason JT, Vindas PS, Alvarez LP, Akpagana K, Gbeassor M, De Souza C, Smith ML. "Inhibition of human pathogenic fungi by ethnobotanically selected plant extracts." *Mycoses.* 2003 Feb;46(1-2):29-37.

79. Ficker CE, Arnason JT, Vindas PS, Alvarez LP, Akpagana K, Gbeassor M, De Souza C, Smith ML. "Inhibition of human pathogenic fungi by ethnobotanically selected plant extracts." *Mycoses.* 2003 Feb;46(1-2):29-37.

80a. Nguefack J, Leth V, Amvan Zollo PH, Mathur SB, "Evaluation of five essential oils from aromatic plants of Cameroon for controlling food spoilage and mycotoxin producing fungi," *Int J Food Microbiol.*, 2004 Aug 1;94(3):329-34.

80b. Jagetia GC, Baliga MS, Venkatesh P, Ulloor JN. "Influence of ginger rhizome (Zingiber officinale Rosc) on survival, glutathione and lipid perxidation in mice after whole-body exposure to gamma radiation." *Radiat Res.* 2003 Nov;160(5):584-92.

80c. Ficker C, Smith ML, Akpagana K, Gbeassor M, Zhang J, Durst T, Assabgui R, Arnason JT, "Bioassay-guided isolation and identification of antifungal compounds from ginger," *Phytother Res.* 2003 Sep;17(8):897-902.

80d. Ficker CE, Arnason JT, Vindas PS, Alvarez LP, Akpagana K, Gbeassor M, De Souza C, Smith ML, "Inhibition of human pathogenic fungi by ethnobotanically selected plant extracts," *Mycoses,* 2003 Feb;46(1-2):29-37.

80e. Martins AP, Salgueiro L, Goncalves MJ, da Cunha AP, Vila R, Canigueral S, Mazzoni V, Tomi T, Casanova J. "Essential oil composition and antimicrobial activity of three Zingiberaceae from S. Tome e Principe." *Planta Med.* 2001 Aug;67(6):580-4.

81. Ankri S, Mirelman D. "Antimicrobial properties of allicin from garlic." *Microbes Infect.* 1999 Feb;1(2):125-9.

82. Arora DS, Kaur J. "Antimicrobial activity of spices." *Int J Antimicrob Agents.* 1999 Aug;12(3):257-62.

83. McLain N, Ascanio R, Baker C, Strohaver RA, Dolan JW. "Undecylenic Acid Inhibits Morphogenesis of Candida albicans." *Antimicrobial Agents and Chemotherapy.* Oct. 2000 p.2873-2875. Vol. 44, No. 10.

84. Ponikau JU, Sherris DA, Kita H, Kern EB. "Intranasal antifungal treatment

in 51 patients with chronic rhinosinusitis." *J Allergy Clin Immunol.* 2002 Dec;110(6):862-6.

85. Goto C Kasuya S, Koga K, Ohtomo H, Kagei N. "Lethal efficacy of extract from Zingiber officinale (traditional Chinese medicine) or [6]-shogaol and [6]-gingerol in Anisakis larvae in vitro." *Parasitol Res.* 1990;76(8):652-6.

86. "Parasites and Health". "Anisakiasis." Web site: Center for Disease Control. Accessed 10/30/2007. <www.dpd.cdc.govdpdx/HTML/Anisakiasis.htm>.

87. *"Anisakis simplex* and related worms." Bad Bug Book. Web site: U.S. Food and Drug Administration. Accessed 10/23/2007. <http://www.cfsan.fda. gov/~mow/chap25.html>.

88. Adwunmi CO, Oguntimein BO, Furu P. "Molluscicidal and antischistosomal activities of Zingiber officinale." *Planta Med.* 1990 Aug;56(4):374-6.

89. "Schistosomiasis." Fact Sheet for the general public. Web site: U.S. Centers for Disease Control and Prevention. Accessed 10/30/2007. <http://www.dpd.cdc. gov>.

90. Datta A, Sukul NC. "Antifilarial effect of Zingiber officinale on Dirofilaria immitis." *J Helminthol.* 1987 Sep;61(3):268-70.

91. Laura H. Kramer, Vladimir V. Kartashev, Giulio Grandi, Rodrigo Morchón, Sergei A. Nagornii, Panagiotis Karanis, and Fernando Simón. "Human Subcutaneous Dirofilariasis, Russia." Volume 13, Number 1-January 2007. Web site: U.S. Centers for Disease Control and Prevention. Accessed 11/15/2007. <www.http://www.2acdc.gov/ncidod/ts/print.asp>.

92. Leo Kartman. "On the Growth of Dirofilaria Immitis in the Mosquito" *Am. J. Trop. Med. Hyg.* 2(6), 1953, pp.1062-1069.

93. Dr. James Howenstine, MD. "The Overlooked Relationship Between Infectious Diseases and Mental Symptoms" September 13, 2004. Article on web site of: James L. Schaller, MD, MAR, DABFM, DABPN, DAAPM, CMI, CMR, PA. Accessed 4/7/2008. <http://www.personalconsult.com/ articles/infectionandmentalsymptoms.html>.

94. Buka SL, Cannon TD, Torrey EF, et al. "Maternal exposure to herpes simplex virus and risk of psychosis among adult offspring." *Biol Psychiatry.* 2008 Apr 15;63(8):809-15. Epub 2007 Nov 5.

95. Yolken RH, Torrey EF. "Are some cases of psychosis caused by microbial agents? A review of the evidence." *Mol Psychiatry.* 2008 May;13(5):470-9. Epub 2008 Feb 12.

96. "Toxoplasmosis > Epidemiology & Risk Factors" Web site: U.S. Center for Disease Control. Accessed 1/25/2009. <http://www.cdc.gov/toxoplosmosis/ epi.html>.

97. *"Toxoplasma gondii* and Schizophrenia". Web site: U.S. Center for Disease Control. Accessed 1/18/2009. <http://www.cdc.gov/ncidod/eid/vol9no11/03-0143.htm>.

98a. Jones-Brando L, Torrey EF, Yolken R. "Drugs used in the treatment of schizophrenia and bipolar disorder inhibit the replication of Toxoplasma gondii." Schizophr Res. 2003 Aug 1;62(3):237-440

98b.   Torrey EF, Yolken RH. "Toxoplasma gondii and schizophrenia." *Emerg Infect Dis.* 2003 Nov;9(11):1375-80.

99.   "*Toxoplasma gondii* and Schizophrenia". Web site: U.S. Center for Disease Control. Accessed 1/18/2009. <http://www.cdc.gov/ncidod/eid/vol9no11/03-0143.htm>.

100.   Xie H, Cook GS, Costerton JW, Bruce G, Rose TM, Lamont RJ. "Intergeneric communication in dental plaque biofilms." *J Bacteriol.* 2000 Dec;182(24):7067-9.

101a. Akoachere JF, Ndip RN, Chenwi EB, Ndip LM, Njock TE, Anong DN. "Antibacterial effect of Zingiber officinale and Garcinia kola on respiratory tract pathogens." *East Afr Med J.* 2002 Nov;79(11):588-92.

101b. Ohara A, Saito F, Matsuhisa. "Screening of Antibacterial Activities of Edible Plants against *Streptococcus mutans.*" *Food Sci. Technol. Res.,* 14 (2). 190-193, 2008.

102.   Featherstone JD. "Prevention and reversal of dental caries: role of low level fluoride." *Community Dent Oral Epidemiol.* 1999 Feb;27(1):31-40.

103.   Chapple IL. "Reactive oxygen species and antioxidants in inflammatory diseases." *J Clin Periodontol.* 1997 May;24(5):587-96.

104.   de Pablo P, Dietrich T, McAlindon TE. "Association of periodontal disease and tooth loss with rheumatoid arthritis in the US population." *J Rheumatol.* 2008 Jan;35(1):70-6. Epub 2007 Nov 15.

105a. Shillinger T, Kluger W, Exner M, et al. "Dental and periodontal status and risk for progression of carotid atherosclerosis: the inflammation and carotid artery risk for atherosclerosis study dental substudy." *Stroke.* 2006 Sep;37(9):2271-6. Epub 2006 Aug 3.

105b. Elter JR, Champagne CM, Offenbacher S, Beck JD. "Relationship of periodontal disease and tooth loss to prevalence of coronary heart disease." *J Periodontol.* 2004 Jun;75(6):782-90.

105c. Ingrid Glurich, Sara Grossi, Boris Albini, et al. "Systemic Inflammation in Cardiovascular and Periodontal Disease: Comparative Study." *Clin Diagn Lab Immunol.* 2002 March; 9(2): 425-432.

105d. Loesche WJ. "Periodontal disease: link to cardiovascular disease." *Compend Contin Educ Dent.* 2000 Jun;21(6):463-6, 468, 470 passim; quiz 484.

CHAPTER 19

Help for Our Heart
and Blood Vessels

THE circulatory system includes the heart, blood, and many miles
of blood vessels. It is estimated that the average adult has about
60,000 miles of blood vessels, most of which are extremely small. Some
vessels are so small that red blood cells (also called platelets) must line
up single file and even fold to a smaller shape in order to pass through.

For most of us, it takes a conscious effort to keep our heart and
blood vessels healthy. Various factors can work against us, including
heredity, diabetes, and our own bad habits—such as smoking, not exercising, and a poor diet (eating too many foods laden with saturated fats,
trans fats, sugar, white flour, and too few fruits, fiber, and vegetables).
All these place an extra burden on our circulatory system. Heart disease
is the leading cause of death in the United States, followed by cancer.[1]
Stroke is the third and fourth leading cause of death (third for women,
fourth for men) but is a leading cause of long-term disability.[2]

DAMAGE FROM FREE RADICALS—AGAIN!

Free radicals attack the fats in our bloodstream, oxidizing them. This
is one of the first steps in the formation of plaque in our blood vessels.[3]
Plaque is made up of oxidized fatty deposits and other substances that
stick to the inner wall of our blood vessels. Plaque can grow large enough
to significantly reduce the flow of blood through the blood vessel. Worse

yet, plaque can break off and travel through the blood vessels until it causes a blood clot, stopping the flow of blood. If the blood clot blocks the flow of blood to the heart, it often results in a heart attack. If the clot blocks the flow of blood to the brain, it can cause a stroke.

Free radicals also cause damage to our blood vessels. In fact, one study states 5 ways free radicals and their resulting oxidation damage our blood vessels.[4] Continuous damage to our blood vessels can lead to the development of atherosclerosis, which is commonly called "hardening of the arteries." Atherosclerosis occurs when blood vessels become hardened and narrowed from the damaging effects of oxidation, inflammation, and buildup of plaque. (*Athero* means "paste" and *sclerosis* means "hardness.")

DAMAGE FROM INFLAMMATION—AGAIN!

Oxidation of fats in our blood causes inflammation to the vessel wall, which is yet another step toward the development of atherosclerosis.[5] Chronic inflammation can also be triggered by bacterial and viral infections, further increasing the risk of atherosclerosis and heart disease.[6] The many processes leading to these diseases of the circulatory system are very complex and are not yet completely understood.

LDL CHOLESTEROL— WHAT WE NEED TO KNOW

The fats we eat are broken down into tiny particles in the small intestine. Next, they are given a protein coating called lipoprotein (*lipo* is another name for "fat"). This protein coating actually makes the tiny fat particles become attracted to the water in our blood. It is amazing that our small intestine knows to provide this protein coating since fats and oils do not normally mix with water. This protein coating is essential for life! (Remember Dr. Budwig stated back in the 1950s to thoroughly mix flaxseed oil with cottage cheese or yogurt—so the oil particles get connected to protein and attracted to blood!)[7]

Once in the bloodstream, the tiny particles of fat and cholesterol are circulated throughout our body and delivered to our cells and tissues. Our cells use the cholesterol for several important processes—it becomes part of our cell walls and is also needed to make hormones, vitamin D, and bile. Amazingly, our liver manufactures bile from cholesterol. Bile, in turn, is needed to break down fats! Since cholesterol is needed by every cell in our body, our liver can even manufacture cholesterol out of carbohydrates if we do not get enough cholesterol in our diet. We get cholesterol by eating animal foods such as meat, eggs, milk, and cheese. Our liver produces about 75% of the cholesterol in our body while 25% comes from the foods we eat.[8] Plants do not produce cholesterol.

LDL (short for low-density lipoprotein) is the protein coating that surrounds a large cluster of fatty acids and some cholesterol. The problem begins when we eat too many fatty foods, often resulting in too much LDL floating around in our bloodstream—much more than our body can use. These clusters of fats within the LDL are easy targets for attack by free radicals, after which they become oxidized (made rancid). Oxidized fats stick to our blood vessel walls. It is widely accepted that a high level of oxidized LDL fats in the blood is an important risk factor in the development of atherosclerosis.[9] The common name LDL cholesterol is not entirely accurate since LDL is actually the type of protein that carries cholesterol and other fatty acids. We will use the name LDL cholesterol, however, since it is most recognized.

CLEANING UP THE EXCESS LDL CHOLESTEROL

Fortunately, our bodies have several ways to clean up some of the excess LDL cholesterol:

- HDL (short for high-density lipoproteins)
- Antioxidants in our bodies
- Exercise and diet

HDL is produced by the liver and acts like a sponge, picking up extra LDL cholesterol from tissues and blood and transporting it back

to the liver. The liver stores the extra LDL cholesterol or may convert it
into bile or body fat. High levels of HDL in our blood, commonly called
HDL cholesterol, are good.

Our bodies also have their own limited supplies of antioxidants
that fight against the oxidation of LDL cholesterol. Many fruits and
vegetables are rich sources of antioxidants and can help build up the
antioxidants in our bodies.

Exercise and diet can help lower LDL cholesterol. Exercise also
increases the level of good HDL cholesterol. It is a huge benefit to lose
weight if you are overweight and stop smoking if you smoke.[10]

Some general guidelines for cholesterol levels are the following:

- An LDL cholesterol level under 130 mg/dL (milligrams
  per deciliter of blood) is very good but over 160 mg/dL
  is considered high and unhealthy. LDL cholesterol is often
  called the "bad cholesterol."
- An HDL cholesterol level over 60 mg/dL is very good and
  helps reduce the risk of heart disease but under 40 mg/dL is
  bad and increases risk of heart disease. HDL is often called
  the "good cholesterol."[11]

HDL HAS TWO MORE TRICKS THAT HELP OUR BODIES

Most people do not know that HDL has antioxidant and anti-
inflammatory actions—two more amazing ways HDL protects our
heart and blood vessels. Keep your HDL levels up!

OTHER WAYS TO REDUCE LDL CHOLESTEROL

Omega-3 EFAs such as flax and fish oil can reduce LDL and help
protect our circulatory system. One study recommends measuring the
shortage of omega-3 EFAs in the blood and using it as a risk factor
for cardiovascular disease. Low levels of omega-3s in the blood would

indicate an increased risk factor for cardiovascular disease.[12] The importance of omega-3 EFAs was discussed in chapter 13.

Foods that help lower bad LDL cholesterol are barley, oat bran, beans, carrots, celery, garlic, nuts, shiitake mushrooms,[13] almonds, apples, avocados, calcium, chili peppers, whole grains, fish, flaxseed, fruit, high-fiber cereals, olive oil, onions, psyllium, soy foods, vegetables, walnuts, and wheat germ.[14]

Prescription medications are another way to reduce LDL cholesterol but may have some undesirable side effects. Commonly prescribed statin drugs block the production of LDL cholesterol by blocking specific enzymes that produce LDL. Interestingly, some researchers speculate that statin drugs "work not so much by lowering cholesterol but rather by reducing arterial inflammation."[15]

GINGER HAS MULTIPLE ACTIONS THAT CAN HELP OUR HEART AND BLOOD VESSELS

Although more controlled human studies are needed, it is interesting that ginger can also benefit our circulatory system.

- One study using mice showed that a standardized extract of ginger helped prevent LDL cholesterol from being oxidized and, in turn, significantly reduced the development of atherosclerosis.[16]
- Another study showed that ginger reduces cholesterol levels by stimulating the conversion of cholesterol into bile acids.[17] Bile acts as a strong detergent to break down fats and cholesterol and is released into the digestive tract after eating foods that contain fat. About 95% of the bile is reabsorbed at the end of the small intestine, where it enters the bloodstream and is circulated back to the liver via the portal vein. The study also stated that curcumin (from turmeric) and capsaicin (abundant

in cayenne pepper) also reduced LDL cholesterol but probably by a different mechanism.

- A study using rabbits that were fed a high-cholesterol diet showed that dried ginger powder significantly reduced the development of atherosclerosis by about 50% over a 75-day period. While the dried ginger did *not* lower cholesterol by any significant amount, the study concluded that ginger's protective actions probably were a result of its antioxidant actions and some blood-thinning actions.[18] (An equivalent human dosage would be about 6 to 7 grams based on the weight of a 150-pound adult as compared to the weight and dosage used in the rabbit study.) Keep in mind that amounts of dried ginger powder over 2 grams per day are considered medicinal/therapeutic doses for which you should first consult your physician.

- On the other hand, one human study (using 4 grams of dried ginger powder per day for 3 months) showed that dried ginger did *not* lower cholesterol and did *not* thin the blood in patients with coronary artery disease; however, 1 single dose of 10 grams of powdered ginger had significant blood-thinning effects.[19]

> Note: When ginger is dried, the gingerols in fresh ginger are transformed into shogaols, which give dried ginger powder different properties from fresh ginger.[20] The variations of gingerols and shogaols in extracts and dried powder may be one reason for conflicting results of various studies. Both fresh and dried ginger are helpful in different ways.

TURMERIC AND CURCUMIN CAN HELP

Turmeric, ginger's botanical cousin, contains the compound curcumin, which was also found to lower oxidized cholesterol and increase HDL in human volunteers. In the study, 500 milligrams of curcumin per day were used for 7 days.[21] Alzheimer's disease has been linked to high levels of cholesterol within neurons (nerve cells).[22] It is interesting that curcumin is being aggressively researched for possible treatment of Alzheimer's.

OPEN UP THE OATMEAL!

It has been proven since the early 1980s that oats and oat bran can reduce LDL cholesterol.[23] Over 40 studies are listed at www.quakeroatmeal.com.[24]

Oatmeal is a unique grain in that its bran and germ are retained in the final rolled-oat product. The bran and germ contain most of the nutrients.[25] Other processed grains such as wheat are commonly stripped of the bran and germ.

For breakfast, I like to eat finely rolled oats with cinnamon sprinkled on top. I shake the bowl so the cinnamon sifts down through the oatmeal, then I add cold water. I prefer it uncooked—it tastes kind of like cookie dough. I like to add fruit such as sliced banana, fresh pineapple, kiwi, or whatever fruit or topping is on hand. Applesauce also can add some flavor.

Here is another way to enjoy oatmeal: First, put some frozen fruit (blueberries, cherries, etc.) in a bowl. Next, add some water and let it sit for 10 to 15 minutes so the fruit thaws out a bit, then add oatmeal and maybe some oat bran and kasha (we will learn more about kasha shortly). Lastly, sprinkle on some cinnamon, give it a shake, then add the rest of the water. Feel free to add some more fruit or fruit topping.

Oat bran works even better at removing LDL cholesterol than rolled oats because the bran contains more water-soluble fiber (called beta-glucan)—the sticky gel that makes cooked oatmeal so gooey. The water-soluble fiber and other compounds in oat bran act like a stickey sponge, picking up extra cholesterol from the digestive tract and moving it out of the body.[26] You may want to sprinkle some oat bran on your cereal, oatmeal, and other foods. Oat bran can also be mixed in with casseroles and ground-meat dishes.

BRING ON THE BARLEY AND BUCKWHEAT!

According to James Duke, author of *The Green Pharmacy*, barley may work even better than oats at lowering LDL cholesterol because it has up to 3 times more water-soluble fiber. Legumes such as lentils and kidney beans also have significant amounts of water-soluble fiber and can help lower cholesterol.[27]

Barley is most well-known for use in soups, but it can also be substituted for rice in some recipes. Barley flour can be substituted for up to one-third of the flour in bread and muffin recipes. Barley is one of the oldest grains known to man. Wheat bran and rice bran, although not water soluble, have many other beneficial properties.

Buckwheat is another superfood because it is loaded with rutin.[28] Rutin is a phytochemical known since the 1940s to help strengthen the blood vessels.[29] More recent studies show that rutin also relaxes the blood vessels[30] and has antitumor actions.[31] Rutin is a potent antioxidant and is also available as a supplement. Quercetin, a similar phytochemical to rutin, also relaxes the blood vessels.[32] Quercetin is abundant in apples, onions and onion skins, berries, tea, grapes, and red wine.

James Duke also recommends rutin for people with varicose veins. Rutin is present in buckwheat, onion skins, violets, and pansies (yes, you can eat these flowers), according to Duke, who heartily recommends eating a few of these flowers each day as colorful additions to salads. Duke also recommends eating kasha, a cereal-type product made by roasting buckwheat. Onion skins can be cooked with soups, then the skins removed before eating.[33] I found kasha at a local natural foods store for under $3 a pound. I enjoy mixing it with my oatmeal and sprinkling it on salads. I also enjoy making and eating buckwheat pancakes from time to time.

When I was a child, my father once planted buckwheat in a portion of our garden in order to make the soil richer. (We did not eat it because we did not know of its tremendous benefits.) My father was a picture of health (other than smoking). Little did I know that buckwheat contained the very phytochemical that might have prevented a sudden aneurysm in his brain. He died at the young age of 51. (An aneurysm occurs when a weakened blood vessel balloons and in many cases, suddenly ruptures). Looking back, I believe the E-F-G approach and a diet containing some buckwheat could have prevented his early death back in 1981.

ANTIOXIDANTS HELP OUR BLOOD VESSELS

In addition to oxidizing fats in our blood and forming plaque, free radicals also attack the blood vessels, causing the plaque to stick to their inner walls. A proper balance between antioxidants and oxidants is required for the proper function of blood vessels.[34] Antioxidants act as fire extinguishers to snuff out free radicals, reducing oxidative damage and the buildup of plaque in our blood vessels.

The gingerols in fresh ginger are very potent antioxidants and appear to be one of the primary mechanisms for ginger's effectiveness in reducing the development of atherosclerosis in animal studies.[35] *Over 50 antioxidants have been identified in ginger, one of nature's richest sources of antioxidants.*[36]

Polyphenols, another important group of phytochemicals found in many natural foods, are also potent antioxidants. Polyphenols have amazing protective actions to strengthen our blood vessels and fight viruses and cancers. Over 200 different polyphenols have been identified. The most well-known polyphenols are found in green tea, apples, potatoes, brewed coffee, grapes, red wine made from grapes, nuts, blueberries, strawberries, cranberry, plums, cherries, peaches, pomegranates, raspberries, pears, and wheat bran.[37]

HIGH BLOOD PRESSURE

Another important risk factor for cardiovascular problems is high blood pressure. High blood pressure is dangerous because it increases the risk of heart attack and stroke. In animal studies, ginger extract was able to lower blood pressure and increase the size of blood vessels.[39]

Some general guidelines from the American Heart Association are the following:

- Normal blood pressure should be less than 120 mm-Hg (systolic) and less than 80 mm-Hg (diastolic). Systolic pressure is measured when the heart is pumping and diastolic when the heart is not pumping. (mm-Hg means millimeters of mercury, or the pressure required to raise a column of mercury in open atmosphere.)
- High blood pressure is above 140 mm-Hg (systolic) and above 90 mm-Hg (diastolic).[40]

Other ways to lower blood pressure are to reduce salt in your diet and to eat more potassium-rich foods, such as bananas, apricots, avocados, beans, cantaloupe, figs, potatoes, seedless raisins, unsalted tomato sauce, and winter squash. Too much sodium (salt) and not enough potassium can also cause *confusion, irritability, fatigue,* muscle cramps, abdominal bloating, and heart disease.[41]

GINGER HAS SOME BLOOD-THINNING ACTIONS

Blood must not be too thick or too thin. If blood is too thick, the platelets coagulate (clump together) too easily as happens when we eat too many fat-laden, unhealthy foods. This increases the risk of blood clots, heart attack, and stroke. (A heart attack occurs when blood to the heart muscle is severely reduced or stopped; a stroke occurs when a blood vessel feeding the brain bursts or becomes clogged, depriving brain cells of blood and oxygen). On the other hand, if blood is too thin it will not coagulate enough to seal off a cut or other injury. Proper balance is necessary.

One human study of 30 healthy adult volunteers showed that 5 grams of dry ginger powder helped protect against the blood-thickening effects of a fatty meal that contained 50 grams of fat.[42] We will consider amounts above 2 grams of dry ginger powder per day to be medicinal doses for which you should consult your physician.

Another human study involving women volunteers showed that just 5 grams of fresh ginger per day for 7 days was effective in reducing blood platelet thromboxane.[43] Thromboxane is a chemical regulator that causes the blood to coagulate (get thicker and clump together) and the blood vessels to constrict (get narrower). Another name for harmful blood clotting is thrombosis, as when a blood clot develops in a vein or artery, often in the leg. (*Thrombus* is another name for a blood clot.) This is a dangerous condition, especially if the blood clot travels to the heart or brain, which can lead to heart attack or stroke.

One research study in 1991 suggested using ginger extract and carbon dioxide for the treatment of Kawasaki disease, a condition in young children caused by a viral or other infection. Antigens from the infection attack the wall of the blood vessel and cause the blood to thicken, resulting in blood clots, heart attack, and aneurysm. (An aneurysm is when a blood vessel expands like a balloon and possibly bursts.) Vasculitis (inflammation and narrowing of the blood vessels) also occurs.[44] Other treatments have been developed for this disease.

There remains some disagreement as to what amounts of ginger begin to thin the blood. More human studies are needed to determine the extent of ginger's effectiveness. The E-F-G approach uses only small amounts (1 to 2 grams of dried powder and up to 15 grams of fresh ginger), which, according to many human studies, should not cause problems with over-thinning for most people. A 1994 study conducted in the United Kingdom showed that up to 2 grams of dried ginger powder in a 24-hour period was unlikely to cause blood platelet dysfunction.[45]

OTHER FOODS HAVE BLOOD-THINNING ACTIONS

Other foods and supplements that also act to thin the blood include garlic, onions,[46] curcumin (in turmeric),[47] olive oil,[48] *Ginkgo biloba* (in some cases, *Ginkgo biloba* caused spontaneous bleeding),[49] ginseng,[50] grape skins and grape seeds,[51] green tea,[52] soy sauce,[53] tomato extract,[54] quercetin (abundant in apples, onions, and onion skins),[55] vitamin E,[56] and, although not a food, moderate exercise can help thin the blood and strengthen the cardiovascular system in healthy people. However, very strenuous exercise has the opposite effect and causes the blood to thicken.[57] An additional advantage of regular exercise is that it can also increase the level of good HDL cholesterol in some people.[58] Omega-3 essential fatty acids including flax and fish oils also have some blood-thinning actions[59] and can improve the overall function of blood vessels.[60]

SOME CAUTIONS TO KEEP IN MIND

Consult your physician if you are pregnant or taking medications before taking ginger. Refer to the cautions in chapter 10. Remember that ginger can increase or decrease the effect of some medications.

- Do not use ginger if you are anticipating surgery.
- Do not attempt to use ginger or the E-F-G approach in place of prescribed blood-thinning medications such as warfarin.
- Consult your physician before taking ginger if you are taking aspirin or other blood-thinning medications. Three studies reported no findings of interactions between warfarin and ginger.[61] (Warfarin is a very common blood-thinning medication. It is a synthetic form of a chemical first identified in sweet clover plants in the 1940s.)[62] However, one study (a database search) did report cerebral hemorrhage (bleeding in the brain) due to interaction between warfarin and *Ginkgo biloba*. The study also reported a few cases of hemorrhage and bleeding in patients taking just *Ginkgo biloba* alone or just garlic alone (with no warfarin).[63]
- One study reported complications while taking ginger products: a 76-year-old white European woman who was using phenprocoumon (a blood thinner commonly used in Europe,

slightly different from warfarin) reported excess blood thinning, but her blood returned to normal after she stopped using ginger products and was given vitamin K1.[64] Since the heart and blood vessels are extremely important, you and your medical practitioner must decide what is best for you.

- Omega-3 EFAs in flaxseed oil and fish oil can also help thin the blood; however, there do not appear to be any clinical trials involving increased blood loss while taking omega-3 supplements.[65]
- Proteolytic enzyme supplements that have an enteric coating have some blood-thinning effects and should not be used by anyone with clotting disorders such as hemophilia, those on dialysis, those who are going to have (or just had) surgery, those on blood-thinning medications, and women who are pregnant or breast-feeding.[66]

IF YOU'RE INTERESTED ...

Here are some studies from around the world relating to ginger's blood-thinning action:

1979, Cornell Medical School (New York)—human study: A medical researcher, while routinely testing his own blood, noticed it did not clump together easily. By a process of elimination, he discovered it had been caused by the ginger marmalade he loved. After further testing, he confirmed that a ginger extract inhibited platelet aggregation.[67]

1984, Srivastava, K. C. (Denmark)—lab study: Aqueous (liquid) extracts of onion, garlic, and fresh ginger were shown to inhibit platelet aggregation. Ginger's effects were the strongest of the 3 foods and were dose dependent. If the same actions take place in the body, then onion, garlic, and ginger could be useful as natural antithrombotic (anticoagulation) supplements.[68]

1986, Srivastava, K. C. (Denmark)—lab study: Aqueous (liquid) components extracted from *fresh* ginger inhibited platelet thromboxane formation and platelet aggregation in the lab.[69] (Thromboxane is released by blood platelets and acts to thicken the blood.)

1989, Srivastava, K. C. (Denmark)—human study: Danish women who consumed 5 grams of *fresh* ginger daily for 7 days had significantly reduced platelet thromboxane production in blood samples.[70]

1993, Verma, S. K., Singh, J., Khamesra, R., and Bordia, A. (India)—human study: Ten healthy individuals were given 5 grams of dry ginger powder daily in 2 divided doses along with 100 grams of butter. The dry ginger powder significantly inhibited chemical-induced platelet aggregation.[71]

1994, Lumb (United Kingdom)—human study: Up to 2 grams of dry ginger powder had no measurable effect on bleeding time and platelet function of 8 healthy male volunteers.[72]

1995, Guh, J. H., Ko, F. N., Jong, T. T., and Teng, C. M. (Taiwan)—animal study: Gingerol (most abundant in *fresh* ginger) inhibited aggregation of blood platelets in rabbits. It is concluded that gingerol inhibits thromboxane formation by the platelets.[73]

1996, Janssen, P. L., Meyboom, S., van Staveren, W. A., de Vegt, F., and Katan, M. B. (Netherlands)—human study: This study could not confirm that eating 15 grams of *fresh* ginger daily for 2 weeks had any effect on platelet thromboxane production in humans. Also, it could not confirm that eating 40 grams of cooked stem ginger every day for 2 weeks had any effect on platelet thromboxane production in humans. The study involved 18 healthy volunteers.[74]

1997, Bordia, A., Verma, S. K., and Srivastava, K. C. (India)— human study: A dose of 4 grams of dried ginger taken daily for 3 months did not affect chemical-induced platelet aggregation in patients with coronary artery disease. However, a single dose of 10 grams of dried ginger powder significantly reduced platelet aggregation that was induced by 2 chemical compounds.[75]

1998, Bhandari, U., Sharma, J. N., and Zafar, R. (India)—animal study: Rabbits fed ginger extract along with a high cholesterol diet for 10 weeks showed a lower degree of atherosclerosis than the rabbits that had not been given ginger extract.[76]

2001, Verma, S. K., and Bordia, A. (India)—human study: A dose of 5 grams of dried ginger powder consumed with a fatty meal (50 grams of fat) not only counteracted the blood-thickening effect of the fatty meal but also significantly increased blood-thinning activity in 30 healthy adult volunteers. This demonstrates the therapeutic potential of ginger.[77]

2001, Koo, K. L., Ammit, A. J., Tran, V. H., Duke, C. C., and Roufogalis, B. D. (Australia)—lab study: Synthetic gingerols helped prevent chemical-induced blood coagulation in a dose range similar to aspirin.[78] (Gingerols are abundant in fresh ginger).

2002, Thomson, M., Al-Qattan, K. K., Al-Sawab, S. M., Alnaqeeb, M. A., Khan, I., and Ali, M. (Kuwait)—animal study: Results suggest that ginger extract (in large enough doses) could be used as a "cholesterol-lowering, antithrombotic, and anti-inflammatory agent."[79]

2003, Nurtjahja-Tjendraputra, E., Ammit, A. J., Roufogalis, B. D., Tran, V. H., and Duke, C. C. (Australia)—lab study: Gingerols, shogaols, and other compounds in ginger are more potent anticoagulation agents than aspirin under the conditions of the study.[80] (Gingerols are most abundant in fresh ginger but are transformed into shogaols upon drying. Shogaols are most abundant in dried ginger powder).

2004, Kruth, P., Brosi, E., Fux, R., Morike, K., and Gleiter, C. H. (Germany)—human study: A 76-year-old white European woman taking the blood-thinning medication phenprocoumon also began using ginger products, which resulted in too much blood thinning. Her blood returned to normal after she stopped using ginger products and was given vitamin K1 supplements.[81] (Vitamin K1 acts to thicken the blood.)

2009, Nicoll R, Henein MY.—review of recent trials: "Human trials have been few and generally used a low dose with inconclusive results, however dosages of 5 g or more demonstrated significant anti-platelet activity. More human trials are needed using an appropriate dosage of a standardized extract. Should these prove positive, ginger has the potential to offer not only a cheaper natural alternative to conventional agents but one with significantly lower side effects."[82]

CHAPTER 19

1.   "Leading Causes of Death in Females, United States, 2003." "Leading Causes of Death in Males, United States, 2003." Web site: Centers for Disease Control. Accessed 8/30/2007. <http://www.cdc.gov/women/lcod,htm>. <http://www.cdc.gov/men/lcod,htm>.

2.   "Stroke Facts and Statistics." Web site: U.S. Center for Disease Control. Accessed 8/31/2007. <http://www.cdc.gov/stroke/stroke_facts.htm>.

3a.   Jialal I, Devaraj S. "The role of oxidized low density lipoprotein in atherogenesis." *J Nutr.* 1996 Apr;126(4 Suppl):1053S-7S.

3b.   Frei B. "Cardiovascular disease and nutrient antioxidants: role of low-density lipoprotein oxidation." *Crit Rev Food Sci Nutr.* 1995 Jan;35(1-2):83-98.

3c.   Schwartz CJ, Valente AJ, Sprague EA, Kelley JL, Nerem RM. "The pathogenesis of atherosclerosis: an overview." *Clin Cardiol.* 1991 Feb;14(2 Suppl 1):I1-6.

3d.   DiCorleto PE, Chisolm GM 3rd. "Participation of the endothelium in the development of the atherosclerotic plaque." *Prog Lipid Res.* 1986;25(1-4):365-74.

4.   Yung LM, Leung FP, Yao X, Chen ZY, Huang Y. "Reactive oxygen species in vascular wall." *Cardiovasc Hematol Disord Drug Targets.* 2006 Mar;6(1):1-19.

5a.   Liao F, Andalibi A, Qiao JH, Allayee H, Fogelman AM, Lusis AJ. "Genetic evidence for a common pathway mediating oxidative stress, inflammatory gene induction, and aortic fatty streak formation in mice." *J Clin Invest.* 1994 August; 94(2): 877-884.

5b.   Mi-Kyung Chang, M.D. "Oxidized lipids and programmed cell death in atherosclerosis." Web site: Tobacco-Related Disease Research Program. Accessed 9/7/2007. <www.trdrp.org/fundedresearch/Views/Grant_Page. asp?grant_id=1552>.

6a.   Aftab J. Ahmed, Ph.D. "C-REACTIVE PROTEIN, a Coronary Trojan Horse." Web site: BuyWobenzym.com. Accessed 10/2/2007. <http://buywobenzym.com/article.cfm?PID=1&AID=39>.

6b.   Tohgi H, Konno S, Takahashi S, Koizumi D, Kondo R, Takahashi H. "Activated coagulation/fibrinolysis system and platelet function in acute thrombotic stroke patients with increased C-reactive protein levels." *Thromb Res.* 2000 Dec 1;100(5):373-9.

7.   Budwig, Johanna . *Flax Oil as a True Aid Against Arthritis, Heart Infarction, Cancer and Other Diseases.* Apple Publishing Co. Ltd. 1994. pp.10-11, 30-31.

8.   "Two Sources of Cholesterol" Web site: American Heart Association. Accessed 2/10/2009.http://www.americanheart.org/print_presenter. jhtml?identifier=3046105>.

9a.   Jialal I, Devaraj S. "The role of oxidized low density lipoprotein in atherogenesis." *J Nutr.* 1996 Apr;126(4 Suppl):1053S-7S.

9b.   Witztum JL. Steonberg D. "Role of oxidized low density lipoprotein in atherogenesis." *J Clin Invest.* 1991 Dec;88(6):1785-92.

9c.   Schwartz CJ, Valente AJ, Sprague EA, Kelly JL, Nerem RM. "The pathogenesis of atherosclerosis: an overview." *Clin Cardiol.* 1991 Feb;14(2 Suppl 1):I1-16.

10.   "High Blood Cholesterol: What You Need To Know". Web site: U.S. Department of Health and Human Services. Accessed 2/13/2009. <http:// www.nhlbi.nih.gov>.

11.   "High Blood Cholesterol: What You Need To Know". Web site: U.S. Department of Health and Human Services. Accessed 2/13/2009. <http:// www.nhlbi.nih.gov>.

12.   William S. Harris, PhD. "Omega-3 Fatty Acids and Cardiovascular Disease: A Case for Omega-3 Index as a New Risk Factor." *Pharmacol Res.* 2007 March 55(3): 217-223.

13.   James A. Duke, Ph.D. *The Green Pharmacy.* Rodale Press, Inc. Emmaus, PA. 1998. pp.256-261.

14.   Richard Trubo, Mary Carroll. *Chloesterol Cures.* Rodale Press, Inc. 1997. pp.17, 25,27, 41, 52, 64, 87, 91, 94, 96, 97, 111, 147, 151, 160, 171, 187, 188, 198, 204.

15.   Michael F. Roizen MD, Mehmet C. Oz MD. "Dangerous Medical Myths" *Bottom Line health.* Volume 19, Number 9, September 2005.

16.   Fuhrman B, Rosenblat M, Hayek T, Coleman R. Aviram M. "Ginger Extract Consumption Reduces Plasma Cholesterol, Inhibits LDL Oxidation and Attenuates Development of Atherosclerosis in Atherosclerotic, Apolipoprotein E-Deficient Mice." *Journal of Nutrition.* 2000;130:1124-1131.

17. Srinivasan K, Sambaiah K. "The effect of spices on cholesterol 7 alpha-hydroxylase activity and on serum and hepatic cholesterol levels in the rat." *Int J Vitam Nutr Res*. 1991;61(4):364-9.

18. Verma SK, Singh M, Jain P, Bordia A. "Protective effect of ginger, Zingiber officinale Rosc on experimental atherosclerosis in rabbits." *Indian J Exp Biol*. 2004 Jul;42(7):736-8.

19. Bordia A, Verma SK, Srivastava KC. "Effect of ginger (Zingiber officinale Rosc.) and fenugreek (Trigonella foenumgraecum L.) on blood lipids, blood sugar and platelet aggregation in patients with coronary artery disease." *Prostaglandins Leukot Essent Fatty Acids*. 1997 May;56(5):379-84.

20. Bhattarai S, Tran VH, Duke CC. "The stability of gingerol and shogaol in aqueous solutions." *J Pharm Sci*. 2001 Oct;90(10):1658-64.

21. Soni KB, Kuttan R. "Effect of oral curcumin administration on serum peroxides and cholesterol levels in human volunteers." *Indian J Physiol Pharmacol*. 1992 Oct;36(4):273-5.

22. Puglielli L, Tanzi RE, Kovacs DM. "Alzheimer's disease: the cholesterol connection." *Nat Neurosci*. 2003 Apr;6(4):345-51.

23a. Anderson JW, Story L, Sieling B, Chen WJ, Petro MS, Story J. "Hypercholesterolemic effects of oat-bran or bean intake for hypercholesterolemic men." *American Journal of Clinical Nutrition*. 1984: Volume 40, pp.1146-1155.

23b. Kirby RW, et al. "Oat-Bran Intake Selectively Lowers Serum Low-Density Lipoprotein Cholesterol Concentrations of Hypercholesterolemic Men." *American Journal of Clinical Nutrition*. 1981: Volume 34, pp.824-828.

24. "Oats and Cholesterol Lowering - Summary of Studies." Web site: Quaker Oatmeal. Accessed 10/3/2007. <http://quakeroatmeal.com/qo_HealthProfessionals/heartHealth/index.cfm>.

25. Salene Yeager. *The Doctors Book of Food Remedies*. Rodale Press, Inc. Emmaus, PA. 1998. p.374.

26. Selene Yeager. *The Doctors Book of Food Remedies*. Rodale Press, Inc. Emmaus, PA. 1998. pp.374-376.

27. James A. Duke, Ph.D. *The Green Pharmacy*. Rodale Press, Inc. Emmaus, PA. 1998. pp.256-261.

28. "Buckwheat" Web site: whfoods.com. Accessed 1/27/2009. <http://www.whfoods.com/genpage...>.

29. Angus L. MacLean and Charles E. Brambel. "Dicumarol and Rutin in Vascular Disorders." *Trans Am Ophthalmol Soc*. 1946; 44 194-213.

30a. Zhou XM, Yao H, Xia ML, Cao CM, Jiang HD, Xia Q. "[Comparison of vasodilation effect between quercetin and rutin in the isolated rat thoracic aorta]" *Zhejiang Da Zue Xue Bao Yi Xue Ban*. 2006 Jan;35(1):29-33.

30b. Xia ML, Zhou XM, Yao H, Jiang HD, Bruce IC, Wei EQ, Xia Q. "Rutin-induced endothelium vasorelaxation in rat aortic Rings and the underlying mechanism." *Conf Proc IEEE Eng Med Biol Soc.* 2005;6:5595-7.

31.   C. Guruvayoorappan and Girija Kuttan. "Antiangiogenic Effect of Rutin and its Regulatory Effect on the Production of VEGF, IL-1beta and TNF-alpha in Tumor Associated Macrophages." *Journal of Biological Sciences.* 7 (8): 1511-1519, 2007.

32.   Zhou XM, Yao H, Xia ML, Cao CM, Jiang HD, Xia Q. "[Comparison of vasodilation effect between quercetin and rutin in the isolated rat thoracic aorta]" *Zhejiang Da Zue Xue Bao Yi Xue Ban.* 2006 Jan;35(1):29-33.

33.   Duke JA. *The Green Pharmacy.* Rodale Press, Emmaus, PA. 1997 pp.446-447.

34a. Rojas A, Figueroa H, Morales MA, Re L. "Facing up the ROS labyrinth-- Where to go?" *Curr Vasc Pharmacol.* 2006 Jul;4(3):277-89.

34b. Aviram M. "Macrophage foam cell formation during early atherogenesis is determined by the balance between pro-oxidants and antioxidants in arterial cells and blood lipoproteins." *Antioxid Redox Signal.* 1999 Winter;1(4):585-94.

35a. Liu N, Huo G, Zhang L, Zhang X. "[Effect of Zingiber Officinale Rosc on lipid peroxidation in hyperlipidemia rats]." *Wei Sheng Yan Jiu.* 2003 Jan;32(1):22-3. [Article in Chinese].

35b. Fuhrman B, Rosenblat M, Hayek T, Coleman R. Aviram M. "Ginger Extract Consumption Reduces Plasma Cholesterol, Inhibits LDL Oxidation and Attenuates Development of Atherosclerosis in Atherosclerotic, Apolipoprotein E-Deficient Mice." *Journal of Nutrition.* 2000;130:1124-1131.

36.   Masuda Y, Kikuzaki H, Hisamoto M, Nakatani N. "Antioxidant properties of gingerol related compounds from ginger." *Biofactors.* 2004;21(1-4):293-6.

37.   Jean Carper. *The Food Pharmacy.* Bantam Books, New York, NY. 1988. pp.84-90.

38.   Not used.

39a. Ghayur MN, Gilani AH, Afridi M, Houghton PJ. "Cardiovascular effects of ginger aqueous extract and its phenolic constituents are mediated through multiple pathways." *Vascul Pharmacol.* 2005 Oct;43(4):234-41. Epub 2005 Sep 12.

39b. Ghayur MN, Gilani AH. "Ginger lowers blood pressure through blockade of voltage-dependent calcium channels." *J Cardiovasc Pharmacol.* 2005 Jan;45(1):74-80.

40.   "What is High Blood Pressure?" Web site: American Heart Association. Accessed 2/13/2009. <http://www.americanheart.org/presenter.jhtml?identifier=2112>.

41.   "potassium" Web site: whfoods.org. Accessed 4/2/2010. <http://www.whfoods.com/genpage...>

42.   Verma SK, Bordia A. "Ginger, fat and fibrinolysis." *Indian J Med Sci.* 2001 Feb;55(2):83-6.

43. Srivastava KC. "Effect of onion and ginger consumption on platelet thromb-axane production in humans." *Prostaglandins Leukot Essent Fatty Acids.* 1989 Mar;35(3):183-5.

44. Backon J. "Implication of thromboxane in the pathogenesis of Kawasaki disease and a suggestion for using novel thromboxane synthetase inhibitors in its treatment." *Med Hypotheses.* 1991 Mar;34(3)230-1.

45. Lumb AB. "Effect of dried ginger on human platelet function." *Thromb Haemost.* 1994 Jan;71(1):110-1.

46. Srivastava KC. "Aqueous extracts of onion, garlic and ginger inhibit platelet aggregation and alter arachidonic acid metabolism." *Biomed Biochim Acta.* 1984;43(8-9):S335-46.

47a. Shah BH, Nawaz Z, Pertani SA, Roomi A, Mahmood H, Saeed SA, Gilani AH. "Inhibitory effect of Curcumin, a food spice from turmeric, on platelet-activating factor- and arachidonic acid-mediated platelet aggregation through inhibition of thromboxane formation and Ca2+ signaling." *Biochem Pharmacol.* 1999 Oct 1;58(7):1167-72.

47b. Srivastava KC, Bordia A, Verma SK. "Curcumin, a major component of food spice turmeric (Curcuma longa) inhibits aggregation and alters eicosanoid metabolism in human blood platelets." *Prostaglandins Leukot Essent Fatty Acids.* 1995 Apr;52(4):223-7.

48. Larsen LF, Jaspersen J, Marckmann P. "Are olive oil diets antithrombotic? Diets enriched with olive, rapeseed, or sunflower oil affect postprandial factor VII differently." *The American Journal of Clinical Nutrition.* 70(6), 1999, pages 976-982.

49. Bent S, Goldberg H, Padula A, Avins A. "Spontaneous Bleeding Associated with Ginkgo biloba." *J Gen Intern Med.* 2005 July; 20(7):657-661.

50. Teng CM, Kuo SC, Ko FN, Lee JC, Lee LG, Chen SC, Huang TF. "Antiplatelet actions of panaxynol and ginsenosides isolated from ginseng." *Biochim Biophys Acta.* 1989 Mar 24;990(3):315-20.

51. Shanmuganayagam D, Beahm MR, Osman HE, Krueger CG, Reed JD, Folts JD. "Grape Seed and Grape Skin Extracts Elicit a Greater Antiplatelet Effect When Used in Combination than When Used Individually in Dogs and Humans." *J. Nutr.* 132:3592-3598, December 2002.

52. Lill G, Voit S, Schror K, Weber AA. "Complex effects of different green tea catechins on human platelets." *FEBS Lett.* 2003 Jul 10;546(2-3):265-70.

53. Tsuchiya H, Sato M, Watanabe I. "Antiplatelet activity of soy sauce as functional seasoning." *J Agric Food Chem.* 1999 Oct;47(10):4167-74.

54. O'Kennedy N, Crosbie L, Whelan S, Luther V, Horgan G, Broom JI, Webb DJ, Duttaroy AK. "Effects of tomato extract on platelet function: a double-blinded crossover study in healthy humans." *Am J Clin Nutr.* 2006 Sep;84(3):561-9.

55a. Hubbard GP, Wolffram S, de Vos R, Bovy A, Gibbins JM, Lovegrove JA.

"Investigation of onion soup high in quercetin inhibits platelet aggregation and essential components of the collagen-stimulated platelet activation pathway in man: a pilot study." *Br J Nutr.* 2006 Sep;96(3):482-8.

55b. Hubbard GP, Wolffram S, Lovegrove JA, Gibbons JM. "Ingestion of quercetin inhibits platelet aggregation and essential components of the collagen-stimulated platelet activation pathway in humans." *J Thromb Haemost.* 2004 Dec;2(12):2138-45.

56a. Stuart MJ, Oski FA. "Vitamin E and platelet function." *Am J Pediatr Hematol Oncol.* 1979 Spring;1(1):77-82.

56b. Freedman JE, Keaney JF Jr. "Vitamin E Inhibition of Platelet Aggregation Is Independent of Antioxidant Activity." *Journal of Nutrition.* 2001;131:374S-377S.

57a. Imhof A, Koenig W. "Exercise and thrombosis." *Cardiol Clin.* 2001 Aug;19(3):389-400.

57b. Koenig W, Ernst E. "Exercise and thrombosis." *Coron Artery Dis.* 2000 Mar;11(2):123-7.

58. "Cholesterol". Web site: American Heart Association . Accessed 9/7/2007. <www.americanheart.org/print_presenter.jhtml?identifier=4488>.

59. Allman MA, Pena MM, Pang D. *Eur J Clin Nutr.* 1995 Mar;49(3):169-78.

60. Abeywardena MY, Head RJ. "Longchain n-3 polyunsaturated fatty acids and blood vessel function." *Cardiovasc Res.* 2001 Dec;52(3):361-71.

61a. Jiang X, Blair EY, McLachlan AJ. "Investigation of the effects of herbal medicines on warfarin response in healthy subjects: a population pharmacokinetic-pharmacodynamic modeling approach." *J Clin Pharmacol.* 2006 Nov;46(11):1370-8.

61b. Weidner MS, Sigwart K. "The safety of a ginger extract in the rat." *J Ethnopharmacol.* 2000 Dec;73(3):513-20.

61c. Vaes LP, Chyka PA. "Interactions of warfarin with garlic, ginger, ginkgo, or ginseng: nature of the evidence." *Ann Pharmacother.* 2000 Dec;34(12):1478-82.

62. Stahmann MA, Huebner CF, Link KP. "Studies on the hemorrhagic sweet clover disease. V. Identification and synthesis of the hemorrhagic agent." *J Biol Chem* . 1941;138:513-27 PDF. Accessed 9/6/2007. <http://www.jbc.org/cgi/reprint/138/2/513>.

63. Vaes LP, Chyka PA. "Interactions of warfarin with garlic, ginger, ginkgo, or ginseng: nature of the evidence." *Ann Pharmacother.* 2000 Dec;34(12):1478-82.

64. Kruth P, Brosi E, Fux R, Morike K, Gleiter CH. "Ginger-associated overanticoagulation by phenprocoumon." *Ann Pharmacother.* 2004 Feb;38(2):257-60. Epub 2003 Dec 19.

65a. Simopoulos AP. "Omega-3 fatty acids in health and disease and in growth and development." *Am J Clin Nutr.* 1991 Sep;54(3):438-63.

65b. Simopoulos AP. "Summary of the NATO advanced research workshop on dietary omega 3 and omega 6 fatty acids: biological effects and nutritional essentiality." *J Nutr.* 1989 Apr;119(4):521-8.

66. Cichoke A. *The Complete Book of Enzyme Therapy.* New York, Avery, 1999. p.44.

67. Dorso CR, Levin RI, Eldor A, Jaffe EA, Weksler BB. "Chinese food and platelets." *N Engl J Med.* 1980 Sep 25;303(13):756-7.

68. Srivastava KC. "Aqueous extracts of onion, garlic and ginger inhibit platelet aggregation and alter arachidonic acid metabolism." *Biomed Biochim Acta.* 1984;43(8-):S335-46.

69. Srivastava KC. "Isolation and effects of some ginger components of platelet aggregation and eicosanoid biosynthesis." *Prosataglandins Leukot Med.* 1986 Dec;25(2-3):187-98.

70. Srivastava KC. "Effect of onion and ginger consumption on platelet thromboxane production in humans." *Prostaglandins Leukot Essent Fatty Acids.* 1989 Mar;35(3):183-5.

71. Verma SK, Singh J, Khamesra R, Bordia. "Effect of ginger on platelet aggregation in man." *Indian J Med Res.* 1993 Oct;98:240-2.

72. Lumb AB. "Effect of dried ginger on human platelet function." *Thromb Haemost.* 1994 Jan;71(1):110-1.

73. Guh JH, Ko FN, Jong TT, Teng CM. "Antiplatelet effect of gingerol isolated from Zingiber officinale." *J Pharm Pharmacol.* 1995 Apr;47(4):329-32.

74. Janssen PL, Meyboom S, van Staveren WA, de Vegt F, Katan MB. "Consumption of ginger (Zingiber officinale roscoe) does not affect ex vivo platelet thromboxane production in humans." *Eur J Clin Nutr.* 1996 Nov;50(11):772-4.

75. Bordia A, Verma SK, Srivastava KC. "Effect of ginger (Zingiber officinale Rosc.) and fenugreek (Trigonella foenumgraecum L.) on blood lipids, blood sugar and platelet aggregation in patients with coronary artery disease." *Prostaglandins Leukot Essent Fatty Acids.* 1997 May;56(5):379-84.

76. Bhandari U, Sharma JN, Zafar R. "The protective action of ethanolic ginger (Zingiber officinale) extract in cholesterol fed rabbits." *J Ethnopharmacol.* 1998 Jun;61(2):167-71.

77. Verma SK, Bordia A. "Ginger, fat and fibrinolysis." *Indian J Med Sci.* 2001 Feb;55(2):83-6.

78. Koo KL, Ammit AJ, Tran VH, Duke CC, Roufogalis BD. "Gingerols and related analogues inhibit arachidonic acid-induced human platelet serotonin release and aggregation." *Thromb Res.* 2001 Sep 1;103(5):387-97.

79. Thomson M, Al-Qattan KK, Al-Sawan SM, Alnaqeeb MA, Khan I, Ali M. "The use of ginger (Zingiber officinale Rosc.) as a potential anti-inflammatory and antithrombotic agent." *Prostaglandins Leukot Essent Fatty Acids.* 2002 Dec;67(6):475-8.

80. Nurtjahha-Thendraputra E, Ammit AJ, Roufogalis BD, Tran VH, Duke CC. "Effective anti-platelet and COX-1 enzyme inhibitors from pungent constituents of ginger." *Thromb Res.* 2003;111(4-5):259-65.

81. Kruth P, Brosi E, Fux R, Morike K, Gleiter CH. "Ginger-associated overanticoagulation by phenprocoumon." *Ann Pharmacother.* 2004 Feb;38(2):257-60. Epub 2003 Dec 19.

82. Nicoll R, Henein MY. "Ginger (Zingiber officinale Roscoe): a hot remedy for cardiovascular disease?" *Int J Cardiol.* 2009 Jan 24;131(3):408-9. Epub 2007 Nov 26.

CHAPTER 20

Ginger's Antinausea Actions

G INGER'S well-known claim to fame throughout history has been its ability to help calm upset stomachs. It is not surprising that ginger was grown aboard ancient Chinese ships[1]—obviously for the benefit of sailors' queasy tummies, although I'm sure its rich supply of vitamin C was an added bonus against scurvy. Because much information is available on ginger's ability to calm upset stomachs, we will limit this chapter to some main points and a few interesting studies.

PREGNANCY-RELATED NAUSEA AND VOMITING

A 2001 survey among obstetricians and gynecologists in the United States reported that 51.8% of those physicians had recommended ginger for treatment of moderate nausea during pregnancy.[2]

From the available literature and the historical use of ginger, it appears that a few small slices of fresh ginger per day during pregnancy is safe for short periods (several days) unless there is a history of miscarriage, in which case ginger should be avoided. Alternately, 1 or 2 cups of ginger tea per day could be taken as allowed by your medical practitioner. One source states that the amount of ginger used in tea is about 250 mg.[3] One reference recommends eating small, frequent meals that are rich in carbohydrates and low in fat. This strategy may help reduce the occurrence of nausea.[4]

The American Herbal Products Association (AHPA) gives *fresh* ginger a class 1 safety rating, meaning it is safe with appropriate use over a wide dosage range. Dried ginger is rated class 2b and 2d. The class 2b rating means it should not be used during pregnancy unless directed by a professional with expertise in the use of ginger during pregnancy. The class 2d rating means there are other restrictions according to professional guidance. [5.]

Here are the results of 2 major overviews of available literature from past studies and trials:

- The first overview concluded "ginger appears to be a fairly low-risk and effective treatment for nausea and vomiting associated with pregnancy" when given in low doses for patients who did not respond to other first-line therapies. The study did express concerns over product quality due to limited regulation of dietary supplements. [6]
- The second overview of 6 controlled trials concluded ginger was either superior to a placebo at relieving nausea and vomiting or as effective as the reference drug vitamin B6. [7] Vitamin B6, also known as pyridoxine hydrochloride, [8] is known to reduce the severity of nausea and vomiting during pregnancy.

Also, one reference cites the bacteria *Helicobacter pylori* as a possible cause of nausea and vomiting during pregnancy. [9] (Remember from chapter 18 that ginger can help fight against this bacteria.)

Most experts agree that larger studies are needed to determine the safety of ginger, the best forms of ginger to use, and proper doses. No adverse conditions have been reported for the small doses used in the studies.

Here are some more studies relating to ginger and pregnancy-related nausea:

- A 1991 landmark study of 30 pregnant women with hyperemesis gravidarum (severe nausea and vomiting) was conducted by the University of Copenhagen in Denmark. The

women were given 250 milligrams of dry ginger powder 4
times a day (equal to 1 gram a day). Ginger was given for only
4 days. Over 70% of the women preferred the time period in
which they received ginger. No adverse effects on pregnancy
outcome were observed as a result of using ginger in the
study.[10]

- In Thailand, a study of 70 pregnant women with nausea and
vomiting was performed by the Chiang Mai University. Of the
group that was given 250 mg of dry ginger powder 4 times a
day for 4 days, 87% reported improvement in nausea symptoms. No adverse effects on pregnancy outcome were detected.
(One 250 mg capsule was given after each meal and one at bed
time). This study was reported in 2001.[11]

- A study in the United States in 2002 involved 26 women with
nausea and vomiting in their first trimester who were given
1 tablespoon of ginger *syrup* 4 times a day mixed with 4 to
8 ounces of water (equivalent to 1 gram of ginger per day).
Other women in the study were given a placebo 4 times a day.
After 6 days, 67% of the women who received the ginger syrup
and water had stopped vomiting. After 9 days, 77% of the
women who received ginger syrup reported decreased nausea.
The study lasted for 2 weeks.[12]

- A larger Australian study involved 120 woman with morning
sickness who were less than 20 weeks pregnant were given 125
milligrams of ginger extract divided and given 4 times a day
for 4 days. (The ginger extract was equivalent to 1.5 grams of
dried ginger per day.) Other women in the study were given a
placebo 4 times a day. Nausea and retching were reduced for
the women who received the ginger extract although vomiting
was not significantly reduced. Follow-up of the babies showed
normal birth weight and no adverse effects. This study was
reported in 2003.[13] (Retching is attempting to vomit without
anything coming up).

- A study of 138 women in Thailand with nausea and vomiting

due to pregnancy were given either 500 mg of ginger in capsules or 10 mg of vitamin B6, 3 times a day for 3 days. Nausea and vomiting were significantly reduced in both groups. Ginger and vitamin B6 produced similar results for reducing nausea and vomiting. This study was reported in 2003.[14] The exact form of ginger used (powder, extract, etc) was not specifically stated in the abstract of this study.

- A Canadian study involving 187 women who took ginger during their first trimester of pregnancy concluded that "ginger does not appear to increase the rates of major malformations above the baseline rate of 1% to 3% and that it has a mild effect in the treatment of NVP" (NVP is short for nausea and vomiting of pregnancy). The women in this study were permitted to use different forms of ginger including dried powder and ginger tea. Birth weights in the ginger group were a bit less than in the group that did not receive ginger. This study was reported in 2003.[15]

- A large Australian study involving 291 women who were less than 16 weeks pregnant showed that ginger was as effective as vitamin B6 in reducing nausea, vomiting, and retching. Women were given either a capsule of 350 mg of ginger 3 times a day (1.05 grams total per day) or 25 mg of vitamin B6, also 3 times a day. The study lasted 3 weeks.[16] The exact form of ginger used (dried powder, extract, etc.) was not specified.

- A study conducted in Thailand in 2005 involved 170 pregnant women who had symptoms of nausea and vomiting. Half of the women received 500 mg of dry ginger powder twice a day. The other half were given 50 mg of dimenhydrinate twice daily. The study lasted 7 days. The study concluded, "Ginger is as effective as dimenhydrinate in the treatment of nausea and vomiting during pregnancy and has fewer side effects."[17] (Dimenhydrinate is an antihistamine medication used to prevent nausea, vomiting, and dizziness caused by motion sickness. Antihistamine medications are also used to reduce

allergy-related reactions such as congestion, sneezing, itching
and runny nose).

- Another study in Thailand involved 126 women who were less
  than 16 weeks pregnant who had nausea and vomiting. They
  were given either 650 mg of dried ginger powder 3 times a
  day or 25 mg of vitamin B6, also 3 times a day, before meals.
  The study lasted 4 days. Both supplements were effective in
  reducing nausea and vomiting but ginger was more effective than vitamin B6. Side effects were very minor. Of the 61
  women who received ginger, 8 reported heartburn, 7 reported
  some sedation, and 1 reported arrhythmia. In the vitamin B6
  group of 62 women, 2 reported heartburn, 11 reported sedation, and 2 reported headache. This study was reported in
  2007.[18]

SEA SICKNESS AND MOTION SICKNESS

Two studies reported ginger to be helpful in reducing the effects of
seasickness. One Danish study in 1988 involved 80 naval cadets who
were unfamiliar with sailing on heavy seas. The sailors were given either
1 gram of dry ginger powder or a placebo. Ginger reduced cold sweating
and vomiting significantly better than the placebo.[19]

A very large Swiss study in 1994 involved 1,741 tourist volunteers
who went for a boat ride (on a whale safari) off the coast of Norway.
Ginger proved to be one of 6 medications that was recommended for
seasickness based on the 1,489 volunteers who followed up with the
study.[20]

Other studies of motion sickness make use of a rotating chair to
induce nausea and vomiting. One study found ginger to be helpful
in delaying nausea and vomiting[21] while several other studies showed
ginger was not helpful.[22]

Generally, it appears ginger is more likely to reduce nausea and
vomiting when it is related to gastric conditions of the stomach but may

not be helpful when nausea originates in the ear or the central nervous system.[23]

NAUSEA AND VOMITING DUE TO LAPAROSCOPIC SURGERY

The use of general anesthesia during surgery often increases the likelihood of nausea and vomiting when waking from the surgery. Laparoscopic surgery involves inserting a tiny video camera (laparoscope) through a small incision in the abdomen. Of 6 studies reviewed, 3 showed ginger to be helpful in reducing nausea and vomiting following surgery[24] while 3 others showed ginger was not helpful.[25] In one of the studies where ginger was successful, patients were given 1 gram of dry ginger powder 1 hour before anesthesia was given.

NAUSEA AND VOMITING DUE TO CHEMOTHERAPY

- A 2004 human study in Thailand showed ginger to be as helpful as the medication metoclopramide for reducing nausea and vomiting caused by the cancer drug cisplatin (1 gram of ginger powder was given for 5 days, starting on the first day of chemotherapy).[26] Cisplatin has been one of the most widely prescribed cancer drugs that acts to inhibit the growth of cancer cells. It is prescribed for cancers of the lung, stomach, bladder, ovaries, and testicles.[27]

- A 1997 study in India used 2 types of ginger extracts for treating cisplatin-induced nausea in dogs. An ethanolic extract of ginger provided significant protection against nausea and vomiting while an aqueous extract of ginger had no effect on nausea and vomiting.[28]

- A follow-up animal study in 1998 showed that *ginger juice* was more effective than the extracts used in the previous study. Ginger juice was also more effective than the prescribed anti-vomiting drug ondansetron. Mice were used in this follow-up study.[29]

It would be interesting to see more studies using ginger juice. As described previously, fresh ginger tea is made by placing a chunk of fresh ginger in a garlic press and squeezing the juice into a cup. Next, add lukewarm water that is heated to less than 140°F (60°C). Add some honey for sweetness if desired. A temperature less than 140°F ensures the delicate enzymes are not destroyed.

REFERENCES FOR CHAPTER 20

1. "Chinese Food History – Timeline". Web site accessed 10/27/2008. <http://www.eatingchina.com/articles/timeline.htm>.
2. Power ML, Holzman GB, Schulkin J. "A survey on the management of nausea and vomiting in pregnancy by obstetrician/gynecologists." *Prim. Care Update Ob Gyns.* 2001 Mar;8(2):69-72.
3. Paul Bergner. "Zingiber: Is ginger safe during pregnancy?" Medical Herbalism 3(3):7. Web site: meddherb.com. Accessed 12/15/2007. <http://medherb.com/Medica/Zingiber_-__Is_ginger_safe_during_pregnancy_.htm>.
4. Vutyavanich T, Wongtrangan S, Ruangsri R. "Pyridoxine for nausea and vomiting or pregnancy: a randomized, double-blind, placebo-controlled trial. *Am J Obstet Gynecol.* 1995 Sep;173(3 Pt 1):881-4.
5. McGuffin M, Hobbs C, Upton R, Goldberg A. *Botanical Safety Handbook.* American Herbal Products Associations Botanical Safety Handbook. CRC Press. Boca Raton. 1997.
6. Boone SA, Shields KM. "Treating pregnancy-related nausea and vomiting with ginger." *Ann Pharmacother.* 2005 Oct;39(10):1710-3. Epub 2005 Aug 30.
7. Borrelli F, Capasso R, Aviello G, Pittler MH, Izzo AA. "Effectiveness and safety of ginger in the treatment of pregnancy-induced nausea and vomiting." Obstet Gynecol. 2005 Apr;105(4):849-56.
8a. Vutyavanich T, Wongtrangan S, Ruangsri R. "Pyridoxine for nausea and vomiting or pregnancy: a randomized, double-blind, placebo-controlled trial. *Am J Obstet Gynecol.* 1995 Sep;173(3 Pt 1):881-4.
8b. Sahakian V, Rouse D, Sipes S, Rose N, Niebyl J. "Vitamin B6 is effective therapy for nausea and vomiting of pregnancy; a randomized, double-blind placebo-controlled study." *Obstet Gynecol.* 1991 Jul;78(1):33-6.
9. Quinla JD, Hill DA. "Nausea and vomiting of pregnancy." *Am Fam Physician.* 2003 Jul 1:68(1):121-8.
10. Fischer-Rasmussen W, Kjaer SK, Dahl C, and Asping, U. "Ginger treatment of hyperemesis gravidarum." *European Journal Obstetrics, Gynecology,and Reproductive Biology* 38, no. 1 (Jan. 1991): 19-24.

11. Vutyavanich T, Kraisarin T, Ruangsri R "Ginger for nausea and vomiting in pregnancy: randomized, double-masked, placebo-controlled trial." *Obstet Gynecol.* 2001; 97(4):577-82.

12. Keating A, Chez RA. "Ginger syrup as an antiemetic in early pregnancy." *Altern Ther Health Med.* 2002 Sep-Oct;8(5):89-91.

13. Willetts KE, Ekangaki A, Eden JA. "Effect of a ginger extract on pregnancy-induced nausea: a randomised controlled trial." *Aust N Z J Obstet Gynaecol.* 2003 Apr;43(2):139-44.

14. Sripramote M, Lekhyananda N. "A randomized comparison of ginger and vitamin B6 in the treatment of nausea and vomiting of pregnancy." *J Med Assoc Thai.* 2003 Sep;86(9):845-53.

15. Portnoi G, Chng LA, Karimi-Tabesh L, Koren G, Tan MP, Einarson A. "Prospective comparative study of the safety and effectiveness of ginger for the treatment of nausea and vomiting in pregnancy." *Am J Obstet Gynecol.* 2003 Nov;189(5):1374-7.

16. Smith C, Crowther C, Willson K, Hotham N, McMillian V. "A randomized controlled trial of ginger to treat nausea and vomiting in pregnancy." *Obstet Gynecol.* 2004 Apr;103(4):639-45.

17. Pongrojpaw D, Somprasit C, Chanthasenanont A. "A randomized comparison of ginger and dimenhydrinate in the treatment of nausea and vomiting in pregnancy." *J Med Assoc Thai.* 2007 Sep;90(9):1703-9.

18. Chittumma P, Kaewkiattikun K, Wiriyasiriwach B. "Comparison of ginger and vitamin B6 for treatment of nausea and vomiting in early pregnancy: a randomized double-blind controlled trial." *J Med Assoc Thai.* 2007 Jan;90(1):15-20.

19. Grontved A, Brask T, Kambskard J, Hentzer E. "Ginger root against seasickness. A controlled trial on the open sea." *Acta Otolaryngol.* 1988 Jan-Feb;105(1-2):45-9.

20. Schmid R, Schick T, Steffen R, Tschopp A, Wilk T. "Comparison of Seven Commonly Used Agents for Prophylaxis of Seasickness." J Travel Med. 1994Dec 1;1(4):203-206.

21. Lien HC, Sun WM, Chen YH, Kim H, Hasler W, Owyang C. "Effects of ginger on motion sickness and gastric slow-wave dysrhythmias induced by circular vection." *Am J Physiol Gastrointest Liver Physiol.* 2003 Mar;284(3):G481-9.

22a. Stewart JJ, Wood MJ, Wood CD, Mims ME. "Effects on ginger on motion sickness susceptibility and gastric function." *Pharmacology.* 1991;42(2):111-20.

22b. Holtmann S, Clarke AH, Scherer H, Hohn M. "The anti-motion sickness mechanism of ginger. A comparative study with placebo and dimenhydrinate." *Acta Otolaryngol.* 1989 Sep-Oct;108(3-4):168-74.

23. Holtmann S, Clarke AH, 'Scherer H, Hohn M. "The anti-motion sickness

mechanism of ginger. A comparative study with placebo and dimenhydrinate." *Acta Otolaryngol.* 1989 Sep-Oct;108(3-4):168-74.

24. Pongrojpaw D, Chiamchanya C. "The efficacy of ginger in prevention of postoperative nausea and vomiting after outpatient gynecological laparoscopy." *J Med Assoc Thai.* 2003 Mar;86(3):244-50.

25a. Morin AM, Betz O, Kranke P, Geldner G, Wulf H, Eberhart LH. "[Is ginger a relevant antiemetic for postoperative nausea and vomiting?]" *Anasthesiol Intensivmed Notfallmed Schmerzther.* 2004 May;39(5):281-5. [Article in German].

25b. Eberhart LH, Mayer R, Betz O, Tsolakidis S, Hilpert W, Morin AM, Geldner G, Wulf H, Seeling W. "Ginger does not prevent postoperative nausea and vomiting after laparoscopic surgery." Anesth Analg. 2003 Apr;96(4):995-8, table of contents.

25c. Visalyaputra S, Petchpaisit N, Somcharoen K, Choavaratana R. "The efficacy of ginger root in the prevention of postoperative nausea and vomiting after outpatient gynaecological laparoscopy." *Anaesthesia.* 1998 May;53(5):506-10.

26. Manusirivithaya S, Sripramote M, Tangjitgamol S, Sheanakul C, Leelahakorn S, Thavaramara T, Tangcharoenpanich K. "Antiemetic effect of ginger in gynecologic oncology patients receiving cisplatin." *Int J Gynecol Cancer.* 2004 Nov-Dec;14(6):1063-9.

27. "Cisplatin". Web site: Chemical & Engineering News. Accessed 12/4/2007. <http://pubs.acs.org/cen/coverstory/83/8325/8325cisplatin.html?print>.

28. Sharma SS, Kochupillai V, Gupta SK, Seth SD, Gupta YK. "Antiemetic efficacy of ginger (Zingiber officinale) against cisplatin-induced emesis in dogs." *J Ethnopharmacol.* 1997 Jul;57(2):93-6.

29. Sharma SS, Gupta YK. "Reversal of cisplatin-induced delay in gastric emptying in rats by ginger (Zingiber officinale)." *J Ethnopharmacol.* 1998 Aug;62(1):49-55.

PART V

The Finish Line!

CHAPTER 21

The Dark Side—The Bright Side

THE DARK SIDE OF HUMAN NATURE

I will put it in writing one last time: Infections, microbes, heavy metals, and other factors can affect our brains, our behavior and degrade our mental abilities and reasoning. Because we are human, everyone of us has some degree of abnormality. Most of us do a good job of managing and containing our abnormalities so we can function in society. However, add a chronic infection, chemical imbalance, or hormonal problem and the job of managing and containing our abnormalities becomes much more difficult. A slight streak of anger can become an outbreak of rage. Negative thoughts and a sharp tongue can become outbreaks of sarcasm and putting others down. When we consider the many factors that can impair our reasoning and judgment, we have a deeper understanding of how a person can give up restraint and "go off the deep end," doing something hurtful and destructive to himself/herself or others. When we consider chronic infections or other imbalances, we can gain some understanding of the dark side of human behavior, especially when the ability to manage and contain destructive behavior is reduced or even lost.

THE HARSH SIDE OF LIFE

Along the same destructive path, a sincere person trying to make it through life with degraded abilities may not perform up to expectations

364

at work and may not be able to give his or her best. Bosses and managers lose patience when performance is below standard and goals and deadlines are not met. Lethargy, indifference, and poor decisions are more likely when thinking is foggy and energy is drained. Life can be difficult when we are at the receiving end of harsh treatment from those who expect better productivity from us. We will be left with emotional scars, adding yet more burdens to carry. Life can be more difficult than it needs to be when we are functioning below our inherited potential.

THE BRIGHT SIDE

Another E-F-G approach is an Everyday Faith in God. We all need wisdom and moral guidance to help us determine right from wrong and do good for our fellow man. We need to know there is a God who loves us and who will guide us "through the valley of the shadow of death" in our times of hopelessness, anger and despair. Perhaps when we feel like going off the deep end, a higher moral law will keep us from giving in to destructive behaviors. Add prayer along with healthy foods, supplements, exercise, and good relationships. We all need these.

CHAPTER 22

Simple Recipes for the E-F-G Approach

GINGER RECIPES

Ginger Slices

HERE'S a simple way to take fresh ginger and feel its head-clearing effect:

1. Using a serrated knife, carve off a thin slice of root about the size of a penny or nickel.
2. Place it in your mouth like a lozenge, chewing slightly from time to time to release more flavor and vapors as desired. These vapors can help clear your head. (If you chew it up all at once, the sudden warmth may be overwhelming!)
3. Slowly exhale through your nose, allowing the soothing vapors to rise up into the passageways of your head. Inhaling through your mouth and slowly exhaling out your nose will allow the vapors to flow into your sinuses.

Fresh Ginger Tea

A great way to get more fresh ginger in your diet is to make a quick and delicious tea. First, heat a cup of water to less than 140°F (60°C). Next, place a chunk of fresh ginger in a garlic press and squeeze the juice into the lukewarm water. Add some honey for sweetness if you like. Do not boil or steep fresh ginger because the delicate, yet powerful enzymes will be destroyed.

Meat Tenderizer

Squeeze fresh ginger using a garlic press and spread juice over meat before cooking.

Teriyaki Marinade

1/4 cup oil
1/4 cup soy sauce
2 tablespoons ketchup
1 tablespoon lemon juice
1 tablespoon vinegar
1/4 teaspoon pepper
1 tablespoon crushed fresh ginger
1 teaspoon garlic powder

Mix ingredients, pour into large plastic bag, add up to 6 steaks, and refrigerate for 8 to 12 hours, turning a couple of times.

Recipe from M. Hunt, "Fresh ginger makes better meat tenderizer," *TwinCities.com Pioneer Press*, February 16, 2004; Accessed 6/1/2004., http://www.twincities.com/mld/twincities/living/7949674.htm.

FLAX RECIPE

Fruit Flax Smoothie

My favorite way to use flaxseeds is to make fruit flax smoothies for my family of 5. These cold drinks make a wonderful dessert because they taste almost like a milk shake. Here is what I do:

1. Put 1/2 cup of flaxseeds (I prefer golden flaxseeds) in an electric blender and grind up (1/2 cup = 90 grams flaxseed = 125 mL).
2. Add 2 to 3 cups of ice water that still has ice in it (750 mL).
3. Add 1/2 cup of low-fat cottage cheese (or 3 times as much yogurt or a combination of both).
4. Add fresh or frozen fruit (such as strawberries, pineapple or an orange) and a banana (I like to use pieces of frozen bananas).
5. Add 1/4 teaspoon of stevia, a natural herbal sweetener; or you can add honey or ice cream (1/4 teaspoon = 1 ml).
6. Blend everything together. The water-soluble fiber from the flaxseeds will cause the drink to thicken almost like a milk shake. This is your super omega-3 drink!

If you have a fresh pineapple on hand, you can make use of the inner core. I cut the core into thin slices first then add it to the smoothie and blend. You will also get the benefit of pineapple's enzyme bromelain! Dr. Johanna Budwig also stated that skim milk or nuts also have sufficient proteins to make the oil from flaxseeds water soluble as discussed in chapter 13.

If you are a chocolate fan, omit the fruit and add 2 tablespoons of dark cocoa and 2 tablespoons of chocolate malt (2 tablespoons = 12 mL). In lieu of the chocolate malt, you can use 1 to 2 tablespoons of inulin which is sweet and provides a rich flavor similar to malt. Inulin contains FOS (fructooligosaccharides). Remember from chapter 12 that FOS is not digested but becomes a source of food for the beneficial bacteria in the digestive tract. Enjoy!

Nutrition Note: Flaxseeds provide omega-3 EFAs. Use dark cocoa for chocolate smoothies because it is rich in antioxidants. Pineapple is a rich source of proteolytic enzymes.

GARLIC RECIPES

Toasted Garlic Bread

My favorite way to use garlic is to crush 3 or 4 cloves using a garlic press and mix with olive oil. Use about 3 or 4 cloves. It is important to let the crushed garlic sit for 10 minutes so the phytochemicals can mix. Next, mix the garlic with 1/4 to 1/3 cup of virgin olive oil. I like to pretoast the bread in the toaster or oven and then spread the garlic/olive oil over the toasted bread. This way, the active phytochemicals in garlic are not destroyed by heating. Next, sprinkle on some Parmesan cheese.

Make plenty because it tastes even better as a leftover and can be cut in small squares and used as croutons on salads. It also makes a great snack—when you are away from other people, of course. This is also a great way to use up bread crusts. My family enjoys using toasted garlic bread for meatball sandwiches with spaghetti sauce.

Nutrition Note: Both garlic and olive oil have antibacterial, antioxidant, and anticancer actions. Garlic is also rich in selenium and sulfur—two important compounds for fighting heavy metal toxicity. Virgin olive oil contains monounsaturated fats, which are very healthy for our heart and blood vessels. Remember to take a couple spoonfuls of extra virgin olive oil each day.

Mashed Potatoes with Garlic

Crush 2 or 3 cloves of garlic and add to basic mashed potatoes.

Cut up potatoes and put in a pan. (If the skin looks good, you can leave the skin on.) Add water enough to cover potatoes. Add a pinch of salt. Cook potatoes until soft. Drain off most of the water but reserve it in case you want to use it later. Add a pinch of pepper and some butter if you like. With a mixer, whip the potatoes, adding milk and some of the cooking water until desired consistency. Add the crushed garlic and mix together.

Nutrition Note: As possible, try to use water that vegetables are cooked in since most of the vitamins end up in the cooking water.

SIMPLE AND INEXPENSIVE RECIPES

Quick, Simple, Low Calorie Breakfast Oatmeal

Place 1/2 to 1 cup of finely rolled oats (quick oats) in a bowl, sprinkle cinnamon on top, then shake bowl so cinnamon falls down into oatmeal. Next, add 1/2 to 1 cup of water. I prefer to eat oatmeal uncooked because it tastes kind of like cookie dough. Add fruit such as bananas, fresh pineapple, kiwi, applesauce, or whatever fruit or topping happens to be on hand. Add some walnuts too. You can also use milk instead of water, especially for growing children.

I enjoy using frozen berries or cherries. First thing in the morning, I put some frozen fruit in my bowl, then add enough water to cover the fruit. After my morning shave and shower, I come back and the berries are thawed. Next, I add the oatmeal, maybe some kasha, oat bran, or raisin bran cereal, then bananas or some fruit topping. This has been my favorite everyday breakfast for over 13 years. I enjoy it cold and uncooked rather than hot and gooey.

Nutrition Note: Oatmeal is a rich supply of digestible fiber, which has been shown to remove cholesterol from the digestive tract. Fresh or frozen fruit provides enzymes and phytochemicals. Cinnamon has antibiotic actions and may also help control blood sugar. Walnuts have omega-3 EFAs and protein.

Sprouted Mung Beans

In the wintertime, I like to sprout mung beans because they sprout very quickly. In chapter 14, we learned that seeds have their highest enzyme content when their sprouts measure 1/4 inch long. Small sprouting kits are inexpensive. A good Web site for buying seeds for sprouting is www.wheatgrasskits.com. Remember, sprouted seeds are a rich source of enzymes.

Pancakes

(Single recipe, for 3 to 4 people, makes about 14 pancakes)

3/4 cup whole wheat flour
3/4 cup white flour
1/2 cup wheat bran
3 teaspoons baking powder
    (I recommend non-aluminum baking powder)
1 or 2 tablespoons sugar (or honey or just 1/2 teaspoon stevia)
1/2 teaspoon salt
1 egg
1/4 cup melted butter (or canola or palm oil)
1 cup milk
1 cup water
1 teaspoon vanilla extract
1/2 cup semi-sweet chocolate chips (optional)

(Double recipe, for 6 to 8 people, makes about 28 pancakes)

1 1/2 cups whole wheat flour
1 1/2 cups white flour
1 cup wheat bran
1/8 cup baking powder
    (I recommend non-aluminum baking powder)
2 to 4 tablespoons sugar (or honey or just 1 teaspoon of stevia)
1 teaspoon salt

2 or 3 eggs
1/2 cup melted butter (or canola, coconut or palm oil)
2 cups milk
2 cups water
2 teaspoons vanilla extract
1 cup semi-sweet chocolate chips (optional)

I like to use a large steel bowl to which I add butter and then place over a burner on very low heat. After the butter has melted, add egg(s), beat with a whisk, and then add remaining ingredients. Add the flour last. Whisk everything together. You may have to add some extra flour if the batter is too thin. Cook on a hot, greased griddle at about 350°F. Use about 1/4 cup batter for each pancake. Cook until bubbles appear then flip over and cook on the other side a few more minutes until slightly brown. Leftover pancakes can be refrigerated and warmed up in the toaster the next morning, eaten as a snack, or packed in a lunch box.

Pancake recipes are very forgiving, so feel free to experiment. You can substitute one-quarter to one-half of the flour for buckwheat or barley flour.

Nutrition Note: Whole wheat and other whole grains are more filling than white flour, so you are satisfied sooner. Whole grains are metabolized slowly and do not produce a quick surge of insulin, which is inflammatory.

Remember, buckwheat is loaded with rutin, which strengthens blood vessels and has no gluten. (Gluten is a protein in wheat and other grains that many people are allergic to. Gluten gives bread its sponginess.) Rutin is also an antioxidant. Barley flour contains water-soluble fiber that can absorb bad LDL cholesterol and move it out of our bodies.

Clam Spaghetti

This is a favorite recipe from my landlady when I was just out of college. It feeds my family of 5 plus makes another meal of leftovers.

1/4 cup olive oil
6 garlic cloves, sliced or crushed
1/4 cup parsley, dried or fresh, chopped
2 cans clams (6 1/2-ounce cans, the same size as a tuna can)
2 pounds spaghetti noodles
mozzarella cheese, grated

Cook spaghetti per directions on box. When done, drain spaghetti and put back into pot. In a separate pan, add olive oil and garlic and heat for a few minutes so garlic flavor blends with olive oil. Add both cans of clams with juice. Bring to a boil, then reduce to a simmer for another 5–10 minutes to fully cook the clams. Add parsley. Pour this into the pot of drained spaghetti. Mix together and let stand at lowest burner setting for about 1/2 hour, stirring from time to time. Serve on individual plates. Top with cheese as desired.